Date: 6/10/11

The Science of Drinking

How Alcohol Affects
Your Body and Mind

Amitava Dasgupta

ROWMAN & LITTLEFIELD PUBLISHERS, INC.
Lanham • Boulder • New York • Toronto • Plymouth, UK

Published by Rowman & Littlefield Publishers, Inc.
A wholly owned subsidary of The Rowman & Littlefield Publishing Group, Inc.
4501 Forbes Boulevard, Suite 200, Lanham, Maryland 20706
http://www.rowmanlittlefield.com

Estover Road, Plymouth PL6 7PY, United Kingdom

British Library Cataloguing in Publication Information Available

Library of Congress Cataloging-in-Publication Data

Dasgupta, Amitava, 1958–
  The science of drinking : how alcohol affects your body and mind /
Amitava Dasgupta.
    p. cm.
  Includes bibliographical references and index.
  ISBN 978-1-4422-0409-6 (cloth : alk. paper) — ISBN 978-1-4422-0411-9
(electronic)
  1. Alcohol—Physiological effect. 2. Drinking of alcoholic beverages—
Psychological aspects. I. Title.
  QP801.A3D37 2011
  615'.7828—dc22

                                                                    2010051613

∞™ The paper used in this publication meets the minimum requirements of
American National Standard for Information Sciences—Permanence of Paper
for Printed Library Materials, ANSI/NISO Z39.48-1992.

Printed in the United States of America

Contents

Preface

What happens when you drink your favorite cocktail? How does it go from beverage to buzz? Or from buzz to blotto? As a practicing toxicologist and researcher in the field of alcohol and drugs, I will present answers for everything you ever wanted to know about drinking—from what creates the high to how you reach a blood alcohol level that gets you into trouble. Did you know that the smell we commonly perceive as alcohol is not alcohol but is from other volatile substances present in a drink? Did you know that alcoholism is an illness and that proper treatment can restore an alcoholic to a normal life? Overwhelming scientific research and evidence points toward the beneficial effects of drinking in moderation, including a lower risk of cardiovascular disease and stroke, a lower risk of developing dementia with advancing age, and some increase in longevity. Many people do not know that drinking red wine protects the heart more than white wine, while beer, margaritas, and hard liquor are less effective in providing such protection.

I want to share the latest scientific facts on the effect of alcohol on one's body and mind. Drinking in moderation is a good way to loosen inhibition in a relationship and let your creativity flow. The key is to distinguish between drinking sensibly and drinking insensibly. Scientific research has provided some guidance on how much and how often we should drink to get the benefits of alcohol and at what point drinking hurts our bodies. In addition, there are clear guidelines about how much alcohol is safe to drink in an evening before driving home to avoid being charged with a DWI. While those with advanced science backgrounds can decipher the technical medical literature written about this subject, my goal is to present these scientific facts in a more accessible fashion that everyone will be able to understand. I want to provide you with clear guidance on what constitutes a healthy drinking habit based on scientific information. In order to understand the effect of alcohol on the human body, I will discuss the pharmacology and toxicology of alcohol so that readers will understand the body's response to alcohol. I also provide guidelines for what amount of alcohol is safe before driving, explain why you should always consume alcohol with food, and why you should sip alcohol rather than drinking it like soda or water. I also discuss the loopholes of alcohol testing so that you'll know if you have been wrongly charged with a DWI. This book will also be useful for lawyers who need to understand the scientific basis of alcohol testing and how the human body handles alcohol.

Most auto accidents are due to a deadly combination of drugs and alcohol. This book will focus on which particular combinations of drugs and alcohol cause the most harm. Alcohol and recreational drugs are deadly combinations and must be avoided at all times. Other than alcohol, methanol and ethylene glycol (antifreeze) abuse is also common, especially in winter, and such overdoses may be more life threatening than an alcohol overdose. Most consumer health books don't even address this issue. I have provided many of the sources of the information covered in this book in the notes at the end of each chapter so that advanced readers, especially health care professionals, can go and read the source material for more in-depth information. I hope readers enjoy this book and get all the information they need on alcohol.

Amitava Dasgupta
Houston, Texas

1

Alcohol Use and Abuse

Past and Present

Alcohol is a drug (pharmaceutical) with medicinal value. One of the first drugs known to mankind, alcohol use can be traced back to 10,000 years ago. In pharmacology class we learn that another name for a drug is "poison." A drug is beneficial if consumed in recommended doses but harmful if taken in excess. Most of the drugs used in medicine do not have any abuse potential except for a few classes of drugs, such as benzodiazepines, which are used for anxiety and insomnia, and opioids, which are used for treating severe pain. Commonly prescribed benzodiazepines include alprazolam, lorazepam, temazepam, and diazepam, while opioids include hydrocodone, hydromorphone, and oxycodone, among others.

Alcohol is the most widely used legal drug available without a prescription. Another legal drug with high abuse potential available without a prescription is tobacco. However, it is important to mention that tobacco has no known health benefits, while drinking alcohol in moderation has many health benefits, including prolonging life. Many studies have concluded that moderate drinkers live longer than nondrinkers and enjoy a better quality of health (see chapter 4). In addition, abuse potential of opioids (both synthetic and natural opiates) is much higher than alcohol. Drinking one drink or less a day may actually keep the doctor away, but consumption of five or more drinks per day for a prolonged period makes a person alcohol dependent. However, women, underage drinkers, the elderly, and people with a genetic predisposition for addiction to alcohol may become alcohol dependent with fewer drinks per day over a long period of time.

Another proof that alcohol is a drug is that it is known to interact with many other drugs. For example, alcohol can be toxic to a person taking

Tylenol (acetaminophen) regularly for pain control, even if that individual consumes alcohol in moderation (see chapter 8). A majority of Americans consume alcohol, but only a small percentage of the population becomes alcohol dependent. However, this small percentage of people (approximately 8 percent of Americans are alcohol dependent) makes a huge impact on society, costing the U.S. economy about $185 billion a year (see chapter 5). In this chapter, alcohol use in both historic and modern times will be discussed, but the emphasis of the chapter is to convince you that alcohol should be treated as a drug. As a practicing toxicologist, I treat drugs with respect. If you treat alcohol with respect, you will reap the benefits of drinking in moderation and enjoy a long, healthy life.

FRUIT RIPENING AND HISTORICAL ORIGINS OF DRINKING: DRUNKEN MONKEY HYPOTHESIS

Originally proposed by Professor Robert Dudley of the University of California, Berkeley, the "drunken monkey hypothesis" proposes that the human attraction to alcohol may have a genetic basis due to the high dependence of early primates on fruit as a food source. For 40 million years, primate diets were rich in fruits, and in the humid tropical climate where the early evolution of humans took place, yeasts on fruit skin and within fruit converted fruit sugars into ethanol (alcohol). Since it is small in size, when the alcohol molecule diffused out of the fruit, an alcoholic smell identified the food as ripe and ready to consume. In tropical forests where early primates (referred to simply as "monkeys" in the hypothesis name) lived, competition for ripe fruits was intense, and those capable of following the smell of alcohol to identify ripe foods and consuming them rapidly survived better than others. Eventually natural selection favored primates who had a keen appreciation for the smell and taste of alcohol. Fossilized teeth show that fruit was a major component in the primate diet between 45 million and 34 million years ago, and some of the closest ancestors of human species—gorillas, chimpanzees, and orangutans—ate diets based on fruit. Primates are known to have a higher olfactory sensitivity to alcohol than other mammals. As human evolution continued, fruits were mostly replaced by roots, tubers, and meat. Although our ancestors stopped relying heavily on fruit, it is possible that the taste for alcohol arose during our long-shared ancestry with primates.[1]

The yeasts that occur on fruits consume sugar molecules as a source of energy and in the absence of oxygen (anaerobic fermentation) produce alcohol. For example, unripe palm contains no alcohol, but ripened palm has about 0.6 percent alcohol content, and overripe palm falling on the ground has approximately 4 percent alcohol. Monkeys usually prefer ripe fruits with approximately 1 percent alcohol content but avoid over-ripe fruits with 4 percent alcohol and lower sugar content. Anecdotally, humans often consume alcohol with food, suggesting that drinking with food is a natural combination. For millions of years, the amount of alcohol consumed by our ancestors was strictly limited, and the situation did not change even 10,000 years ago when humans became agriculturists and could produce plenty of barley and malt, the raw material for fermentation. Yeasts stop producing alcohol when the alcohol level reaches between 10 and 15 percent because yeasts start dying at this alcohol concentration. Ancient beers and wines probably contained only 5 percent alcohol until alcohol distillation was invented in Central Asia around AD 700. Then drinks with a higher alcohol content became available and the history of alcohol abuse by humans began.[2]

ALCOHOL FROM A HISTORICAL PERSPECTIVE

The first historical evidence of alcoholic beverages came from an archaeological discovery of Stone Age beer jugs from approximately 10,000 years ago. The first palm date wine was probably brewed in Mesopotamia. Evidence of wine appeared in Egypt about 5,000 years ago—Osiris was worshipped as a wine god throughout the nation. The first beer was probably brewed in ancient Egypt and both wine and beer were offered to the gods. Egyptians used alcoholic beverages for pleasure and rituals, and for medical and nutritional purposes. However, even in ancient times the Egyptians were aware of the harmful effect of excess consumption of alcohol and emphasis was on moderate use. The earliest evidence of alcohol use in China dates back to 5000 BC when alcohol was mainly produced from rice, honey, and fruits. A Chinese imperial edict ca. 1116 BC made it clear that the use of alcohol in moderation was the key and was prescribed from the heavens. In ancient India, alcoholic beverages were known as "sura," a favorite drink of Indra, the king of all gods and goddesses. Use of such drinks was known in 3000–2000 BC, and ancient Ayurvedic texts concluded that alcohol was a medicine if consumed in moderation but a poison if consumed in excess. Beer was known to Babylonians as early as 2700 BC. In ancient Greece winemaking was common in 1700 BC. Hippocrates (ca. 460–370 BC) identified numerous medicinal properties of wine but was critical of drunkenness.[3]

In ancient civilizations, alcohol was used to quench thirst because water was often contaminated with bacteria. Hippocrates specifically cited that only water from springs, deep wells, and rainfall was safe for drinking. In the event that water was contaminated, alcohol was preferred for drinking because alcoholic beverages were free from bacteria and other pathogens (alcohol is an antiseptic agent). When alcoholic beverages were added to contaminated water, the alcohol killed most pathogens and made water safer for drinking. In ancient Western civilization, people consumed beer and wine more than water for quenching thirst. Beer was a drink for common people, while wine was reserved for elites. Around 30 BC, wine became available to common Romans due to the expansion of vineyards.

During ancient times, beer and wine produced from fermentation of cereals, grapes, or fruits had much lower alcohol content than today's beer or wine and were safer for human consumption in larger quantities. Nevertheless, some folks drank too much alcohol, and drunkenness was greatly condemned in ancient Western cultures. In the New Testament Jesus approved alcohol consumption by miraculously transforming water into wine. His followers extended the balance between use and abuse of wine and practiced moderation. In ancient Eastern civilization, drinking alcoholic beverages to quench thirst was less common than in Western civilization because drinking tea was very popular in Eastern countries. During boiling to prepare tea, all pathogens died, thus making tea drinking very safe.[4]

Yeast can produce alcoholic beverages with up to 15 percent alcohol content. In order to produce a higher alcohol content, a process known as distillation is needed. Distilled spirits originated in China and India ca. 800 BC, but the distillation process became common in Europe only during the eleventh century and later. Alcohol consumption was common during the Middle Ages, and monasteries produced alcoholic beverages to nourish their monks and to sell to the public. Before the Renaissance most Europeans had mastered the art of brewing, and distillation produced not only beers and wines but also hard liquor.

During early American history, colonials showed little concern over drunkenness, and production of alcoholic beverages was a major source of commerce. In 1791, however, a tax, popularly known as the "whiskey tax," was imposed on both privately and publicly brewed distilled whiskey. The whiskey tax was repealed by President Thomas Jefferson in 1802, but a new alcohol tax was imposed between 1814 and 1817 to help pay for the War of 1812. In 1862 President Abraham Lincoln introduced a new tax (which included taxing whiskey) to help defray Civil War costs. The same act also created the office of the commissioner of Internal Revenue. In 1906 the Pure Food and Drug Act was passed, which regulated the labeling of products containing alcohol, opiates, cocaine, and cannabis (marijuana), among others. The law became effective in January 1907. In 1920 alcohol was prohibited in the United States, but Congress repealed the law in 1933. In 1978 President Jimmy Carter signed a bill to legalize home brewing of beer for personal use for the first time since prohibition.[5]

SCIENCE OF FERMENTATION AND DISTILLATION

Fermentation is a process by which yeasts convert sugar into alcohol in the absence of oxygen, a process first scientifically understood by Louis Pasteur. There are different types of sugar, such as glucose, fructose (fruit sugar), galactose (milk sugar), and sucrose (cane sugar, which contains two sugar molecules: glucose and fructose joined together). Glucose and fructose are monosaccharides or simple sugar, while sucrose (table sugar) is a disaccharide and is more structurally complex than monosaccharides. Yeast is capable of converting simple sugars like glucose and fructose into alcohol. Yeast converts glucose into pyruvate and finally ethanol (alcohol) is produced from acetaldehyde. Yeast converts simple sugars to alcohol through a complex biochemical enzymatic pathway involving yeast enzymes (fig. 1.1). The overall reaction is, however, quite simple.

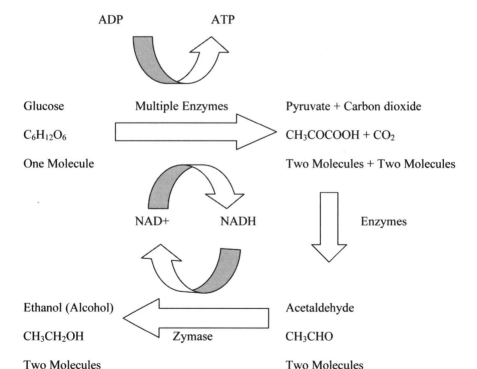

Figure 1.1.   Fermentation of glucose by yeast-producing alcohol

Key: ADP: Adenosine diphosphate; ATP: Adenosine triphosphate; NAD: Nicotinamide adenine dinucleotide, a cofactor for reduction (loss of hydrogen from the molecule) of acetaldehyde to alcohol; NADH: Reduced form of NAD

Overall reaction:

$$C_6H_{12}O_6 \longrightarrow 2\ CH_3CH_2OH + 2\ CO_2$$

Fermentation is a natural process where various species of wild yeasts and bacteria convert fruit sugars to alcohol. Overripe fruits and rotten fruits contain a much higher alcohol content than ripe fruits. Yeasts are classified as fungus, and there are more than 1,500 different species found in nature. The yeast species *Saccharomyces cerevisiae* has been used for thousands of years for baking and fermenting alcoholic beverages. Other species of yeast, for example, *Candida albicans*, are pathogenic and cause yeast infections in humans. For preparing bread, the amylase present in flour breaks down starch into maltose. During baking maltase enzymes present in baking yeast split maltose into two glucose molecules, which are then fermented into alcohol and carbon dioxide. The released carbon dioxide causes dough to rise, while the little alcohol produced adds to bread's flavor, although most alcohol is evaporated during the baking process. The yeast species used for baking, although classified broadly as "brewer's yeast," is a different type from that used for beer manufacturing.

Brewing Beer

Beer is the most popular alcoholic beverage in the world. In the first step of beer brewing (malting), malted barley is soaked in hot water, allowing malt to germinate, thus releasing amylases, the enzymes needed for converting the starch that is present in grains into sugars. Different roasting times and temperatures produce different colors of malt from the same grain; the darker the malt, the darker the beer. Although barley is the main grain used for brewing beer, other sources of starch, such as rye, wheat, and even rice, may also be used. The malting process can be broken down into three parts: steeping, where barley (or other grains) are added to the vat and water is added for soaking; then a five-day period for germination, where grains may be spread on the floor; and finally kilning, where germinating malt is dried under higher temperature to produce the final product, "malt." The malt is then cracked in a process called "milling," followed by "mashing," where supplementary grains such as corn, rye, or sorghum may be added to the malt. The next step is "lautering," where liquid containing sugar is separated from grains. Then the malt extract is boiled to ensure sterility. During this step hops are added as a flavoring agent, which gives the beer its characteristic bitter taste. This step may last for one to two hours, and this produces the "wort." The wort is cooled to bring it back to fermenting temperature and yeast is added, which produces alcohol from the sugars present in the wort (which is produced by a complex process starting from the starch present in barley).

Brewers classify yeasts for beer manufacturing into "top-fermenting" and "bottom-fermenting" yeasts. Top-fermenting yeasts form foam at the top of the fermenting vessel; these yeasts can produce a higher alcoholic content, and the fermentation process is carried out at relatively higher temperatures (61°F–75°F). Beers produced by these yeasts are commonly called "ale-type" beers, which are fruitier, sweeter beers. An example of a top-fermenting yeast is *Saccharomyces cerevisiae*. Bottom-fermenting yeasts, which are used for the production of the majority of beers, ferment sugars at lower temperatures (50°F–64°F). Bottom-fermenting yeasts are larger yeast strains that tend to settle at the bottom as the fermentation process is progressing to completion. Beer-fermenting yeasts can tolerate up to 5 or 6 percent alcohol concentration before they start to die.

The fermentation process is carried out anaerobically (in the absence of air containing oxygen) in a fermentor that is sealed off during the process, except for a vent pipe through which liberated carbon dioxide gas can escape from the vessel. The fermentation process may take a week or longer. When fermentation is nearly complete, most yeasts will settle at the bottom (if the beer is brewed using bottom-fermenting yeast), and the carbon dioxide vent is sealed off so that residual carbon dioxide may stay within the beer, making it carbonated. Alternatively, carbon dioxide may be added to the beer. Then beer is pumped off, cooled, and bottled for shipment.[6] For commercial production of beer, strict quality control procedures are adopted in each step of production to ensure quality, such as measuring specific gravity and other parameters to ensure that the final product meets all classifications determined by the manufacturer.

Producing Wine

Wine is brewed using a different strain of yeast capable of tolerating more alcohol than brewer's yeast. Wine-producing yeasts can tolerate up to 12 to 15 percent of alcohol content.

Wines are primarily made from grapes, although other fruits such as plums, peaches, and apples may also be used for winemaking. Usually wines are made from harvesting ripe grapes in a vineyard. Wild yeasts are present in ripe grapes. Although wild yeast can produce wine, the fermentation process may be unpredictable. Usually, cultured yeasts are added to the crushed grapes and expressed juice, which is called the "must." For producing red wine, grape skins are added to the must and contribute to the reddish color of the wine. For making white wine, grape skins are removed prior to the fermentation process. Red wine is fermented at a higher temperature (up to 85°F) than white wine (64°F–68°F). After fermentation, solid residues are allowed to settle and wine is pumped off to a new container for storage, sometimes in wooden oak barrels. Then wine is allowed to age for a year or more while a complex chemical reaction takes place, producing small molecular weight compounds that add to the distinct taste and flavor of a particular wine. Sake, Japanese wine, is fermented from rice, while mead is made from honey, and hard cider is made from apples. Again, strict quality control procedures are adopted by commercial breweries in each step of wine manufacturing to ensure high quality of the end product. Acidity and specific gravity of wine is carefully controlled by the manufacturers to meet their specifications.

The formation of flavor in wine is from original compounds present in grapes, some of which may be transformed biochemically during fermentation. In addition, during the aging process, if the wine is stored in oak barrels, trace chemicals present in the wood may leach into the wine and participate in a complex chemical process that produces other molecules. Phenolic compounds present in grapes are responsible for wine color and its distinct taste. These compounds include anthocyanins, gallic acid, catechin, and so on.[7]

The aroma of wine consists of 600 to 800 volatile compounds mostly characteristic of grapes used for wine production. Various monoterpene compounds and sulfur-containing thiol compounds are responsible for the characteristic aroma of various wines. During wine production compounds such as esters (ethyl acetate, amyl acetate, phenyl ethyl acetate, etc.), higher alcohols (higher molecular weight than alcohol or ethyl alcohol), volatile fatty acids (acetic acid, isovaleric acid), and other complex compounds such as mercaptans and ketones are generated, contributing to the aroma of wine. During aging, a complex chemical process may take place that modifies the structures of certain compounds already present in the wine.[8] Usually, residual carbon dioxide is not allowed to stay in wine. However, champagne is supplemented with carbon dioxide in order to achieve its bubbly appearance. Carbon dioxide is also added to produce sparkling wine. In port wine alcohol is added after production in order to increase its alcoholic content.

Preparation of Distilled Spirits

Beverages produced by fermentation followed by distillation are known as spirits. After fermentation alcohol content is usually 14–16 percent, but in order to make alcoholic beverages with 45–75 percent alcohol content, vaporizing the alcohol from the original preparation (which contains approximately 85 percent water) and then condensing alcohol vapor in specialized equipment is needed. This is possible because the boiling point of alcohol is 78°C (172.4°F), while the boiling point of water is 100°C (212.0°F). When water is boiled, the temperature rises until it reaches

Table 1.1. Fermenting Materials Used for Preparing Some Popular Spirits

Alcoholic Beverage	Fermenting Material	Alcohol Content
Brandy /cognac	Grapes (distilled wine)	40–50%
Bourbon	Corn	40–55%
Gin	Malt, other grains and juniper berry	38–45%
Rum	Sugarcane or molasses	40–57%
Schnapps	Fermented grains or fruits	30–40%
Tequila	Tequila agave (blue agave) stem	40–45%
Vodka	Malt, molasses or potatoes	40–50%
Whiskey*	Barley	40–55%

*There are different types of whiskeys, such as Scotch whiskey, Irish whiskey, Canadian whiskey, American whiskey, and so on. Scotch whiskeys are usually distilled twice or three times, distilled in Scotland, and aged for a minimum three years in oak cases.

100°C, and then water starts evaporating and temperature no longer increases. Similarly, when an alcohol and water mixture is boiled, alcohol starts evaporating at 78°C, and the vapor is mostly composed of alcohol. Then the vapor is allowed to pass through a tube called a condenser, which is cooled, and alcohol vapor is converted into liquid alcohol again. The instrument in which alcohol distillation is carried out is called a still. The still can be a pot, which is usually used for home distillation (in the United States a license is required for distilling alcohol), while the column still is used for industrial production of various spirits. Bourbon, gin, vodka, whiskey, and rum are all made through the distillation process using various fermenting materials (table 1.1).

NUTRITIONAL VALUE OF ALCOHOLIC BEVERAGES

Alcoholic drinks consist primarily of water, alcohol, and variable amounts of sugars and carbohydrates (residual sugar and starch left after fermentation). Sometimes sugars are also added before fermentation to enhance the alcohol content of the beverage. Alcoholic drinks contain negligible amounts of other nutrients, such as proteins, vitamins, or minerals. Therefore, any calories derived from drinking alcoholic beverages come mostly from alcohol content and some from the carbohydrate and sugar, which are present in the drink. However, distilled liquors, such as cognac, vodka, whiskey, and rum, contain no sugars. Red wine and dry white wines contain 2 to 10 gm of sugar per liter, while sweet wines and port wines may contain up to 120 gm of sugar per liter of wine. Beer and dry sherry contain 30 gm of sugar per liter. Usually a standard drink contains approximately 14 gm of pure alcohol (see chapter 2). Burning 1 gm of alcohol produces more calories than burning carbohydrate. Therefore, drinking one can of beer provides approximately 100 calories.[9]

CURRENT USE AND ABUSE OF ALCOHOL

According to a survey by the U.S. government of adults ages eighteen and older, approximately 50 percent of adults are currently drinkers (at least twelve drinks in the past year) and 14 percent are infrequent drinkers (one to eleven drinks in the past year). In addition, 6 percent are former regular drinkers, 9 percent are former infrequent drinkers, while 21 percent are lifetime abstainers. Among current drinkers 61 percent are men and 42 percent are women. Women and Asian Americans are more likely to be lifetime abstainers than are men. In general, older adults drink less frequently than young adults.[10] Only a small percentage of Americans who drink on a regular basis are heavy drinkers.

Unfortunately, underage drinking in the United States is a serious problem because the adolescent brain is more susceptible to alcohol-related damage than the adult brain. According to a 2006 report by the National Institute of Alcohol Abuse and Alcoholism, each year approximately 5,000 young people under the age of twenty-one die as a result of underage drinking (approximately 1,900 deaths from motor vehicle accidents, 1,600 as a result of homicide, 300 from suicide, and others from injuries such as falls, burns, and drowning).[11] According to the National Survey on Drug Use and Health Report published in November 2008, more than one-quarter of people ages twelve to twenty (28.1 percent) used alcohol in the past month, 51.1 percent of ages eighteen to twenty, 25.9 percent of ages fifteen to seventeen, and 6.1 percent of ages twelve to fourteen. This is a shocking statistic because alcohol has a devastating effect on the developing brain of a twelve-year-old person. Nearly one-third of the current underage alcohol drinkers (30.6 percent) paid for the last alcoholic drink they consumed, 14.6 percent got it free from another underage person, 8.5 percent received it from another relative, and an alarming 5.9 percent received their last drink from a parent or guardian. Current alcohol users ages twelve to twenty consumed more drinks on average (six drinks) if they paid for the drink than those who received their drinks free (an average of nearly four drinks). Underage women more often received their last drink free compared to men and more men consumed alcohol than did women.[12]

Binge drinking is also very problematic for adolescents, and statistics for binge drinking among underage drinkers, as well as adverse effects of drinking on adolescents' brains, are discussed in chapter 3. Underage drinking is a major public health and safety issue, because young people who start drinking at an early age have a much greater risk of becoming alcohol dependent later in life than individuals who start drinking at age twenty-one or older.

WHY ALCOHOL IS A DRUG

According to the American Council for Drug Education, alcohol is the oldest and most widely used drug in the world. Nearly half of all Americans consume alcohol. Although most drink only occasionally and sensibly, there are 10 to 16 million alcoholics and problem drinkers (this number is lower than the estimated 18 million given as a recent estimate by a U.S. government study; see more on this in chapter 5), which includes 4.5 million adolescents with drinking problems. Alcohol intoxication results in crime, violence, and disturbances that consume more resources than other aspects of police operations, and the health consequences of alcohol abuse are a huge economic burden on the nation. Although illegal drugs cause addiction more rapidly than alcohol, and in much smaller doses, according to the American Council for Drug Education, alcohol is America's most serious drug problem.[13]

Alcohol can be considered a psychoactive drug because it has complex interactions with various neurotransmitters and receptors in the brain, producing pleasurable effects when consumed in moderation. However, with excess consumption, the positive effects of drinking are replaced by negative effects, such as anxiety and depression. If consumed in moderation, alcohol can protect against age-related dementia and Alzheimer's disease, but if consumed in excess it can cause severe brain damage. In addition, alcohol shares many pathways of various psychoactive drugs for its pharmacological actions (see chapter 3). Therefore, alcohol can be considered a drug. The Substance Abuse and Mental Health Services Administration (SAMHSA) has published many reports on substance abuse where alcohol and drugs are placed in the same category.

Alcohol, like any drug, has prophylactic effects in preventing many diseases, including coronary heart disease (the number one killer in America), stroke, various cancers, diabetes, arthritis, and other diseases, as well as increasing longevity (see chapter 4). However, if consumed in excess, it is detrimental to health (see chapter 5). Therefore, like a drug, alcohol is effective in low doses and toxic in higher doses. Like a drug, alcohol is metabolized by liver enzymes, and a toxic metabolite of alcohol known as "acetaldehyde" is generated. If acetaldehyde is accumulated in the body due to excess alcohol intake, it can cause liver damage.

Many individuals with a genetic makeup susceptible to alcohol abuse are also susceptible to drug abuse, indicating that alcohol can be compared to an illicit drug, but with lower abuse potential. According to a current survey (Dick and Agarwal 2008), 8.5 percent of American adults met the criteria for an alcohol use disorder, 2 percent met the criteria for a drug abuse disorder, while 1.1 percent met the criteria for both, indicating that many abusers of illicit drugs are also dependent on alcohol. People ages eighteen to twenty-four had the highest rates of co-occurring alcohol and illicit drug abuse disorders. Researchers have established that some of the risk of addiction to both drugs and alcohol are inherited. Children of alcoholics are 50 to 60 percent more likely to abuse alcohol, while children of parents abusing illicit drugs are 45 to 79 percent more likely to abuse illicit drugs. This suggests that risk factors for alcohol and illicit drug dependence are rooted in the genes.[14] In their study Dick and Agarwal concluded that some of the same genes that increase a person's risk for problems with alcohol might also put him or her at greater risk for illicit drug dependence. Moreover, the same genes might increase the risk of other psychiatric problems, such as conduct disorders, adult antisocial behavior, borderline personality disorder, and so on (fig. 1.2). Studies with twins suggest that the overlap between dependence on alcohol and other drugs largely results from shared genetic factors. There are various genes that make a person susceptible to alcohol and drug abuse. Certain genes control metabolism of alcohol, while other genes reinforce the effect of alcohol in the brain.[15]

CONCLUSION

Alcohol is the oldest drug known to mankind. Human fondness for alcohol may have originated from the genetic makeup of early primates 30 to 40 million years ago who lived on a diet of ripe fruits (drunken monkey hypothesis). Ancient alcoholic beverages were low in alcohol content, but with the discovery of distillation, alcohol content surged. Modern beers and wines have a higher alcohol content than ancient beer and wine. Alcohol was recognized as a drug by physicians of ancient Greece and other ancient civilizations as well as by Muslim doctors and Indian Ayurvedic doctors. Alcohol has many health benefits if consumed in moderation, but it is toxic if consumed in excess.

NOTES

1. R. Dudley, "Ethanol, Fruit Ripening, and the Historical Origins of Human Alcoholism in Primate Frugivory," *Integrative and Comparative Biology* 44, no. 4 (August 2004): 315–23.

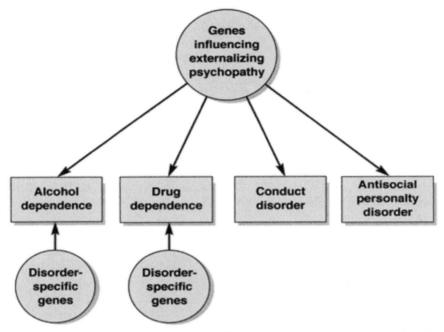

Figure 1.2. A schematic representation illustrating common influences of genetic factors on alcohol and drug dependence, personality, and conduct disorders. Some of the proposed genetic factors are considered to have a general influence on all types of externalizing personality, whereas others are thought to have disorder-specific influence. Externalizing psychopathy is defined as psychiatric disorders characterized by disinhibition behavior, antisocial personality disorder, attention deficit/hyperactivity disorder, and conduct disorder.

Source: Reference 14, a U.S. government publication; information in public domain.

2. D. Stephens and R. Dudley, "The Drunken Monkey Hypothesis: The Study of Fruit-Eating Animals Could Lead to an Evolutionary Understanding of Human Alcohol Abuse," *Natural History* magazine, December 2004.

3. David Hanson, *Preventing Alcohol Abuse: Alcohol Culture and Control* (Westport, CT: Greenwood, 1995).

4. B. L. Vallee, "Alcohol in the Western World," *Scientific American*, June 1998.

5. "History of Alcohol Use," *Heads Up!* Loyola Marymount University, Los Angeles, http://www.lmu.edu/pages25071.aspx.

6. Barrie Pepper, *The International Book of Beer: A Guide to the World's Most Popular Drink* (New York: New Line Books, 2006).

7. J. S. Jensen, S. Demiray, M. Egebo, and A. S. Myers, "Prediction of Wine Color Attributes from Phenolic Profiles of Red Grapes (*Vitis vinifera*)," *Journal of Agriculture and Food Chemistry* 56, no. 3 (February 2008): 1105–15.

8. P. Polásková, J. Herszage, and S. E. Ebeler, "Wine Flavor: Chemistry in a Glass," *Chemical Society Review* 37, no. 11 (November 2008): 2478–89.

9. C. S. Liber, "Relationships Between Nutrition, Alcohol Use and Liver Disease," *Alcohol Research and Health* 27, no. 3 (2003): 220–31.

10. Summary of Health Statistics for U.S. Adults: National Interview Survey 2008, National Center for Health Statistics, United States, Hyattsville, ND.

11. Alcohol Alert #67, "Underage Drinking," National Institute on Alcohol Abuse and Alcoholism, January 2006, http://pubs.niaaa.nih.gov/publications/aa67/aa67.htm.

12. "Underage Alcohol Use: Where Do Young People Get Alcohol?" National Survey on Drug Use and Health Report, November 20, 2008, Office of Applied Studies, Substance Abuse and Mental Health Services Administration (SAMHSA).

13. "Basic Facts about Drugs," American Council for Drug Education, http://www.acde.org/common/Alcohol.htm.

14. Alcohol Alert #76, "Alcohol and Other Drugs," National Institute on Alcohol Abuse and Alcoholism, January 2006, http://pubs.niaaa.nih.gov/publications/aa76/aa76htm.

15. D. M. Dick and A. Agarwal, "The Genetics of Alcohol and Other Drug Dependence," *Alcohol Research and Health* 31, no. 2 (2008): 111–18.

2

How the Human Body Handles Alcohol

A Guide to Drinking Sensibly and Avoiding a DWI

Alcoholic beverages can be classified under three broad categories: beer, wine, and spirits. Beer and wine are fermented beverages produced from sugar- or starch-containing plant materials. The normal fermentation process, which uses yeast, cannot produce alcoholic beverages with an alcohol content higher than 14 percent. Therefore, hard liquors or spirits are produced using fermentation followed by another process called distillation. Alcohol is full of calories, and heavy drinking is a serious health hazard, including premature death due to liver cirrhosis. However, drinking in moderation has many health benefits, including protection against cardiovascular disease, stroke, type 2 diabetes, a lower risk of forming gallstones, and possibly a longer life (see chapter 4). Therefore, the key is to drink in moderation and drink sensibly. This chapter discusses how the body handles alcohol and provides clear guidance regarding drinking in moderation so that after a pleasant evening of good food and wine, you will not be stopped by the police for a suspected DWI (driving with impairment/driving while intoxicated; in some states DUI, driving under the influence). The guidelines provided in this chapter are conservative guidelines, because I believe it is better to be safe than sorry.

DEFINITION OF A STANDARD DRINK

The alcohol content of various alcoholic beverages varies widely. The average alcohol content of beer is 5 percent, wine is 10 percent, and whiskey is 40 percent. However, the serving sizes also vary according to the type of beverage. For example, beer usually comes in a 10- or 12-ounce bottle, while a shot of tequila in a mixed drink is only 1.5 ounces. Therefore, regardless of the alcoholic beverage, a standard drink contains roughly the same amount of alcohol. In the United States, a standard drink is defined as a bottle of beer (12 ounces) containing 5 percent alcohol, 8.5 ounces of malt liquor containing 7 percent alcohol, a 5-ounce glass of wine containing 12 percent alcohol, 3.5 ounces of fortified wine (like sherry or port) containing about 17 percent alcohol, 2.5 ounces of cordial or liqueur containing 24 percent alcohol, or 1.5 ounces of distilled spirits such as gin, rum, vodka, or whiskey. Each standard drink contains approximately the same amount of alcohol. For example, beer contains an average 5 percent alcohol, so the total alcohol content of 12 ounces of beer is $12 \times 0.05 = 0.6$ ounce of alcohol, which is equivalent to 14 gm of alcohol. In general, the average bottle of beer contains 0.56 ounce of alcohol and a standard wine drink may contain 0.66 ounce of alcohol, but distilled spirits may contain up to 0.89 ounce of alcohol. Therefore, 0.6 ounce of alcohol in a standard drink is a reasonable approximation.[1]

In a mixed drink or cocktail, if one shot of distilled spirits is used, the alcohol content should be 0.6 ounce. In a bar, a bartender uses a "jigger" for preparing mixed drinks. A jigger is a measuring device used to pour precisely 1.5 ounces of alcohol. A jigger may also have a smaller 1-ounce cup called a pony shot. For simple mixed drinks such as rum and coke or gin and tonic, each cocktail comes with one shot of liquor, and consuming one such drink is equivalent to drinking one bottle of beer, as far as blood alcohol level is concerned. However, in some mixed drinks, two shots are used, so the alcohol content of that mixed drink equals two standard drinks. A cocktail usually contains one or more types of distilled spirits, fruit juice, honey, milk, or other ingredients. If a mixed drink is prepared from more than one distilled spirit, then one mixed drink may be equivalent to two to three standard drinks. For example, a margarita is prepared from tequila and triple sec orange-flavored liquor containing 30 percent alcohol and is often served with salt on the glass rim. Depending on the alcohol content, drinking a 10-ounce margarita may be equivalent to two to three standard drinks.

Because blood alcohol level depends on the number of standard drinks, it is often difficult to calculate blood alcohol level if you are consuming mixed drinks prepared from more than one type of liquor. The alcohol content may also vary from bar to bar because of the use of different recipes. Malt liquor is a North American term referring to a type of beer with higher alcohol content. Malt liquors are often cheaper than beer and contain an average of 7 percent alcohol. Some malt liquors are available in a 40-ounce bottle. Therefore, drinking one such bottle of malt liquor is equivalent to consuming 2.8 ounces of alcohol, which is equivalent to 4.6 standard drinks, or drinking more than four bottles of beer.

Historically, the alcohol content of various drinks was expressed as "proof," which is a measure of the alcohol content. The term originated in the eighteenth century when British sailors were paid with rum as well as money. In order to ensure that the rum was not diluted with water, it was "proofed" by dousing gunpowder with it and setting it on fire. If the gunpowder failed to ignite, it indicated that the rum had too much water and was considered "under proof." A sample of rum that was 100 proof contained approximately 57 percent alcohol by volume (43 percent water). In the United States, proof to alcohol by volume is defined as a ratio of 1:2. Therefore, a beer that has 4 percent alcohol by volume is defined as 8 proof. In the United Kingdom, alcohol by volume to proof is a ratio of 4:7. Therefore, multiplying alcohol by volume content with a factor of 1.75 would provide the proof of the drink.

Currently in the United States, the alcohol content of a drink is measured by the percentage of alcohol by volume. The code of Federal Regulations (27CFR [4-1-03 edition] §5.37 Alcohol Content) requires the label of alcoholic beverages to state the alcohol content by volume. The regulation permits, but does not require, the "proof" of the drink to be printed on the label as well. In the United Kingdom and in European countries, the alcohol content of a beverage is also expressed as the percentage of alcohol in the drink. The alcohol content of various popular beverages is given in table 2.1. It is important to note that a standard drink contains approximately the

Table 2.1. Alcohol Content of Various Drinks

Beverage	One Standard Drink	Alcohol Content
Standard American beer	12 ounces (355 mL)	4–10%
Anchor Porter		5.6%
Budweiser		5%
Budweiser Light		4%
Coors		4.9%
Coors Light		4.2%
Flying Dog Horn Dog		10.5%
Michelob		5%
Michelob Light		4.3%
Michelob Ultra Light		4.1%
Miller		4.7%
Miller Light		4.2%
Table wine	5 ounces (148 mL)	7–14%
Sparkling wine	5 ounces (148 mL)	8–14%
Fortified wine	2–5 ounces (59–148 mL)	14.0–24%
Whiskey	0.6 ounce (18 mL)	40–75%
Vodka	0.6 ounce (18 mL)	40–50%
Gin	0.6 ounce (18 mL)	40–49%
Rum	0.6 ounce (18 mL)	40–80%
Tequila	0.6 ounce (18 mL)	45–50%
Brandies	0.6 ounce (18 mL)	40–44%

same amount of alcohol (roughly 0.6 ounces). Therefore, regardless of the type of drink, your "body burden" of alcohol depends mostly on the number of drinks consumed, as well as your body weight, gender, and whether or not you consume food while drinking.

HOW THE BODY HANDLES ALCOHOL

When you drink, alcohol is absorbed from your stomach and small intestine. It then undergoes a chemical transformation by the liver through a process called "metabolism," and eventually the body gets rid of all alcohol consumed. A small amount of alcohol that is not absorbed is found in your breath and is the basis of breath analysis of drivers suspected of driving with impairment. Factors that affect how your body handles alcohol include:

Age
Gender
Race and ethnicity
Body weight
Amount of food consumed
How quickly alcohol is ingested
Alcoholism

In general, alcoholics metabolize alcohol faster than a nonalcoholic person. Age, gender, body weight, and genetic makeup all affect how your body handles alcohol. Drinking faster may cause much higher blood alcohol levels because absorption and elimination of alcohol from the body take place simultaneously.

Absorption

When alcohol is consumed, about 20 percent is absorbed by the stomach and the rest is absorbed from the small intestine. When alcohol is consumed on an empty stomach, blood alcohol levels peak between fifteen and ninety minutes after drinking. Food substantially slows down the absorption of alcohol, and can even reduce the rate of absorption of alcohol for four to six hours. Sipping alcohol versus drinking it like soda or water also slows absorption.

Always consume food when you are drinking. Sip and enjoy your alcohol. Do not consume more than one drink in one hour.

The effect of food on absorption and metabolism of alcohol has been widely studied and reported in the medical literature. In one study (Jones and Jönsson 1994), ten healthy men drank a moderate dosage of alcohol (0.80 gm of alcohol per kg of body weight) in the morning after an overnight fast or immediately after breakfast (two cheese sandwiches, one boiled egg, orange juice, and fruit yogurt). Subjects who drank alcohol on an empty stomach felt more intoxicated than the subjects who drank the same amount of alcohol after eating breakfast. The blood alcohol analysis revealed the cause. The average peak blood alcohol concentration in subjects who drank on an empty stomach was 104 mg/dL (0.104 percent), which was above the legal level of intoxication (0.08 percent). In contrast, the average peak blood alcohol concentration in subjects who drank alcohol after eating breakfast was 67 mg/dL (0.067 percent). The time required to metabolize all alcohol was on average two hours less in subjects who drank alcohol after eating breakfast compared to subjects who drank on an empty stomach. The authors concluded that food in the stomach before drinking not only reduces the peak blood alcohol concentration but also boosts the rate at which the body gets rid of alcohol.[2]

Studies have also been conducted using different types of food, such as high-fat versus high-protein or high-carbohydrate, to see what effect they have on alcohol absorption. Drinking after eating a meal, regardless of the types of foods eaten, decreases the absorption of alcohol.[3] Therefore, drinking alcohol with any food type will reduce alcohol's effects and concentration in the blood. Food intake slows gastric emptying time, and the alcohol dehydrogenase enzyme, which metabolizes alcohol in the liver, is also present in the gastric mucosa (the mucous membrane of the stomach). Part of the alcohol ingested is metabolized in the stomach by this enzyme before the alcohol reaches the small intestine and duodenum for further absorption. Food prolongs the time alcohol spends in your stomach, giving the enzyme a chance to metabolize more alcohol.

Distribution and Metabolism

A small amount of alcohol is metabolized by the enzyme present in the gastric mucosa; also, a small amount of alcohol is metabolized by the liver before it can enter the main bloodstream. This process is known as "first-pass metabolism" or "pre-systematic metabolism." After alcohol is ingested, it is absorbed from the gut and enters the hepatic portal system (a portal vein carries the alcohol to the liver), and some of the alcohol is metabolized. Then the rest of the alcohol enters the bloodstream, which is known as systematic circulation. If a person drinks a certain amount of alcohol, the peak blood alcohol level would be significantly lower than the same amount of alcohol being injected into the same person. This is because alcohol undergoes first-pass metabolism only when ingested.

Also, a man drinking the same amount of alcohol would have a lower peak blood alcohol level compared to a woman with the same body weight. This gender difference in the blood alcohol level is related to the different body water content between a man and a woman. Alcohol loves water and distributes into the aqueous part of the blood known as serum. Because a woman has less body water content (52 percent on average) than a man (61 percent average), less water is available to dissolve the same amount of alcohol compared to a man. Some studies also report that women are more susceptible than men to alcohol-related impairment of cognitive functions.[4]

Women also metabolize alcohol more slowly than do men because the concentration of alcohol dehydrogenase (ADH) is usually lower in women compared to men. Hormonal changes also play a role in the metabolism of alcohol in women, although this finding has been disputed in the medical literature. Some studies suggest that women metabolize alcohol at a higher rate during the luteal phase of the menstrual cycle (days 19–22 of the cycle), but a few days before menstruating, a woman's alcohol metabolism may slow down.[5] Though more studies need to be conducted to confirm this, it has been well documented in medical literature that alcohol addiction causes disturbances in the menstrual cycle, and that such disturbances are more prominent during the middle part of the cycle.[6]

A woman may be more susceptible to the effect of alcohol right before her menstrual cycle.

Your liver metabolizes alcohol using zero-order kinetics, which means that no matter what amount of alcohol is present in the body, the liver gets rid of it at a constant rate. In contrast, most drugs follow first-order kinetics, meaning that the greater burden of a drug in the body, the faster the liver works to transform the drug into a metabolite for excretion in the urine. Consider this analogy: Students will usually party and enjoy life at the beginning of the semester, and study hard before a final exam. They will also work much harder as the deadline of a project approaches. This is like first-order kinetics, where the liver works harder when more drugs (stress) are present in the body. On the other hand, zero-order kinetics is like a student who starts studying at a steady rate from day one but does not study any harder before the finals.

In the liver, at very low (<20 mg/dL; 0.02 percent) or very high (>300 mg/dL; 0.3 percent) concentrations, ethanol elimination follows first-order kinetics; however, for the concentrations between, metabolism is independent of the dose due to enzyme saturation and thus follows zero-order kinetics.

Several enzyme systems are involved in the metabolism of ethanol (ethyl alcohol, or commonly termed "alcohol"), namely, alcohol dehydrogenase (ADH), the microsomal ethanol oxidizing system (MEOS), and catalase.[7] These enzymes also metabolize other similar compounds, such as methanol (wood spirit), isopropyl alcohol (rubbing alcohol), and ethylene glycol (antifreeze).

The first and most important of these, alcohol dehydrogenase, is a family of enzymes found primarily in hepatocytes (liver cells) (equation 2.1).

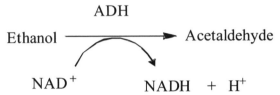

ADH

Ethanol $\longrightarrow$ Acetaldehyde

NAD^+ $\qquad$ $NADH + H^+$

NAD: Nicotinamide adenine dinucleotide is a coenzyme that is found in all living cells.
NADH: NADH is essential for enzymatic transformation of ethanol (alcohol) into acetaldehyde.

At least five classes of ADH are found in humans. ADH activity is greatly influenced by the frequency of ethanol consumption. Adults who consume two to three alcoholic beverages per week metabolize ethanol at a rate much lower than alcoholics. For medium-sized adults, the blood ethanol level declines at an average rate of 15 to 20 mg/dL/h (0.015 to 0.020 percent/hour) or a clearance rate of approximately 3 ounces of ethanol per hour.

The major drug-metabolizing family of enzymes found in the liver is the cytochrome P450 mixed-function oxidase. Many members of this family of enzymes, most notably CYP3A4, CYP1A2, CYP2C19, and CYP2E1 isoenzyme, play vital roles in the metabolism of many drugs. For nonalcoholics, this metabolic pathway is considered a minor, secondary route, but it becomes much more important in alcoholics. In addition to ADH, CYP2EI isoenzyme plays a major role in metabolizing alcohol because it helps alcoholics rid their bodies of alcohol faster than nonalcoholics (equation 2.2).

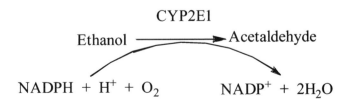

CYP2E1

Ethanol $\longrightarrow$ Acetaldehyde

$NADPH + H^+ + O_2$ $\qquad$ $NADP^+ + 2H_2O$

The acetaldehyde produced due to the metabolism of alcohol, regardless of the pathway, is subsequently converted to acetate as a result of the action of mitochondrial aldehyde dehydrogenase (ALDH2). Acetaldehyde is fairly toxic compared to ethanol and must be metabolized quickly (equation 2.3).

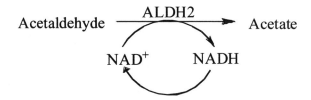

Acetate or acetic acid then enters the citric acid cycle, which is a normal metabolic cycle of living cells, and is converted into carbon dioxide and water. From the chemical point of view, the body burns (oxidizes) alcohol into carbon dioxide and water, and this process generates calories. Therefore, alcoholic drinks are high in calories.

EFFECT OF AGE ON ALCOHOL METABOLISM

In general, a child will metabolize a drug faster than a younger or middle-aged adult, and an elderly person (older than sixty-five) will metabolize a drug more slowly than a younger or middle-aged adult. Metabolism of alcohol changes with advancing age because the activity of the enzymes involved in alcohol metabolism diminish with age. Water volume also reduces with advancing age. An elderly person would have a higher blood alcohol level from consumption of the same amount of alcohol compared to a younger person of the same gender. Moreover, elderly people consume more medications than do younger people, and a medication may interact with alcohol (see chapter 8). It is safe for elderly people to consume one drink a day provided it does not interact with any medication they are taking.[8] If an elderly person doesn't take medication or takes a medication that does not interact with alcohol, drinking in moderation has several health benefits for the elderly. Compared to abstention, consumption of one to six drinks weekly is associated with a lower risk of dementia among older adults.[9] Moderate consumption of alcohol by elderly people also improves cardiovascular health and social behavior. Moderate alcohol consumption on a regular basis is associated with increased quality of life and mood in both older men and women.[10] Among women undergoing menopause, moderate alcohol consumption, along with other lifestyle factors, has a positive effect on their sense of well-being.[11]

GENETIC FACTORS IN ALCOHOL METABOLISM

Alcohol is metabolized by the liver, where it is converted first to acetaldehyde by the enzyme alcohol dehydrogenase. Acetaldehyde is then converted to acetate by the enzyme aldehyde dehydrogenase. Acetaldehyde is the most toxic metabolite of alcohol (both alcohol and acetate are relatively nontoxic). Acetaldehyde produces unpleasant physiological reactions even at low concentration and is responsible for the dreaded alcohol hangover. When acetaldehyde is not rapidly converted into acetate, the results are dramatic: a rapid increase in blood flow to the skin of the face, neck, and chest, rapid heartbeat, headache, nausea, and extreme drowsiness can occur. These unpleasant reactions from drinking, collectively called flushing, may occur more frequently in certain ethnic groups. Approximately half of the Asian population are considered deficient in the alcohol dehydrogenase enzyme and may experience flushing even after consumption of one or two drinks. Such unpleasant reactions also deter people from drinking and may protect against alcoholism. The alcohol-deterrent drug disulfiram works as a deterrent by producing a similar "flush reaction." Disulfiram inactivates aldehyde dehydrogenase in a person who carries the normal gene for that enzyme, in effect producing the same situation as in the Asians who have the inactive, mutant form of the gene. Some East Indians, American Indians, and Alaskan Natives may also have genetic variations that affect metabolism of alcohol. American Indians and Alaskan Natives are five times more likely than other ethnic groups in the United States to die of alcohol-related causes. Caucasian populations usually do not have any significant genetic variation that affects alcohol metabolism. Please see chapter 5 for an in-depth discussion on this important subject.

DRINKING SENSIBLY

In order to reap the beneficial effects of alcohol, one needs to drink in moderation. It is important to drink sensibly during a party or dinner to avoid a DWI charge if you plan to drive home the same night.

Moderate Alcohol Consumption

The following recommendations are from the U.S. government's "Dietary Guidelines for Americans":[12]

Men: No more than two standard alcoholic drinks per day
Women: No more than one standard alcoholic drink per day
Adults over 65 (both male and female): No more than one drink per day

Alcoholic beverages should not be consumed by some individuals, including those who cannot restrict their alcohol intake, women of child-bearing age who may become pregnant, pregnant and lactating women, children and adolescents, individuals taking medications that can interact with alcohol, and those with specific medical conditions. Alcoholic beverages should be avoided by individuals engaging in activities that require attention, skill, or coordination, such as driving or operating machinery.

Alcohol has beneficial effects when consumed in moderation. The lowest all-cause mortality occurs at an intake of one to two drinks per day. The lowest coronary heart disease mortality also occurs at an intake of one to two drinks per day (see chapter 4). The well-established relationship between regular alcohol consumption in moderation and a reduced risk of cardiovascular disease may benefit women at a much younger age than men. In both sexes, however, these beneficial effects of alcohol use can be negated when alcohol is consumed in a heavy episodic drinking pattern, especially for middle-aged and older men.[13] People who are moderate drinkers have friends who are also nondrinkers or moderate drinkers and have hobbies and other interests in common. Moderate drinkers always have blood alcohol well below 0.05 percent (50 mg/dL) and do not get into trouble with the law (at least due to alcohol consumption).

In the United States, a standard drink (12 ounces of beer, 5 ounces of wine, or 1.5 ounces of 80 proof distilled spirits) contains approximately 0.6 ounces or 14 gm of alcohol. Various other countries also have guidelines for drinking in moderation. In Canada, a standard drink is defined as containing approximately 13.5 gm of alcohol. Drinking in moderation means not drinking more than seven drinks a week for both men and women. In the United Kingdom a standard drink contains 8 gm of alcohol, and the guideline for drinking in moderation is 8–16 gm of alcohol per day for both men and women (table 2.2).

Heavy Drinking

Drinking more than recommended can invite problems, because the health benefits of drinking in moderation quickly disappear. Theoretically, drinking more than three drinks a day by men and more than two drinks a day by women can be considered heavy drinking. For all practical purposes, the National Institute of Alcohol Abuse and Alcoholism sets this threshold at more than fourteen drinks per week for men (or more than four drinks per occasion) and more than seven drinks per week for women (or more than three drinks per occasion). Individuals whose drinking exceeds these guidelines are at increased risk for adverse health effects. Hazardous drinking is defined as the quantity or pattern of alco-

Table 2.2. Guidelines for Drinking in Moderation in Various Countries

Country	Amount of Alcohol (One Drink)	Men	Women
United States	14 gm	Up to 28 gm/day (2 drinks)	Up to 14 gm/day (1 drink)
Canada	13.5 gm	Up to 94.5 gm/week (Up to 7 drinks/ week)	Up to 94.5 gm/week (Up to 7 drinks/week)
Australia	10 gm	Up to 40 gm/day Two days/week no drinking	Up to 40 gm/day Two days/week no drinking
UK	8 gm	8–16 gm/day (Up to 2 drinks)	8–16 gm/day (Up to 2 drinks)
France	12 gm	60 gm/day (Up to 5 drinks)	36 gm/day (Up to 3 drinks)
Japan	19.8 gm	Two drinks of sake per day at the most (39.6 gm of alcohol/day maximum)	
Spain	10 gm	Up to 30 gm/day (Up to 3 drinks/ day)	Up to 30 gm/day (Up to 3 drinks/day)
Italy	10 gm	Up to 40 gm/day Elderly Up to 30 gm/day	Up to 30 gm/day Elderly Up to 25 gm/day
New Zealand	10 gm	Up to 210 gm/week No more than 60 mg in one occasion	Up to 140 gm/week No more than 40 mg in one occasion
Ireland	8 gm	Up to 24 gm/day (Up to 3 drinks)	Up to 16 gm/day (Up to 2 drinks)

hol consumption that places individuals at high risk from alcohol-related disorders. Usually hazardous drinking is defined as twenty-one or more drinks per week by men or more than seven drinks per occasion at least three times a week. For women, more than fourteen drinks per week or drinking more than five drinks in one occasion at least three times a week is considered hazardous drinking.[14]

Alcohol use is a leading cause of mortality and morbidity internationally and is ranked by the World Health Organization (WHO) as one of the top five risk factors for disease. Without treatment, approximately 16 percent of all hazardous or heavy alcohol consumers will become alcoholics.[15] Heavy consumption of alcohol leads not only to increased domestic violence, decreased productivity, increased risk of motor vehicle and job-related accidents, but also to increased mortality from liver cirrhosis, stroke, and cancer (see chapter 5 for a more detailed discussion).

Fortunately, alcohol consumption is going down in the United States. Compared to fifty years ago, Americans consume less alcohol now. The per capita consumption of alcohol is much higher in European countries, such as Hungary, the Czech Republic, Germany, France, the United Kingdom, and Denmark, compared to the United States. Fortunately, the perception of the mean reported number of drinks to feel drunk reduced significantly between each survey conducted between 1979 and 2000 in the United States. This may be explained partly by the increase in education, the decline in per capita alcohol consumption, and changes in alcohol policy toward lower blood alcohol levels for determining impairment.[16]

Binge Drinking

"Binge drinking" means heavy consumption of alcohol within a short period of time with the intention of becoming intoxicated. Although there is no universally accepted definition for binge drinking, usually consumption of five or more drinks by males and four or more drinks by females is considered binge drinking. Such drinking patterns always result in blood alcohol levels above 0.08 percent, the legal limit for driving. Despite having a legal drinking age of twenty-one in the United States, binge drinking is very popular among college students. In one study (Naimi et al. 2004), the authors found that 74.4 percent of binge drinkers consumed beer exclusively or predominantly, and 80.5 percent of binge drinkers consumed at least some beer. Wine accounted for only 10.9 percent of binge drinks consumed.[17] Predictably, college binge drinkers are more likely than their nondrinking counterparts to experience one or more alcohol-related problems while in college. In another study (Jennisom 2004), the author observed in a ten-year follow-up of binge drinkers that such drinkers have a much higher risk of becoming dependent on alcohol later in life. Binge drinking also caused early departure from college and less favorable labor market outcomes.[18]

BLOOD ALCOHOL CONCENTRATION AND DWI

DWI stands for "driving with impairment." The charge differs from state to state in the United States and includes DUI or "driving under the influence," OUI or "operating [a vehicle] under the influence," and OWI or "operating [a vehicle] while impaired." In some states DWI stands for "driving while intoxicated." Although impairment may also be drug related, alcohol is the major cause of DWI, not only in the United States but worldwide. Alcohol-related motor vehicle accidents kill approximately 17,000 Americans annually and are associated with more than $51 billion in total costs annually. A strong correlation exists between binge drinkers and alcohol-impaired drivers in the United States. In one study (Flowers et al. 2008), the authors found that overall, 84 percent of all alcohol-impaired drivers are binge drinkers; non–heavy drinkers are also involved in alcohol-related motor vehicle accidents.[19]

Currently, in all states in the United States, the legal limit for driving is 0.08 percent alcohol concentration in the blood. This translates to 80 mg of alcohol in 100 milliliter of whole blood (80 mg/dL). Blood is composed of an aqueous part and various blood cells. Red blood cells contain hemoglobins and carry oxygen throughout the body, a biological process essential for living, whereas white blood cells perform other important functions, including protecting our body from invading organisms. In addition, various other cells, such as neutrophils, eosinophils, basophils, and so on are also found in whole blood. When blood is centrifuged for five to ten minutes, it separates into two levels: the upper aqueous layer (water-containing layer) called "serum" and the bottom red blood cell (RBC) layer. Alcohol is soluble in the aqueous part of blood. In some laboratories, blood alcohol is measured in the serum after separating blood cells from the whole blood. Serum concentration of alcohol is more than whole blood concentration of alcohol. In order to calculate whole blood concentration of alcohol, the measured serum concentration must be multiplied by a factor that is generally considered as 0.85. Therefore, if serum alcohol concentration is 100 mg/dL (0.1 percent), then the whole blood concentration is 85 mg/dL (0.085 percent). In most states, the legal limit of intoxication is defined as 0.08 percent alcohol in whole blood rather than serum alcohol concentration. However, for young adults, many states have a zero-tolerance policy for drivers. After drinking, alcohol enters into the circulatory system and distributes mostly into the aqueous component of blood. The blood alcohol level is determined by the number of drinks consumed and the time elapsed since the beginning of drinking. In general, the blood alcohol concentration reduces by 0.015 percent (15 mg/dL) per hour.

In the United Kingdom and Canada, the legal limit for driving is also 0.08 percent, but in other countries, lower levels of alcohol are mandated as the acceptable upper limit of driving under the influence of alcohol. In Switzerland, Denmark, Italy, the Netherlands, Austria, Australia, China, Thailand, and Turkey, the upper limit is 0.05 percent alcohol. In Japan, the upper acceptable limit is only 0.03 percent, and in certain countries, such as various Middle Eastern countries, Hungary, Romania, and Georgia, there is zero tolerance for blood alcohol limits in drivers.

Although the legal limit of blood alcohol in adult drivers in the United States is 0.08 percent, some driving impairment may occur at an even lower blood alcohol level. There is a general agreement that some impairment of the ability to drive takes place at a blood alcohol level of 0.05 percent. Even

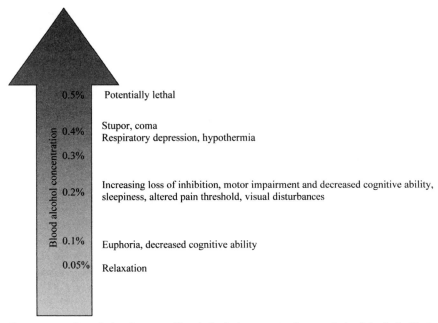

Figure 2.1.   Correlation between blood alcohol concentrations and physiological effects

blood alcohol levels of 0.03 percent affect some cognitive functions that rely on perception and the processing of visual information.[20] Ingestion of one drink generally leads to a blood alcohol level of 0.025 percent. Low blood alcohol levels of 0.05 percent usually produce more relaxation and more social interactions with other individuals. However, intoxication can occur at a blood alcohol level of 0.1 percent, and levels higher than 0.5 percent are potentially lethal (fig. 2.1). The drunkest reported driver in Sweden had a blood alcohol level of 0.55 percent.[21]

CALCULATION OF BLOOD ALCOHOL CONCENTRATION: WIDMARK FORMULA

In 1932, the Swedish scientist Eric P. Widmark developed a formula that is still used today for the calculation of the amount of alcohol ingested and for assessing the concentration of alcohol prior to a blood alcohol analysis.[22] The Widmark formula suggests estimating blood alcohol level on a given amount of alcohol administration by factoring in the subject's body weight and gender. By using this formula, one can estimate the amount of alcohol consumed by a person.

$$A = C \times W \times r$$

The letter A represents the total amount of alcohol consumed by the person in grams, C is the blood alcohol concentration in grams per liter, W is the body weight of the person expressed in kilograms, and r is a constant, which is assumed to be roughly 0.7 for men and 0.6 for women. Although these values are based on a Caucasian population, Tam et al. (2005) calculated that the average r value for Chinese men is 0.68 and average r value for Chinese women is 0.59, which are very close to average r values of Caucasian men and women.[23]

The modern form of the formula to calculate blood alcohol concentration from the amount of alcohol consumed by an individual by figuring in body weight and gender is as follows:

$C = (A/W \times r) - 0.015\ t$, where t represents time passed since the beginning of drinking

In the United States, one standard drink of alcohol has 0.6 ounce of alcohol and the weight of a person is expressed in pounds. However, blood alcohol concentration is expressed as mg per 100 mL of blood. Taking into account all these factors, this formula can be modified for calculating blood alcohol concentration as follows:

C = (Total amount of alcohol consumed in ounces $\times$ 5.14/weight in pounds $\times$ r) $- 0.015\ t$

C is the percentage of blood alcohol. Assuming each drink contains 0.6 ounce of alcohol, this equation can be further modified to:

C = (Number of drinks $\times$ 3.1/weight in pounds $\times$ r) $- 0.015\ t$

Because most standard drinks contain approximately the same amount of alcohol, it is only important to know how many drinks one person consumes. The type of drink does not matter, which makes the calculation easy. For example, if a 150-pound man drinks five beers in a two-hour period, his blood alcohol at the end of drinking would be:

$$\begin{aligned}
C &= (5 \times 3.1/150 \times 0.7) - 0.015 \times 2 \\
&= 0.147 - 0.030 \\
&= 0.117 \text{ percent}
\end{aligned}$$

If a 150-pound woman consumes five beers in two hours, her blood alcohol would be:

$$C = (5 \times 3.1/150 \times 0.6) - 0.015 \times 2$$
$$= 0.172 - 0.030$$
$$= 0.142 \text{ percent}$$

The blood alcohol level in women would be higher than men of the same weight. These calculations show that regardless of gender, drinking five beers or any five drinks within a two-hour time frame would result in a blood alcohol level much higher than the legal limit for driving.

There are many Internet sites that will calculate the blood alcohol level for you when you insert the number of drinks you have consumed, your gender, your body weight, and the time elapsed since you started drinking. In addition, there are also many charts available on Internet sites that provide approximate blood alcohol levels based on your body weight, gender, and number of drinks consumed. You need to subtract 0.015 percent per hour from that number in order to get an approximate blood alcohol level when you are ready to go home. In table 2.3, I have calculated the projected blood alcohol levels for men weighing between

Table 2.3. Projected Blood Alcohol in Males Consuming between 1 and 8 Drinks Using Widmark Formula

Body Weight	Number of Drinks							
	1	2	3	4	5	6	7	8
Male	Blood Alcohol Concentration (%)							
100 lb	0.044	0.088	0.132	0.176	0.220	0.264	0.308	0.352
125 lb	0.035	0.070	0.105	0.140	0.175	0.210	0.245	0.280
150 lb	0.030	0.060	0.090	0.120	0.150	0.180	0.210	0.240
175 lb	0.025	0.050	0.075	0.100	0.125	0.150	0.175	0.200
200 lb	0.022	0.044	0.066	0.088	0.110	0.132	0.154	0.176
225 lb	0.020	0.040	0.060	0.080	0.100	0.120	0.140	0.160
250 lb	0.018	0.036	0.054	0.072	0.090	0.108	0.126	0.144
275 lb	0.016	0.032	0.048	0.064	0.080	0.096	0.112	0.128
Female								
90 lb	0.057	0.114	0.171	0.228	0.285	0.342	0.399	0.456
100 lb	0.051	0.102	0.153	0.202	0.255	0.306	0.357	0.408
125 lb	0.041	0.082	0.123	0.164	0.205	0.246	0.287	0.328
150 lb	0.034	0.068	0.102	0.136	0.170	0.204	0.238	0.272
175 lb	0.030	0.060	0.090	0.120	0.150	0.180	0.210	0.240
200 lb	0.026	0.052	0.078	0.104	0.130	0.156	0.182	0.208
225 lb	0.023	0.046	0.069	0.092	0.105	0.128	0.161	0.184
250 lb	0.020	0.040	0.060	0.080	0.100	0.120	0.140	0.160

100 and 275 pounds and women weighing between 90 and 250 pounds. In these calculations, I assumed that all alcohol was consumed rapidly, so these values represent blood alcohol levels at an equilibrium state. I did not take into account any metabolism of alcohol. You need to subtract 0.015 percent per hour from this number from the time you started drinking. For example, if you are a 125-pound women who consumed four drinks in four hours, then your estimated blood alcohol level is 0.164 percent minus 0.015 multiplied by four, which is 0.060, accounting for the burning of alcohol. Therefore, your estimated blood alcohol level is 0.104 percent, which is above the legal limit for driving. Therefore, even following the rule of one drink per hour is not valid if you consume more than two drinks in one occasion and still plan to drive. For a 150-pound man consuming four drinks in four hours, the estimated blood alcohol level would be 0.120 minus 0.060, which is 0.060, a value below the legal limit for driving; however, this blood alcohol level may still cause some impairment in driving.

In general, you should not consume more than one drink per hour (beer, wine, or dinner wine, but not a cocktail) and not more than two drinks in one occasion. You should wait for at least two hours from the beginning of drinking before you drive, unless your body weight is below 100 pounds or you belong to an ethnic group that has difficulty in metabolizing alcohol due to genetic predisposition. No guideline can be provided for drinking mixed drinks and cocktails, because alcohol content may vary widely at different bars. For example, depending on how it is prepared, one margarita may be equivalent to two or three standard drinks. Always consume alcohol with food.

Again, the guidelines provided are very conservative, and if you drink no more than two standard drinks in two hours, your blood alcohol should likely be below 0.05 percent and you should have little or no impairment for driving. If you weigh between 175 and 200 pounds, then you can consume up to three standard drinks in two to two and half hours and it will probably still be safe to drive. For people between 175 and 200 pounds, one margarita or a double-shot mixed drink should not cause blood alcohol levels over the legal limit for driving, provided at least two hours have passed since initiating drinking and before beginning to drive. A petite woman with a body weight around 100 pounds or less who consumes one beer or one five-ounce glass of wine should wait for two hours before driving. If you are an average woman with a body weight between 125 and 150 pounds, drinking one margarita or mixed drink is fine, provided you wait one and a half to two hours from the initiation of drinking until you drive. For petite women, with a body weight around 100 pounds or less, it is better not to drink mixed drinks, such as margaritas, and then drive, unless at least two and a half to three hours have passed from when you started drinking. Always consume alcohol with food.

ALCOHOLIC ODOR AND BLOOD ALCOHOL

There is a perception that if your breath smells like alcohol, you must have a blood alcohol level exceeding the legal limit for driving. In reality, alcohol is almost odorless, and the alcoholic smell perceived by people is due to the presence of many complex, organic, volatile compounds in alcoholic beverages. Wine aroma is attributed to a large range of molecules from different chemical families, including esters, aldehydes, ketones, terpenes, tannins, and sulfur compounds. Some of these compounds originate from grapes and others are formed during fermentation or aging. In general, more volatile substances are present in white wine compared to red wine.[24] Therefore, there is no correlation between blood alcohol level and alcoholic odor. Such odor may also be present in an individual drinking nonalcoholic beer.

CAN OUR BODIES PRODUCE ALCOHOL?

This is a very popular DWI defense: the defendant never drank alcohol but felt tipsy after eating a big meal, and that caused the accident. I have encountered this defense strategy several times in my twenty years of experience as an expert witness for the state on alcohol- and drug-related cases. Although substantial alcohol may be produced endogenously in a decomposed body by the action of various microorganisms, living bodies do not produce enough endogenous alcohol to be used as a defense in the case of accidents or impaired judgment. In healthy individuals who do not drink, endogenous alcohol levels are usually way below the detection level of instruments used in laboratories for measuring blood alcohol. There are reports of measurable endogenous ethanol production in patients with liver cirrhosis. In one report (Madrid et al. 2002), after a meal in such patients, negligible alcohol levels of 11.3 mg/dL (0.01 percent) and 8.2 mg/dL (0.008 percent) were detected in two out of eight patients. Small intestinal bacterial overgrowth generates such small amounts of endogenous alcohol. Patients with liver cirrhosis often have small intestinal bacterial overgrowth.[25]

CONCLUSION

Drinking in moderation—two drinks a day for men, one drink a day for women, and one drink a day for people older than sixty-five—has health benefits, but heavy drinking is associated with many diseases and also increases mortality from alcohol-related causes. If you drink moderately, then you will not get into trouble with the law, because your blood alcohol should be significantly below the legal limit of 0.08 percent. A good rule of thumb is to drink only one drink in one hour, not exceeding two drinks in two hours if you plan to drive home. Drinking more than that may get you into trouble. Certain ethnic groups, such as Asians, American Indians, and Alaskan Natives have a genetic predisposition that leads to impaired alcohol metabolism. Such individuals may experience flushing due to a buildup of acetaldehyde, a toxic metabolite of alcohol in blood, even from a single drink.

NOTES

1. W. C. Kerr, T. K. Greenfield, J. Tujague, and S. E. Brown, "A Drink Is a Drink? Variation in the Amount of Alcohol Contained in Beer, Wine and Spirits Drinks in a U.S. Methodological Sample," *Alcohol Clinical and Experimental Research* 29, no. 11 (November 2005): 2015–21.

2. A. W. Jones and K. Å. Jönsson, "Food-Induced Lowering of Blood-Ethanol Profiles and Increased Rate of Elimination Immediately after a Meal," *Journal of Forensic Sciences* 39, no. 4 (July 1994): 1084–93.

3. A. W. Jones, K. Å. Jönsson, and S. Kechagias, "Effect of High-Fat, High-Protein, and High-Carbohydrate Meals on the Pharmacokinetics of a Small Dose of Ethanol," *British Journal of Clinical Pharmacology* 44, no. 6 (December 1997): 521–26.

4. S. Mumenthaler, J. L. Taylor, R. O'Hara, and J. A. Yesavage, "Gender Differences in Moderate Drinking Effects," *Alcohol Research and Health* 23, no. 1 (January 1999): 55–64.

5. J. Gill, "Women, Alcohol, and the Menstrual Cycle," *Alcohol and Alcoholism* 32, no. 4 (April 1997): 435–41.

6. B. Augustyńska, M. Ziółkowski, G. Odrowąż-Sypniewska, A. Kiełpiński, M. Gruszka, and W. Kosmowski, "Menstrual Cycle in Women Addicted to Alcohol during the First Week Following Drinking Cessation: Changes in Sex Hormones Levels in Relation to Detected Clinical Features," *Alcohol and Alcoholism* 42, no. 2 (February 2007): 80–83.

7. S. Zakhari, "Overview: How Is Alcohol Metabolized by the Body?" *Alcohol Research and Health* 29, no. 4 (December 2006): 245–54.

8. P. Meier and H. K. Seitz, "Age, Alcohol Metabolism and Liver Disease," *Current Opinion in Clinical Nutrition and Metabolic Care* 11, no. 1 (January 2008): 21–26.

9. K. J. Mukamal, L. H. Kuller, A. L. Fitzpatrick, W. T. Longstreth Jr., Murray A. Mittleman, and David S. Siscovick, "Prospective Study of Alcohol Consumption

and Risk of Dementia in Older Adults," *Journal of American Medical Association* 289, no. 11 (November 2003): 1405–13.

10. A. M. Chan, D. von Muhlen, D. Kritz-Silverstein, and E. Barrett-Connor, "Regular Alcohol Consumption Is Associated with Increased Quality of Life and Mood in Older Men and Women: The Rancho Bernardo Study," *Maturitas* 63, no. 3 (March 2009): 294–300.

11. R. Alati, N. Dunn, D. M. Purdie, A. M. Roche, et al., "Moderate Alcohol Consumption Contributes to Women's Well-Being through the Menopausal Transition," *Climacteric: The Journal of the International Menopause Society* 10, no. 6 (December 2007): 491–99.

12. "Dietary Guidelines for Americans: Chapter 9—Alcoholic Beverages," United States Department of Agriculture and United States Department of Health and Human Services (Washington, D.C.: U.S. Government Printing Office, 2005), 43–46. Available at http://www.health.gov/DIETARYGUIDELINES/dga2005/document/html/chapter9.htm.

13. W. M. Snow, R. Murray, O. Ekumo, S. L. Tyas, et al., "Alcohol Use and Cardiovascular Health Outcome: A Comparison across Age and Gender in the Winnipeg Health and Drinking Survey Cohort," *Age and Aging* 38, no. 2 (March 2009): 206–12.

14. M. C. Reid, D. A. Fiellin, P. G. O'Connor, "Hazardous and Harmful Alcohol Consumption in Primary Care," *Archives of Internal Medicine* 159, no. 8 (August 2008): 1681–89.

15. S. Coulton, "Alcohol Misuse," *Clinical Evidence Handbook, American Family Physician*, April 15, 2009, 79(8): 692–94.

16. W. A. Kerr, T. K. Greenfield, L. T. Midanik, "How Many Drinks Does It Take to Feel Drunk? Trends and Predictors for Subjective Drunkenness," *Addiction* 101, no. 10 (October 2006): 1428–37.

17. T. S. Naimi, R. D. Brewer, J. W. Miller, C. Okoro, and C. Mehrotra, "What Do Binge Drinkers Drink? Implications for Alcohol Control Policy," *American Journal of Preventive Medicine* 33, no. 3 (August 2004): 188–93.

18. K. M. Jennisom, "The Short-Term Effects and Unintended Long-Term Consequences of Binge Drinking in College: A 10-Year Follow-Up Study," *American Journal of Drug and Alcohol Abuse* 30, no. 3 (August 2004): 659–84.

19. N. T. Flowers, T. S. Naimi, R. D. Brewer, R. W. Elder, R. A. Shults, and R. Jiles, "Patterns of Alcohol Consumption and Alcohol-Impaired Driving in the United States," *Alcohol: Clinical and Experimental Research* 32, no. 4 (April 2008): 639–44.

20. D. Breitmeier, I. Seeland-Schulze, H. Hecker, and U. Schneider, "The Influence of Blood Alcohol Concentrations around 0.03 Percent on Neuropsychological Functions: A Double-Blind, Placebo-Controlled Investigation," *Addiction Biology* 12, no. 2 (June 2007): 183–89.

21. A. W. Jones, "The Drunkest Drinking Driver in Sweden: Blood Alcohol Concentration 0.545% W/v.," *Journal of Studies in Alcohol* 60, no. 3 (May 1999): 400–406.

22. I. G. Brouwer, "The Widmark Formula for Alcohol Quantification," *South African Dental Association Journal* 59, no. 10 (November 2004): 427–28.

23. T. W. M. Tam, C. T. Yang, W. K. Fung, K. K. Mok Vincent, "Widmark Factors for Local Chinese in Hong Kong: A Statistical Determination on the Effects of Various Physiological Factors," *Forensic Science International* 151, no. 1 (June 2005): 23–29.

24. J. Torrens, M. Riu-Aumatell, E. Lopez-Tamames, and S. Buxaderas, "Volatile Compounds of Red and White Wines by Headspace: Solid-Phase Microextraction Using Different Fibers," *Journal of Chromatographic Science* 42, no. 6 (July 2004): 310–16.

25. A. M. Madrid, C. Hurtado, S. Gatica, I. Chacon, et al., "Endogenous Ethanol Production in Patients with Liver Cirrhosis, Motor Alteration and Bacterial Overgrowth," *Revista Medica de Chile* 130, no. 12 (December 2002): 1329–34.

3

How Alcohol Affects
the Human Mind

The human brain, the part of the central nervous system where autonomic functions, such as motor responses, heartbeat, respiration, and other activities take place, totally controls the human mind, the part of ourselves that *Webster's* defines as "the element or complex of elements in an individual that feels, perceives, thinks, wills, and especially reasons" (*Webster's Collegiate Dictionary*, 11th ed.). In order to understand how alcohol affects the human mind, we need to understand how alcohol affects the brain. Alcohol (ethanol) is the oldest of all drugs that humans consume for pleasure. Alcohol can affect different parts of our brain, providing relaxation, pleasure, loss of inhibition, and euphoria. The details of the molecular mechanism of how alcohol affects the human brain is still subject to research, but extensive study in this field for more than fifty years has unlocked many key mechanisms by which alcohol affects our mind. Chronic alcohol use is detrimental to brain cells and may cause them to die.

The effect of alcohol on the human mind depends on blood alcohol level and drinking habits. Drinking in moderation (not more than two drinks a day for men, one drink a day for women, and one drink a day regardless of gender in people older than sixty-five) can help an individual to relax after a hard day's work and can also enhance social interactions with others. In addition, moderate drinking has health benefits (see chapter 4 for more detail).

If you want to experience the pleasurable and beneficial effects of alcohol, always drink in moderation. Consuming excess alcohol is detrimental to both the human body and mind.

BLOOD ALCOHOL: EFFECT ON THE HUMAN MIND

Alcohol is a central nervous system depressant that reduces our inhibitions. Therefore, after one drink a person may talk more and feel more relaxed. In addition, alcohol releases neurotransmitters like dopamine, which can elevate our mood through the same positive reinforcement pathway that gives us pleasure after we eat our favorite food or enjoy intimate moments with our loved ones. Alcohol makes your brain feel less inhibited, which can result in exchanging feelings on deeper levels with friends and/or family.

Substantial research has established that the effect of alcohol on the human mind largely depends on the blood alcohol concentration. At a very low blood alcohol level (0.02–0.03 percent) people usually feel relaxation and mild euphoria and some loss of inhibition or shyness. At moderate blood alcohol levels (0.04–0.06 percent), a person may experience euphoria and the pleasurable effects of alcohol, such as being happy and satisfied. Inhibition may completely disappear, and he or she may interact more easily with other people. However, at higher blood alcohol levels, a person becomes impaired with compromised reflexes and motor skills. Such impairments become significant at the legal limit of blood alcohol, or 0.08 percent. Significantly higher blood alcohol levels that exceed the legal limit for driving cause depression instead of elation, complete loss of motor skills, and impaired judgment. At a blood alcohol level of 0.3 percent and higher, complete loss of consciousness may occur, and a blood alcohol level of 0.4 percent and higher may even cause death (see table 3.1).

People like to drink alcohol because of its ability to modify emotional states. Alcohol has a euphoric effect at low to moderate blood alcohol concentrations and can also cause relaxation, disinhibition, and reduced anxiety and stress levels. Rewarding and anxiolytic effects of alcohol are well documented in the medical literature.[1] However, elation caused by alcohol is dependent on blood alcohol concentration. At low to moderate blood alcohol levels, a person experiences the positive stimulatory effects of alcohol, but at higher blood alcohol levels, the negative effects of alcohol on mood (depression) become evident.[2] Alcohol is known to cause reduction in inhibition in a person, probably due to the reduction of frontal lobe functions of the brain. A recently published article (Hoppenbrouwers et al. 2010) concluded that loss of inhibition after drinking is more significant

Table 3.1. Blood Alcohol Level and the Effect on the Human Body and Mind

Blood Alcohol Level %	Effects on Human Body and Mind
0.01 to 0.019 (10 to 19 mg/dL)	Normal appearance of an individual
0.02 to 0.039 (20 to 39 mg/dL)	Feeling of mild euphoria, sense of well-being, and decreased inhibition or shyness. Usually no loss of muscle coordination observed at this blood alcohol level.
0.04 to 0.059 (30 to 59 mg/dL)	Euphoria with feelings of self-satisfaction and loss of most inhibition, making a person more talkative and interactive socially with everyone in the group. Emotions of an individual may be more intense and some behavior may be exaggerated. Some mild impairment may be observed in one's alertness and judgment.
0.06 to 0.79 (60 to 79 mg/dL)	Some impairments may be evident at this blood alcohol level, such as self-control, motor function, judgment, and ability to operate a motor vehicle. Peripheral vision and glare recovery may also be impaired and a person may lose all inhibition.
0.08 to 0.109 (80 to 109 mg/dL)	Balance, speech, hearing, and reaction time are all affected at this blood alcohol level and ability to drive a motor vehicle is severely impaired (legal limit for driving is 0.08 percent blood alcohol). Emotional swings and depression may also be observed at this blood alcohol level.
0.11 to 0.129 (110 mg/dL to 129 mg/dL)	Motor function, speech, judgment, and perception are all severely impaired at this high blood level. Staggering and slurred speech are also common, and a person may feel more angry and aggressive.
0.13 to 0.159 (130 mg/dL to 159 mg/dL)	Feelings of euphoria are totally replaced by feelings of depression and uneasiness. At such high blood alcohol levels a person may not be able to stand or walk without help from others, and vision may become totally blurry.
0.16 to 0.199 (160 mg/dL to 199 mg/dL)	Severe feelings of illness and depression and a person may become nauseous. At such elevated levels of blood alcohol, a person appears drunk.
0.20 to 0.249 (200 mg/dL to 249 mg/dL)	Nausea, vomiting, and some blackouts, and a person cannot move without the assistance of others. Some loss of consciousness may also occur.
0.25 to 0.299 (250 mg/dL to 299 mg/dL)	Stupor, impaired sensation, total memory blackout, and loss of consciousness occur at such severely elevated blood alcohol level.
0.3 to 0.4 (300 mg/dL to 400 mg/dL)	Severe alcohol toxicity, coma, and even death may occur.

in women than in men.[3] Another study (Clarisse et al. 2004), based on 184 degree-level and postgraduate students (ninety-four females and ninety males), indicated that alcohol at a level of approximately 50 mg/dL (0.05 percent) facilitated social interaction and communication.[4] Alcohol also has a calming effect and is capable of reducing anxiety.[5]

The behavioral actions of alcohol on brain neurochemistry are very much dependent on blood alcohol levels. Genetic factors and gender play an important role in the action of alcohol on the human mind, because at certain modest blood alcohol levels, some individuals may feel the pleasurable effects of alcohol, while others may not feel anything at all.[6] In order to understand the mechanism by which alcohol affects our mind, we need to understand how the human brain works.

> In the level of brain chemistry, alcohol is capable of selectively affecting functions of gamma-aminobutyric acid (GABA) receptors. In addition, alcohol can also affect functions of other receptors, such as glutamatergic, serotonergic, dopaminergic, cholinergic, and opioid systems, thus producing a feeling of joy and well-being.

HOW HUMAN BRAINS WORK

The human brain is the control center of the human body that coordinates the ability to move, touch, smell, taste, and hear. The brain also controls mood, level of consciousness, and alertness. The brain is a very complex organ that consists of the cerebrum, the cerebellum, and the brain stem, which are protected by the skull and internal lining, which is called the dura mater. The cerebrum is the largest part of the brain and is divided into two halves, the left and right cerebral hemispheres. The hemispheres are connected by nerve fibers that form a bridge (corpus callosum) through the middle of the brain, and each hemisphere is further divided into frontal, parietal, occipital, and temporal lobes (fig. 3.1). The right hemisphere is believed to control emotion, creativity, and intuitive and subjective judgment, while the left hemisphere is involved in logic, analytical thinking, and mathematical skill.

The cerebrum consists of dense masses of tissues, and the outer layer is called the cerebral cortex, also known as gray matter, which contains most of the nerve cells. The human brain has approximately 100 billion neurons that are specifically designed to receive, process, and transmit information, and are integral for the function of the brain. Similar to the other cells of the body, neurons have a nucleus and cytoplasm but also have characteristic features called axon and dendrite. Axon allows a neuron to send signals to

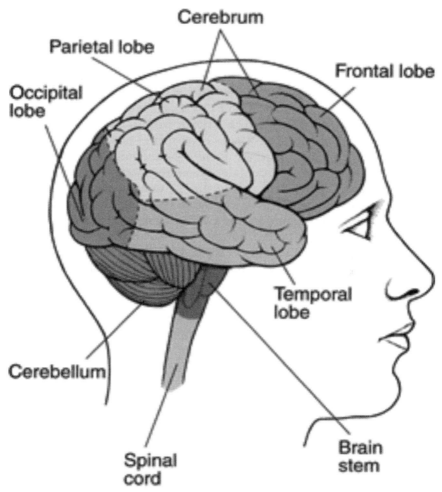

Figure 3.1. Various parts of the human brain from *The Merck Manual of Medical Information*, home ed., edited by Robert S. Porter (Whitehouse Station, NJ: Merck, 2007). Available at http://www.merck.com/mmhe/index.html. Reprinted with permission.

the neighboring neurons, while dendrites serve as the antenna to receive signals from other cells. Neurotransmitters are specific chemicals found in neurons that allow the transmission of the signal from one neuron to the next through synapse, a small gap between neurons. Neurotransmitters are stored in the axon part of the nerve cell (bulbous end), and when an electrical signal reaches the end part of the neuron, a specific neurotransmitter is released that travels through the synaptic gap and reaches the next neuron, either promoting or inhibiting the electrical signal along the next neuron. When a neurotransmitter crosses the synapse gap, it is accepted by the next neuron at a specialized site called a receptor (there are specialized receptors for different neurotransmitters), and it is the interaction between the receptor and the neurotransmitter that dictates the fate of the electrical impulse.

Neurotransmitters not only transmit information throughout the brain but are also capable of transmitting information from the brain to the rest of the body. For example, the first neurotransmitter, acetylcholine, discovered in 1921, sends information to skeletal muscle, sweat glands, and the heart. There are more than 200 known neurotransmitters, but three major categories of substances that act as neurotransmitters are amino acids (primarily glutamic acid, gamma-aminobutyric acid [GABA], aspartic acid, and glycine), peptides (vasopressin, somatostatin, neurotensin, to name a few), and monoamines (norepinephrine, dopamine, and serotonin). The major neurotransmitters of the brain are glutamic acid (also known as glutamate) and GABA, while monoamines and acetylcholine perform specialized functions. GABA is the major inhibitory neurotransmitter, and it can inhibit the action of other neurotransmitters, for example, dopamine. The neuropeptides, which are also categorized as neurotransmitters, perform specialized functions in the hypothalamus. A detailed discussion of how the brain works is beyond the scope of this book, but in table 3.2 functions of different parts of the brain are listed. In this chapter the reward system of the brain, which is responsible for the pleasurable effects of alcohol and drugs, will be discussed in detail, because this center is the key by which alcohol controls the human mind.

HOW THE BRAIN'S REWARD (PLEASURE) SYSTEM WORKS

The human mind seeks pleasure in daily life, and if certain amounts of pleasure or reward are not experienced every day, a person can become

Table 3.2. Function of Different Parts of the Human Brain

Part of the Brain	Major Functions
Frontal lobe	Controls facial expression and gesture
	Coordinates gestures with mood
	Voluntary actions such as looking at an object
	Relaxes bladder to urinate
	Controls motor skills, speech, and thoughts
Parietal lobe	Controls body movement and processes sensory stimulation
	Controls body parts and stores spatial memory
	Controls mathematical skill and language comprehension
Temporal lobe	Stores information and controls memory
	Comprehends sounds and images so that people can recognize a person, object, and so on
Occipital lobe	Controls vision and enables people to have visual memory
Mesolimbic system	Pleasure/reward center of the brain

depressed and may experience what is known as "reward deficiency syndrome." A broad range of activities stimulate our reward pathways, including food, positive social interactions, and/or positive feedback from work, sex, and exercise. In addition, many chemicals, such as alcohol, cocaine, opiates, and marijuana, can also stimulate our reward system. Addiction to drugs or alcohol occurs when the brain's reward system is hijacked by excessive use of drugs or alcohol.

The main center of the brain's reward pathway is at the ventral tegmental area (VTA) of the midbrain, and it is connected to the limbic system through the nucleus accumbens, amygdala, hippocampus, and the medial frontal cortex. There are two major pathways in the reward system that are modulated by the neurotransmitters dopamine and serotonin. The dopamine pathways produce reward, euphoria, and pleasure, while the serotonin pathway produces mood, memory, and sleep (fig. 3.2).

When the cortex of the prefrontal lobe receives and processes a sensory stimulus indicating reward, it sends a signal, announcing the reward to the VTA, which then releases dopamine into the entire reward system network. This region of the brain is also known as the pleasure or reward

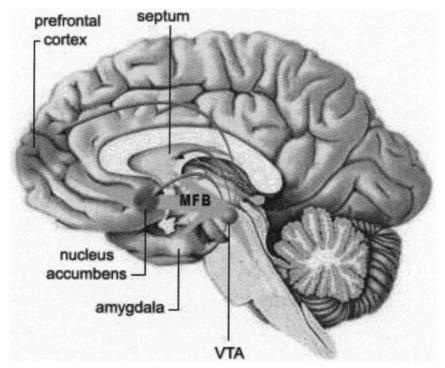

Figure 3.2. Diagram of mesolimbic system, the brain's pleasure structure

Source: Brain Pleasure Center, The Brain from Top to Bottom website, http://thebrain.mcgill.ca/flash/
index_d.html. Information in the public domain. Canadian Institute of Health Research.

bundle, which is part of the medial forebrain bundle (MFB), whose activation leads to repeated feelings of gratification. This structure is also known as the reward circuit of the brain and is distinct from the punishment circuit of the brain. The punishment circuit of the brain helps an individual with coping skills in unpleasant situations and with fighting skills. This circuit includes various brain structures, such as the hypothalamus, thalamus, and some area of the gray matter. The main neurotransmitter of the punishment circuit is acetylcholine. Consequently, the reward and punishment circuits control most of human behavior on a daily basis. The behavioral inhibition system is the third circuit, which comes into play when neither flight nor fight work and the person must passively submit to the environment. Serotonin plays an important role in this circuit. The pathophysiology of chronic depression can be explained partly from the function of this circuit.[7]

ALCOHOL AND THE BRAIN'S PLEASURE SYSTEM

The brain is protected by a thin barrier known as the blood-brain barrier, which limits the substances that can reach the brain. For example, penicillin and many other drugs cannot pass the blood-brain barrier, while alcohol, caffeine, nicotine, abused drugs, and various other drugs, such as drugs used for treating depression, can pass the blood-brain barrier.

Both alcohol and abused drugs stimulate the pleasure center of the brain (mesolimbic system) through similar molecular mechanisms. In general, drugs that are not abused (but that can cross the blood-brain barrier) do not increase dopamine levels in the brain's pleasure circuit, but abused drugs significantly increase dopamine levels, thus providing the euphoria following drug abuse. For example, stimulants such as amphetamines and cocaine increase dopamine levels in the brain's pleasure circuit (mesolimbic system) by inhibiting reuptake of dopamine into nerve terminals via dopamine transporters.[8] Opiates act by activating both dopamine neurons as well as specific opioid receptors on the GABA neurons at the VTA region of the midbrain. Nicotine from tobacco exerts its pleasurable effect by acting on the specific type of receptor for the neurotransmitter acetylcholine. These receptors are known as nicotine receptors. Interestingly, alcohol activates multiple neurotransmitter systems in the brain, but dopamine release in the mesolimbic system is one of the major pathways by which alcohol exerts its rewarding effect.[9]

Euphoria is experienced during the early phase of alcohol consumption (the first ten to fifteen minutes) when the blood alcohol concentration is on the rise. The exact mechanism of euphoria caused by alcohol is still the subject of active investigation, but in addition to the release of dopamine in the mesolimbic system, other neuronal mechanisms involving GABA, opiate, and serotonin receptors may also play some role in alcohol-induced euphoria. Alcohol may reinforce its intake by activating GABA receptors, thus indirectly modulating dopamine levels in the mesolimbic system. GABA receptors are present throughout the brain, and alcohol acts on GABA receptors to inhibit neurons. When a neuron is inhibited, it cannot fire electrical stimulus anymore, and therefore no neurotransmitter is released. Because alcohol inhibits GABA receptors, less neurotransmitter GABA is released and this increases the concentration of dopamine. Because dopamine receptors are also present in the brain's pleasure center, these receptors become activated and fire more rapidly and also result in the release of more dopamine. Therefore, alcohol increases dopamine concentrations by both direct stimulation and indirect stimulation (by inhibiting GABA receptors), and with higher dopamine concentrations, a person experiences euphoria after alcohol consumption. Although the serotonin pathway has also been suggested as a possible factor for alcohol-induced euphoria, Morgan and Badway (2009) demonstrated that it is unlikely that serotonin is involved in the euphoric effect of alcohol.[10]

In addition to the GABA pathway, alcohol can modulate dopamine levels in the mesolimbic system by modulating receptors for other neurotransmitters such as glycine receptors and acetylcholine receptors in the VTA area. At higher blood alcohol levels, euphoria is replaced by depression and other negative effects. Interestingly, dopamine in the mesolimbic system is involved in both the positive and negative reinforcement effect of alcohol depending on the blood alcohol level. Chronic abuse of alcohol can produce functional alteration in the mesolimbic system, and thus may cause permanent damage to this important brain function.[11]

MODERATE ALCOHOL CONSUMPTION AND THE HUMAN BRAIN: BENEFICIAL EFFECTS

Although chronic heavy alcohol consumption damages the human brain and may cause memory loss and severe dementia, light to moderate alcohol consumption may reduce the risk of dementia. The famous Rotterdam Study investigated the effect of alcohol consumption in subjects fifty-five years and older in preventing age-related dementia. The study included 7,983 individuals (3,105 men and 4,878 women) who were monitored every few years regarding health issues. The investigators concluded that light to moderate alcohol consumption (one to three drinks per day) was associated with a lower risk of developing any form of dementia, and such effects appeared to be unchanged by the type of drink consumed.[12] In their study on alcohol and dementia, Pinder and Sandler (2004) demonstrated that moderate alcohol consumption, especially red wine, may lower the risk of developing Alzheimer's disease. The specific anti-oxidant properties of wine's polyphenolic compounds (complex organic molecules found in the skin of grapes) may be particularly important in preventing Alzheimer's disease. However, due to substantially unpre-dictable risk of progression to problem drinking, the authors concluded that the most sensible advice to the general public is that "heavy drinkers should drink less or not at all, that abstainers should not be indiscrimi-nately encouraged to initiate drinking for health reasons and the light to moderate drinkers need not change their drinking habits for health rea-sons except in exceptional circumstances."[13]

It has been demonstrated that beta-amyloid peptide, a neurotoxic substance, can cause the death of brain cells in Alzheimer's disease. Res-veratrol, a natural polyphenolic compound mostly found in red wines, can protect neurons from amyloid-induced toxicity, which may help protect individuals from getting Alzheimer's disease.[14] Interestingly, light to moderate consumption of alcohol in older adults results in a lower risk of developing age-related dementia and Alzheimer's disease than nondrinkers, but frequent drinkers are at high risk for developing alcohol-related dementia. In addition, leisure time physical activities also produce protective effects against dementia, while smoking elevates the risk of Alzheimer's disease. Consuming vegetables and fish has beneficial effects in preventing dementia, but consuming foods high in saturated fats increases the risk.[15] Solfrizzi et al. (2007) studied the impact of alcohol consumption on the incidence of mild cognitive impairment and its pro-gression to dementia in 1,445 patients between sixty-four and eighty-four years old. The authors observed that patients with mild cognitive impair-ment who were moderate drinkers (one drink a day) had a lower rate of progression to dementia than abstainers. Furthermore, wine drinkers showed an even slower rate of progression to dementia than abstainers.[16]

> In patients with mild cognitive impairment, up to one drink per day, especially wine, may decrease the rate of progression to dementia.

CHRONIC ALCOHOL ABUSE AND THE HUMAN BRAIN

Chronic alcohol abuse has devastating effects on the human brain, but there is a difference between how alcohol affects adolescent brains versus adult brains, because in adolescence the mesolimbic system and other parts of the brain are still developing.

How Alcohol Affects the Adolescent Brain

Unfortunately, alcohol is one of the first choices among adolescents, and heavy binge drinking (five or more drinks in one occasion; see chapter 2 for definition) is becoming frequent among high school students in the United States and many other countries. Reports from the European School Survey Project on Alcohol and Other Drugs, which was conducted in thirty-five European countries, indicated that adolescents today drink more in order to get drunk compared to earlier generations.[17] Toumbourou et al. (2009), comparing alcohol use and related harm in school students in the United States and Australia, reported that in Washington State, 10.3 percent of boys and 5.2 percent of girls in fifth grade (age eleven) used alcohol in the past year. In contrast, in Victoria, Australia, 34.2 percent of boys and 21.2 percent of girls used alcohol in the past year, despite having a zero-tolerance policy in both countries for adolescent use of alcohol. Use of alcohol at age eleven is not just shocking, it's a serious health hazard as well.[18]

Underage drinking contributes to the three leading causes of death (unintentional injury, suicide, and homicide) among young people between the ages of twelve to twenty years. The most adverse health hazard of underage drinking is binge drinking. Overall, 44.9 percent of high school students in the United States reported some alcohol use and 28.9 percent reported episodes of binge drinking during the past thirty days of the survey. Binge drinking rates increased with age and school grade. Students who binge drank were more likely than those who didn't binge drink (or those who drank moderately) to report poor academic performance and involvement in other risky behaviors, such as riding with drivers who had been drinking, using illicit drugs, being sexually active, being a victim of dating violence, and attempting suicide.[19] Another study indicates that the rate of lifetime alcohol dependence was 40 percent when an individual started drinking at age fourteen or younger, whereas only 10 percent of individuals who started drinking at age twenty-one were dependent on alcohol in the later part of their lives. Therefore, a long-lasting consequence of alcohol consumption during adolescence is the higher risk of alcohol dependence in adulthood.[20]

Magnetic resonance imaging (MRI) studies have indicated that the human brain continues to develop throughout adolescence and undergoes significant structural and functional changes in synaptic plasticity (the ability of the connection between two neurons to change under various conditions) and neural connectivity, and such refinements with modifications in certain neurotransmitter systems are critical for normal functioning as an adult. Alcohol exposure during the juvenile/adolescent period overactivates developing mesolimbic systems, which then induce certain

adaptations that can trigger long-term behavioral patterns of alcohol addiction and abuse.[21]

> Although, on average, juveniles take their first drink at the age of
> twelve years, individuals who use alcohol before age fourteen are at
> an increased risk of developing alcohol use disorders.

Underage drinkers are also susceptible to immediate ill effects of alcohol
use—such as blackouts, hangovers, and alcohol poisoning—compared
to their adult counterparts. These individuals are also at higher risk of
neurodegeneration (progressive loss of the function of neurons, including neuron death, particularly in the regions of the brain responsible
for learning and memory), impairment of functional brain activity, and
neurocognitive deficits (impairment of cognitive function). Underage
drinking is associated with impaired intellectual development due to
brain damage, and such damage carries through to adulthood. Because
adolescent drinking induces brain structure abnormalities, these changes
lead to poor memory, impaired study habits, poor ability to learn, and
poor academic performance.[22] In a ten-year study using data from 8,661
respondents, Harford et al. (2006) concluded that education beyond high
school has a protective effect against alcohol abuse and dependence. In
addition, people who do not attend college may also have a higher risk
of alcohol abuse than people who attend college.[23] Studies also show that
children of alcoholics constitute a population at risk for skipping school
days, poor performance, and dropping out of school. Children of alcoholics also have a higher incidence of repeating a grade.[24]

There is a difference between how alcohol damages the male versus
female adolescent brain and the extent of damage. In general a female
adolescent brain is more vulnerable to alcohol exposure than is a male
brain. Adolescents with alcohol abuse disorder have smaller prefrontal
cortex volumes compared to healthy adolescents. The prefrontal cortex
is located in the cortical region of the frontal lobe and is a crucial area of
the brain that is involved in planning complex cognitive behavior, such
as learning, critical thinking, working with mentally stored information,
rational judgment, expression of personality, and appropriate social behavior. Consistent with adult literature, alcohol use during adolescence
is associated with prefrontal volume abnormality, including differences
in white matter, but girls are more affected than boys by adverse effects
of alcohol. The prefrontal cortex volume of alcohol-dependent female
adolescents is smaller than that of alcohol-dependent male adolescents.[25]

How Alcohol Affects the Adult Brain

Although the onset of drinking at an early age carries a much higher risk of alcohol dependence and brain damage, with long-lasting effects into adulthood, the onset of drinking at age twenty-one (legal age for drinking) followed by chronic abuse of alcohol can also cause significant damage to the human brain. The two major alcohol-related brain disorders are alcoholic Korsakoff's syndrome and alcoholic dementia. Korsakoff's syndrome is a brain disorder caused by a deficiency of thiamine (vitamin B1), and major symptoms include severe memory loss, false memory, lack of insight, poor conversation skills, and apathy. Some heavy drinkers may also have a genetic predisposition to developing this syndrome. In Korsakoff's syndrome, loss of neurons is a common feature, including microbleeding in certain regions of gray matter.[26] In an alcoholic, when Wernicke's encephalopathy appears along with Korsakoff's syndrome, it is called Wernicke-Korsakoff syndrome.

Wernicke's encephalopathy and Korsakoff syndrome are two related diseases, both caused by thiamine deficiency, but accompanying clinical symptoms may be different. Alcoholics with Korsakoff syndrome always have severe amnesic syndrome (severe memory loss) but may not have classical symptoms of Wernicke's encephalopathy, which include ophthalmoplegia (paralysis or severe weakness of one or more of the muscles that control eye movement), ataxia (lack of coordination during voluntary muscle movement, such as walking), and confusion. However, patients with Wernicke-Korsakoff syndrome show most of the symptoms found in both diseases.

Damage to the anterior nucleus of the thalamus is commonly found in patients with Korsakoff syndrome but may also be present in patients suffering from Wernicke's encephalopathy. The anterior nucleus of the thalamus is involved in learning and memory, as well as the alertness of an individual. The Royal College of Physicians in London recommends that patients admitted to the hospital who show evidence of chronic misuse of alcohol and poor diet should be treated with B vitamins.[27] Paparrigopoulos et al. (2010) reported a case where a fifty-two-year-old man with a ten-year history of heavy alcohol abuse was admitted to the hospital and was treated aggressively for Wernicke-Korsakoff syndrome with 600 mg per day of oral thiamine in addition to 300 mg of thiamine, which was delivered intravenously every day, and he was fully recovered two months after therapy.[28]

Other than developing Korsakoff's syndrome or Wernicke-Korsakoff syndrome, thiamine deficiency in chronic alcohol abusers is a major cause of alcohol-induced brain damage. Thiamine is a helper molecule (cofactor) required by three enzymes involved in carbohydrate metabolism, and brain cells can only use sugar as a fuel. In addition, intermediate products of carbohydrate metabolism pathways are needed for generation of essential molecules for cellular functions (such as brain chemicals, building blocks for proteins, and DNA), and a reduction in thiamine can interfere with many of these important biochemical processes. Chronic alcohol consumption can result in thiamine deficiency by causing inadequate nutritional thiamine uptake, reduced absorption of thiamine from the gastrointestinal tract, and impaired thiamine utilization by the cells.[29] Ke et al. (2009) indicate that although thiamine deficiency causes neurodegeneration (loss of neurons) in the brain, alcohol uses this effect directly because it can cross the blood-brain barrier and diffuse in the brain.[30]

> Alcoholics in general have a reduced brain weight compared to nondrinkers.

Prefrontal white matter is the area in the brain that is most severely affected in alcoholics, and there is a correlation between the degree of loss and daily consumption of alcohol. Loss of white matter is a major cause of cognitive impairment in alcoholics.[31] Significant loss of neurons has also been documented in the cortex, hypothalamus, and cerebellum of alcoholics. The types of neurons that are damaged in chronic alcohol users are the larger neurons from the frontal cortex. These neurons are also damaged in patients with Alzheimer's disease. However, there is no direct link between alcoholic brain damage and Alzheimer's disease. Alzheimer's patients are more impaired on recalling names, recognition memory, and orientation, while subjects with alcohol-induced dementia are impaired in fine motor control, initial letter fluency, and free recall.[32]

Chronic abuse of alcohol results in brain damage to both men and women, but women are more susceptible to alcohol-induced brain damage than are men. At the same mean daily alcohol consumption, blood alcohol levels in women may be higher than men because the woman's body burns alcohol slower than the man's. Based on a study of forty-three alcoholic men and women, and comparing them with thirty-nine healthy controls, Hommer et al. (2001) demonstrated that alcoholic women had a significantly smaller volume of gray and white matter than healthy subjects. Although alcoholic men also had lower amounts of gray matter and white matter compared to the healthy controls, the difference in magnitude was smaller in men than in women. Direct comparison of alcoholic men and women showed that the proportion of the intracranial contents occupied by gray matter was smaller in alcoholic women than alcoholic men when all other factors were adjusted. In addition, the magnitude of difference between the brain volume of alcoholic women and nonalcoholic women was greater than the magnitude of the difference of brain volume between alcoholic and nonalcoholic men. The authors concluded that women's brains are more susceptible to alcohol-related damage than are men's brains.[33]

Binge drinkers, both men and women, are at a higher risk of developing alcohol-related brain damage. Chronic exposure to the high amounts of alcohol that are ingested during binge drinking leads to the stimulation of N-methyl-D-aspartate (NMDA) and calcium receptors, which results in increased release of glucocorticoids (stress molecules such as cortisol, which affect carbohydrate metabolism). NMDA-mediated mechanisms and glucocorticoid actions on the hippocampus are associated with brain damage. In addition, ethanol withdrawal becomes more difficult for binge drinkers.[34] Interestingly, alcohol at low levels inhibits NMDA receptors instead of stimulating them and may exert some beneficial effects.

Alcohol-related brain damage and loss of cognitive functions may be reversible, at least in part, if the brain damage is not permanent and the alcoholic successfully completes a rehabilitation program and practices complete abstinence. Chronic alcoholism is often associated with brain shrinkage, but this may be partially reversed if abstinence is maintained, as demonstrated by Trabert et al. (1995), based on a study of twenty-eight male patients with severe alcohol dependence. Even with three weeks of abstinence, increased brain tissue densities were observed in these subjects.[35] Asada et al. (2010) reported a case where a forty-year-old patient was unable to perform his office duties because of slowly progressive amnesia (severe memory loss). The initial evaluation of the patient indicated severe verbal memory loss, and early stage Alzheimer's disease was suspected because the patient did not disclose his habit of heavy alcohol consumption and no thiamine deficiency was found. Later the patient disclosed his habit of heavy alcohol consumption in the past, and with complete abstinence, his memory and cognitive functions improved markedly. Initial studies with FDG-PET (fluorodeoxyglucose-positron emission tomography), an advanced imaging technique, indicated that glucose metabolism was slower in the brain of the patient, and, as mentioned earlier in this chapter, glucose is the only fuel that brain cells can use. A five-year follow-up study using PET imaging indicated that glucose metabolism in the brain was recovered to the normal level, and the patient showed dramatically improved cognitive functions.[36]

CONCLUSION

Alcohol is a double-edged sword with a neuroprotective effect among low to moderate consumers but a detrimental effect in alcoholics. Drinking in moderation has many health benefits (see chapter 4) and may reduce the risk of dementia and Alzheimer's in the elderly. However, brain development in adolescents is at high risk for permanent damage if exposed to alcohol, especially at a very young age. In addition, adolescents who start drinking around age fourteen or younger are at a very high risk of becoming alcoholics in their adulthood. Underage drinking is a very serious public health and safety concern because the lives of these adolescents may change forever due to drinking, including poor performance in school, dropping out of school, difficulty transitioning to adulthood, and other social adjustment problems. Therefore, no one below the age of twenty-one (the legal age for drinking) should drink. Moderate drinking in adulthood has health benefits, but drinking should be limited to one to two drinks per day at the maximum for men and one drink per day for women. Drinking even less than that (two to three times a week, one glass or drink per occasion) can deliver the most beneficial effects of alcohol (which will be discussed further in chapter 4). However, drinking more for the sake of health is unjustified, because such a practice may cause more harm than good. Women are more affected by adverse effects of alcohol than are men. Fortunately, some of the brain damage caused by alcohol may be reversible. Therefore, friends and family members of a chronic abuser of alcohol must intervene and ensure that the person receives appropriate help for alcohol rehabilitation. It is not too late to help an alcoholic resume a normal life after treatment.

NOTES

1. R. J. Blanchard, L. Magee, R. Veniegas, and D. C. Blanchard, "Alcohol and Anxiety: Ethopharmacological Approaches," *Progress in Neuropharmacology and Biological Psychiatry* 17 (2003): 171–82.

2. J. A. Tucker, R. E. Vuchinich, and M. B. Sobell, "Alcohol's Effects on Human Emotions: A Review of the Stimulation/Depression Hypothesis," *International Journal of Addiction* 17, no. 1 (January 1982): 155–80.

3. S. S. Hoppenbrouwers, D. Hofman, and D. J. Schutter, "Alcohol Breaks Down Interhemispheric Inhibition in Females but Not in Males: Alcohol and Frontal Connectivity," *Psychopharmacology* (Berlin) 208, no. 3 (February 2010): 469–74.

4. R. Clarisse, F. Testu, and A. Reinberg, "Effects of Alcohol on Psycho-Technical Tests and Social Communication in a Festive Situation: A Chronopsychological Approach," *Chronobiology International* 21, nos. 4–5 (July 2004): 721–38.

5. C. A. Moberg and J. J. Curtin, "Alcohol Selectively Reduces Anxiety but Not Fear: Startle Response during Unpredictable versus Predictable Threat," *Journal of Abnormal Psychology* 118, no. 2 (May 2008): 335–47.

6. M. J. Eckardt, S. E. File, G. L. Gessa, K. Grant, et al., "Effects of Moderate Alcohol Consumption on the Central Nervous System," *Alcoholism: Clinical and Experimental Research* 22, no. 5 (August 1998): 998–1040.

7. Brain Pleasure Center, The Brain from Top to Bottom website, http://thebrain.mcgill.ca/flash/index_d.html.

8. G. F. Koob, P. P. Sana, and F. F. Bloom, "Neuroscience of Addiction," *Neuron* 21 (1998): 467–76.

9. D. M. Tomkins and E. M. Sellers, "Addiction and the Brain: The Role of Neurotransmitters in the Cause and Treatment of Drug Dependence," *Canadian Medical Association Journal* 164, no. 6 (March 2001): 817–21.

10. C. J. Morgan and A. Badway, "Alcohol-Induced Euphoria: Exclusion of Serotonin," *Alcohol and Alcoholism* 36, no. 1 (January 2001): 22–25.

11. B. Söderpalm, E. Löf, and M. Ericson, "Mechanistic Studies of Ethanol's Interaction with the Mesolimbic Dopamine Reward System," *Pharmacopsychiatry* 42, no. 1 (May 2009): S87–94.

12. A. Ruitenberg, J. C. van Swieten, J. C. M. Witterman, K. M. Mehta, et al., "Alcohol Consumption and Risk of Dementia: The Rotterdam Study," *Lancet* 359, no. 9303 (January 2002): 281–86.

13. R. M. Pinder and M. Sandler, "Alcohol, Wine and Mental Health: Focus on Dementia and Stroke," *Journal of Psychopharmacology* 18, no. 4 (December 2004): 449–56.

14. E. Savaskan, G. Olivieri, F. Meier, E. Seifritz, et al., "Red Wine Ingredient Resveratrol Protects from β-Amyloid Neurotoxicity," *Gerontology* 49, no. 6 (November–December 2003): 380–83.

15. Y. Lee, J. H. Back, J. Kim, S. H. Kim, et al., "Systematic Review of Health Behavioral Risks and Cognitive Health in Older Adults," *International Psychogeriatric* 22, no. 2 (March 2010): 174–87.

16. V. Solfrizzi, A. D'Introno, A. M. Colacicco, C. Capurso, et al., "Alcohol Consumption, Mild Cognitive Impairment, and Progression to Dementia," *Neurology* 68, no. 1 (May 2007): 1790–99.

17. E. Kuntsche, J. Rehm, and G. Gmel, "Characteristics of Binge Drinkers in Europe," *Social Science and Medicine* 59 (2004): 113–27.

18. J. W. Toumbourou, S. A. Hemphill, B. J. McMorris, R. F. Catalano, et al., "Alcohol Use and Related Harms in School Students in the USA and Australia," *Health Promotion International* 24, no. 4 (December 2009): 373–82.

19. J. W. Miller, T. S. Naimi, R. D. Brewer, and S. E. Jones, "Binge Drinking and Associated Health Risk Behaviors among High School Students," *Pediatrics* 119, no. 1 (January 2007): 76–85.

20. B. F. Grant and D. A. Dawson, "Age at Onset of Alcohol Use and Its Association with DSM-IV Alcohol Abuse and Dependence: Results from the National Longitudinal Alcohol Epidemiological Survey," *Journal of Substance Abuse* 9 (1997): 103–10.

21. M. Pascual, J. Boix, V. Felipo, and C. Guerri, "Repeated Alcohol Administration during Adolescence Causes Changes in the Mesolimbic Dopaminergic and Glutamatergic System and Promotes Alcohol Intake in the Adult Rat," *Journal of Neurochemistry* 108, no. 4 (February 2009): 920–31.

22. D. W. Zeigler, C. C. Wang, R. A. Yoast, B. D. Dickinson, et al., "The Neurocognitive Effects of Alcohol on Adolescents and College Students," *Preventive Medicine* 40 (2005): 23–32.

23. T. C. Harford, H. Y. Yi, and M. E. Hilton, "Alcohol Abuse and Dependence in College and Noncollege Samples: A Ten-Year Prospective Follow-Up in a National Survey," *Journal of the Study of Alcohol* 67, no. 6 (November 2006): 803–9.

24. M. J. Casas-Gil and J. L. Navarro-Guzman, "School Characteristics among Children of Alcoholic Parents," *Psychology Reports* 90, no. 1 (February 2002): 341–48.

25. K. L. Medina, T. McQueeny, B. J. Nagel, K. L. Hanson, et al., "Prefrontal Cortex Volumes in Adolescents with Alcohol Use Disorders: Unique Gender Effects," *Alcoholism: Clinical and Experimental Research* 32, no. 3 (March 2008): 386–94.

26. M. D. Kopelman, A. D. Thomson, I. Guerrini, and E. J. Marshall, "The Korsakoff Syndrome: Clinical Aspects, Psychology and Treatment," *Alcohol and Alcoholics* 44, no. 2 (March–April 2009): 148–54.

27. C. Harper, "The Neurotoxicity of Alcohol," *Human and Experimental Toxicology* 26, no. 3 (March 2007): 251–57.

28. T. Paparrigopoulos, E. Tzavellas, D. Karaiskos, A. Kouzoupis, et al., "Complete Recovery from Undertreated Wernicke-Korsakoff Syndrome Following Aggressive Thiamine Treatment," *In Vivo* 24, no. 2 (March–April 2010): 231–33.

29. P. R. Martin, C. K. Singleton, and S. Hiller-Sturmhofel, "The Role of Thiamine Deficiency in Alcoholic Brain Damage," *Alcohol Research and Health* 27, no. 2 (February 2003): 134–42.

30. Z. J. Ke, X. Wang, Z. Fan, and J. Luo, "Ethanol Promotes Thiamine Deficiency–Induced Neuronal Death: Involvement of Double-Stranded RNA-Activated Protein Kinase Activity," *Alcoholics: Clinical and Experimental Research* 33, no. 6 (June 2009): 1097–1103.

31. H. Mochizuki, T. Masaki, S. Matsushita, Y. Ugawa, et al., "Cognitive Impairment and Diffuse White Matter Atrophy in Alcoholics," *Clinical Neurophysiology* 116, no. 1 (January 2005): 223–28.

32. J. Saxton, C. A. Munro, M. A. Butters, C. Schramke, et al., "Alcohol, Dementia, and Alzheimer's Disease: Comparison of Neuropsychological Profiles," *Journal of Geriatric Psychiatry and Neurology* 13, no. 3 (Fall 2000): 141–49.

33. D. Hommer, R. Momenan, E. Kaiser, and R. Rawlings, "Evidence for a Gender-Related Effect of Alcoholism on Brain Volumes," *American Journal of Psychiatry* 158, no. 2 (February 2001): 198–204.

34. W. A. Hunt, "Are Binge Drinkers More at Risk of Developing Brain Damage?" *Alcohol* 10, no. 6 (November–December 1993): 559–61.

35. W. Trabert, T. Betz, M. Niewald, and G. Huber, "Significant Reversibility of Alcohol Brain Shrinkage within 3 Weeks of Abstinence," *Acta Psychiatry Scandinavia* 92, no. 2 (August 1995): 87–90.

36. T. Asada, S. Takaya, Y. Takayama, H. Yamauchi, et al., "Reversible Alcohol-Related Dementia: A Five-Year Follow-Up Using FDG-PET and Neuropsychological Tests," *Internal Medicine* 49, no. 4 (April 2010): 283–87.

4

Health Benefits of Moderate Alcohol Consumption

Human beings have been consuming alcohol from prehistoric times, and there is still an ongoing debate about whether drinking is beneficial or detrimental to your health. Based on our current knowledge, it can be stated that alcohol, like any drug, is beneficial at a low dose but is a poison if consumed in excess. The beneficial effect of alcohol in preventing heart disease came to media attention with the publication of papers that indicated that in most countries, intake of saturated fats (animal fats) is related to high mortality from coronary heart disease.

The situation in France is paradoxical because the French population consumes high amounts of saturated fats but experiences low mortality from coronary heart disease. Coronary heart disease is caused by atherosclerosis, the narrowing of coronary arteries that supply blood to the heart due to fatty buildup of plaques. This process can cause chest pain (angina pectoris) and eventually heart attack (myocardial infarction). Epidemiological studies have indicated that consumption of alcohol at the level of intake in France (20–30 gm/day, with one drink containing 14 gm of alcohol) can reduce the risk of coronary heart disease by 40 percent. Other than increasing good cholesterol, wine, which is the drink of choice in France, may be able to inhibit platelet aggregation (preventing blood clots from forming in arteries, which stops the flow of blood to the heart), providing further protection against coronary heart disease.[1]

Cardiovascular disease is the major cause of death worldwide, claiming more lives than cancer. In the United States alone, each year approximately 1 million people die from cardiovascular disease, accounting for approximately one-third of all deaths. Cardiovascular disease is a broad term that includes diseases that involve the heart (cardio) and blood vessels (coronary arteries and veins). Coronary heart disease is a category within the broad definition of cardiovascular disease. Other than coronary heart disease, cardiovascular diseases also include heart failure, complications of the heart due to high blood pressure, heart failure, stroke, and related diseases. In the United States, for all categories of major cardiovascular diseases, men had a higher age-adjusted death rate than women. According to the latest statistics available from the U.S. government, the death rate in men in 2007 was 42 percent higher than women (297.7 compared to 209.9 deaths per 100,000). The death from coronary heart disease alone was 69 percent higher in men than women (174.5 compared to 103.4 deaths per 100,000).[2]

In the medical literature, moderate drinking is associated with a reduced risk of coronary heart disease; this is also true for cardiovascular disease. Moderate drinking appears to reduce the risk of atherosclerotic plaque buildup, heart attack, heart failure, and stroke. Moderate drinking is defined as not more than two standard drinks a day for men younger than sixty-five, one drink per day for women, and one drink per day for men who are older than sixty-five. A standard drink is defined as 12 ounces of beer, 5 ounces of wine, or 1.5 ounces of an 80 proof spirit (containing 40 percent alcohol). A standard drink contains 14 gm of pure alcohol (see chapter 2). The consumption of a small amount of alcohol on a regular basis is more helpful than occasional binge drinking (five or more drinks in one occasion) on a weekend. The benefits of moderate drinking are listed in table 4.1.

Moderate alcohol consumption may increase longevity and protect against many diseases, including cardiovascular diseases.

Table 4.1. Benefits of Drinking in Moderation

Increased longevity
Reduced risk of coronary heart diseases (heart attack, angina pectoris)
Better survival chance after a heart attack
Reduced risk of stroke
Reduced risk of other cardiovascular diseases such as heart failure
Reduced risk of developing diabetes
Reduced risk of forming gallstones
Reduced risk of developing arthritis
Reduced risk of developing age-related dementia and Alzheimer's disease
Reduced risk of certain types of cancer
Possibly lowers the chances of getting the common cold

In contrast, chronic heavy consumption of alcohol increases the risk of heart disease, high blood pressure, stroke, various types of cancer, severe liver disease (including liver cirrhosis), sudden death from heart disease, and, for women, risk of miscarriage and fetal alcohol syndrome. Ceratin people who have a family history of alcohol abuse or those taking certain prescription medications, and women who are pregnant or plan to be pregnant, should not consume alcohol at all.

MODERATE ALCOHOL CONSUMPTION AND
REDUCED RISK OF CORONARY HEART DISEASE

Although coronary heart disease is one of the leading causes of death in developed countries, a recently published article indicates that coronary heart diseases are a growing epidemic in developing countries too due to longer life spans and the acquisition of lifestyle-related risk factors.[3] A review of literature up to 1999 by the National Institute of Alcohol Abuse and Alcoholism found that with few exceptions, epidemiological studies from at least twenty countries from North America, Europe, Asia, and Australia demonstrated 20 to 40 percent lower incidences of coronary heart disease among moderate drinkers than nondrinkers. In addition, large-scale prospective studies (representing a total population of more than 1 million men and women of different ethnicities) in which participants provide information on their drinking habits and health-related practices before the onset of disease also indicate a relationship between preventing coronary heart disease and drinking in moderation. The average follow-up period for these studies was eleven years, but the longest was the Framingham Heart Study, which was conducted over a period of twenty-four years. The two largest of these studies, conducted by the American Cancer Society, included one with 276,802 men and another with 490,000 men and women.[4]

The relationship between alcohol consumption and coronary heart disease was examined in the original Framingham Heart Study (so named because the study originated in Framingham, Massachusetts), which was initiated in 1948 with a twenty-four-year follow-up exam using 2,106 men and 2,639 women. Alcohol consumption demonstrated a U-shaped curve over the years, with a reduced risk of developing cardiovascular diseases with moderate drinking but a high risk of developing such diseases with heavy drinking. While smoking is a risk factor for developing coronary heart disease, the Framingham Study revealed that moderate alcohol consumption may also provide protection against coronary heart disease among smokers.[5]

In nonsmokers, beer and wine drinking provided greater reductions in coronary heart disease mortality than drinking spirits.

Smokers who smoke one pack of cigarettes per day have twice the risk of developing coronary heart disease than nonsmokers. Alcohol consumption actually lowered the incidence of coronary heart disease in participants of the Framingham Study, but in a study by Castelli (1990), when alcohol was consumed in greater amounts than two drinks per day, a rise in mortality from cancer and stroke was observed.[6]

In the American Cancer Society prospective study of 276,802 American men over a period of twelve years, the authors determined that the relative risk (RR) of total mortality was 0.88 for occasional drinkers, 0.84 for those drinking one drink per day, and 1.38 in people drinking six or more drinks per day compared to nondrinkers. However, RR of death from coronary heart disease was lower than one in all groups of drinkers compared to nondrinkers (table 4.2). The RR is defined as the ratio of the chance of a disease developing among members of a population exposed to a factor compared with a similar population not exposed to the factor. An RR value less than one indicates that the chance of developing a disease is less in a population that is exposed to the factor than the population not exposed to the factor, while a value higher than one indicates that the chance of developing a disease is higher in the population exposed to the factor than the population not exposed. In this study, the factor is alcohol. Interestingly, the risk of cardiovascular disease was mostly reduced in people who consumed one alcoholic drink per day (RR: 0.79), meaning people who drank one drink per day had a 21 percent lower chance of death from coronary heart disease, and the risk of all causes of mortality was also lowest (RR: 0.84) in that group, meaning that the risk of death from all other causes was 16 percent lower in people who consumed one alcoholic drink per day than nondrinkers.[7]

Table 4.2. Relative Risk Factors for Total Mortality in Drinkers and Nondrinkers

Number of Drinks per Day	Total Mortality	Relative Risk Factor (RR) from Coronary Heart Disease
Occasional drinkers	0.88	0.86
One drink	0.84	0.79
Two drinks	0.93	0.80
Three drinks	1.02	0.83
Four drinks	1.08	0.83
Five drinks	1.22	0.85
Six drinks	1.38	0.92

One drink per day is probably the best practice for obtaining health benefits from consuming alcohol.

In another large prospective study using 490,000 men and women (mean age 56 years, range 30 to 104 years) who reported their alcohol and tobacco use with a nine-year follow-up (46,000 people died during that period), the authors reported that the rate of death from cardiovascular diseases was 30 percent lower in men and 40 percent lower in women who consumed at least one drink per day. The overall death rates were lowest among men and women who consumed one drink daily.[8] Although moderate drinking is associated with reduced risk for heart disease, this benefit disappears in individuals who consume high amounts of alcohol. In a ten-year follow-up study in Sweden of 5,769 adults (ages thirty-five to seventy-five) without cardiovascular disease, Foerster et al. (2009) demonstrated that by increasing the amount of alcohol consumption to more than twenty-five drinks per week, blood pressure increased in heavy drinkers and all beneficial effects of alcohol consumption disappeared. In addition, wine drinking increased good cholesterol (high-density lipoprotein cholesterol or HDL), while drinking beer and spirits resulted in increased concentrations of triglycerides.[9] Sesso et al. (2000) studied the risk of hypertension (high blood pressure) in 28,848 women and 13,455 men who consumed alcohol and observed that light to moderate drinking increased the risk of developing hypertension in men but actually reduced the risk of developing hypertension in women. However, the threshold above which alcohol became deleterious for hypertension risk emerged at four or more drinks for women and more than one drink per day for men.[10]

It is beneficial to drink one drink per day or at least six drinks per week to reduce the risk of coronary heart disease and heart attack. A study by Sesso et al. (2000) using 18,445 men (ages forty to eighty-four) and a seven-year follow-up, revealed that when those individuals consuming one drink per week or less increased their consumption to more than one to six drinks per week, a further 29 percent reduction in the risk for developing cardiovascular disease was observed compared to individuals who did not increase their alcohol consumption at all. The authors concluded that among men with initial low alcohol consumption (one or less drink per week), a subsequent moderate increase in alcohol consumption may lower their risk of developing coronary heart disease.[11]

Diabetic patients are at a higher risk of developing cardiovascular disease. Moderate consumption of alcohol can help these patients lower their chances of getting heart disease. In the Physician's Health Study of 87,938

U.S. physicians (2,970 diagnosed with diabetes mellitus), the authors observed that weekly consumption of alcohol reduced the risk of heart disease by 33 percent, while daily consumption of alcohol reduced the risk by 58 percent among diabetics. For the nondiabetic, weekly consumption of alcohol reduced the risk of heart disease by 18 percent, while daily consumption of alcohol reduced the risk by 40 percent.[12]

Interestingly, women may get beneficial effects from alcohol by consuming lower amounts less frequently than men. In one study (Tolstrup et al. 2006) with 28,448 women and 25,052 men between fifty and sixty-five who were free from cardiovascular disease at enrollment in the study, during a 5.7-year follow-up, the authors observed that women who consumed alcohol at least one day per week had a lower risk of coronary heart disease than those who drank alcohol less than one day a week. However, little difference was found between women who consumed at least one drink per week compared to women who consumed two to four drinks per week, five to six drinks per week, or seven drinks per week. However, for men the lowest risk was found in individuals who consumed one drink per day. The authors concluded that for women, alcohol consumption can reduce the risk of heart disease, and the frequency of drinking may not be an important factor, but for men, drinking frequency, not alcohol intake, is the determining factor in preventing heart disease.[13]

Studies have shown that individuals who consume one alcoholic drink every one to two days have a lower risk of a first myocardial infarction (heart attack) than both nondrinkers and heavy drinkers. In addition, people who drink in moderation also have a higher chance of survival after myocardial infarction. In one study (Mukamal et al. 2001) using 1,913 adult patients who were hospitalized in forty-five different hospitals for heart attack, it was observed that 696 patients consumed less than seven alcoholic drinks per week, 321 consumed seven or more drinks per week, and 896 patients were nondrinkers. Compared with nondrinkers, patients who consumed less than seven drinks per week had a much lower death rate (6.3 deaths per 100 patients versus 3.4 deaths per 100 patients). Those who consumed seven or more drinks per week also showed less mortality (2.4 deaths per 100 patients) compared to nondrinkers (6.3 deaths per 100 patients). The association was similar between men and women as well as among different types of alcoholic beverages. The authors concluded that moderate alcohol consumption was associated with a lower rate of mortality after heart attack.[14] A recently published European study by Brugger-Andersen et al. (2009) using 5,477 patients who had heart failure following myocardial infarction reported that during 2.7 years of follow-up, 946 patients died, but patients with moderate alcohol consumption (one to seven drinks per week) showed 24 percent lower risk of all-cause death, 26 percent lower risk of dying from heart disease, and 8 percent lower risk of hospitalization compared to nondrinkers. The authors concluded that there was a string of positive associations between moderate alcohol consumption and survival after complicated myocardial infarction. However, heavy drinkers had a poor prognosis.[15] In another report, De Lorgeril et al. (2002) analyzed the relationship between drinking wine after myocardial infarction and the risk of recurrence in a patient population of 437. Among these patients 104 complications from heart disease occurred over a period of four years. The authors observed that in comparison to nondrinkers, the risk of developing complications was reduced by 59 percent in patients who drank approximately two alcoholic beverages per day, mostly wine.[16]

Congestive heart failure, another potentially lethal heart disease, occurs when the heart cannot pump blood to the body's organs. This may occur due to narrowing arteries (from plaque buildup), a past heart attack with scar tissues in the heart that interfere with normal function of the heart, high blood pressure, primary disease of the heart, such as cardiomyopathy, as well as birth defects. Moderate alcohol consumption not only reduces the risk of myocardial infarction but also provides protective effects against heart failure. In the Cardiovascular Health Study using 5,595 subjects, Bryson et al. (2006) observed that the risk of heart failure was reduced by 18 percent in individuals who drank one to six drinks per week and 34 percent in individuals who drank seven to thirteen drinks per week. In addition, the authors observed that moderate alcohol consumption lowered the risk of heart failure even in individuals who had experienced a heart attack.[17]

Snow et al. (2009), who conducted a study using 1,154 participants (580 men and 574 women) in Winnipeg, Manitoba, Canada, indicated that the well-established relationship between a reduced risk of cardiovascular disease and moderate consumption of alcohol may not be evident until middle age (thirty-five to forty-nine) or older (fifty to sixty-four) in men. However, women may benefit from moderate consumption of alcohol at a much younger age (eighteen to thirty-four). The beneficial effects of alcohol consumption are negated when alcohol is consumed in heavy episodic drinking patterns (eight or more drinks per occasion), especially for middle-aged and older men.[18]

HOW ALCOHOL PROTECTS AGAINST HEART DISEASE

There are several hypotheses on how moderate drinking can reduce the risk of developing heart disease (table 4.3). It has been well established that cholesterol plays a major role in the formation of plaque in coronary arteries. Narrowing of arteries may result in disruption in blood flow to

Table 4.3. Hypotheses by Which Moderate Alcohol Consumption Reduces Risk of Heart Diseases

Increasing the concentration of good cholesterol (high-density lipoprotein cholesterol)
Decreasing the concentration of bad cholesterol (low-density lipoprotein cholesterol)
Reduces narrowing of coronary arteries by reducing plaque formation
Reduces risk of blood clotting
Reduces level of fibrinogen (a blood-clotting factor)
Increases coronary blood flow
Reduces blood pressure, especially in women

the heart, causing coronary heart disease. There are two main coronary arteries that branch off from the aorta. These two arteries and their branches deliver blood to the heart. When a plaque ruptures, it triggers a complex event of platelet aggregation (the clumping together of platelets in blood), which is a part of the sequence of events that leads to formation of a blood clot (thrombus) in the artery. When a thrombus is formed, it may severely disrupt the blood flow to the heart, causing heart cells to die. This pathological process is called myocardial infarction or heart attack.

It has been demonstrated that when cholesterol is associated with low-density lipoprotein (LDL), it promotes plaque formation in the arteries. This is the reason LDL cholesterol is called "bad cholesterol." However, when cholesterol is associated with high-density lipoprotein (HDL), it prevents plaque buildup and is thus called "good cholesterol." Blood clotting also plays an important role in the pathophysiology of heart attacks. The omega-3 fatty acids found in abundance in fish such as lake trout, sardines, herring, salmon, albacore tuna, and mackerel can reduce the event of blood clotting and may provide protection against a heart attack.

Research has shown that moderate consumption of alcohol reduces the risk of heart disease by increasing blood levels of HDL cholesterol, and that this effect is independent of the type of alcoholic beverages consumed. The American Heart Association and other organizations recommend limiting alcohol consumption to no more than two drinks a day for men and one drink a day for women. Heavy consumption of alcohol, on the other hand, causes heart disease (see chapter 5).[19]

In general, maximal benefit and safety from consuming alcohol appears to be at the level of approximately one drink per day.

Many studies have demonstrated that HDL cholesterol levels in drinkers are higher than nondrinkers. The Honolulu Heart Study showed that men who drank alcoholic beverages had higher blood levels of HDL cholesterol than nondrinkers. Gordon et al. (1981) reviewed data from ten different studies, including the Honolulu Heart Study, and observed that there was a positive correlation between amounts of alcohol consumed and the serum (aqueous part of blood) level of HDL cholesterol. In the male population between ages fifty and sixty-nine, the average HDL cholesterol level was 41.9 mg/dL (dL: 100 milliliters) in people who consumed no alcohol, 47.6 mg/dL in people consuming up to 16.9 gm of alcohol per day (a single drink is 14 gm of alcohol), 50.7 mg/dL in people consuming between 16.9 and 42.2 gm of alcohol per day (one to three drinks), and 55.3 mg/dL in people drinking between 42.3 and 84.5 gm of alcohol per day (three to six drinks). Interestingly, in the Albany, Framingham, and San Francisco studies on the effect of alcohol on HDL levels, the HDL cholesterol levels of men between the ages of fifty and sixty-nine who consumed the highest amount of alcohol per day (42.3 to 85.5 gm/day or approximately three to six drinks per day) were 54.6 mg/dL, 50.1 mg/dL, and 57.8 mg/dL (HDL cholesterol levels among nondrinkers were 46.3 mg/dL, 41.4 mg/dL, and 44.4 mg/dL).[20] In another study (Hulley et al. 1981), the authors observed that the HDL cholesterol level in blood was increased by up to 33 percent in social drinkers as opposed to nondrinkers. A small experiment also revealed an average 15 percent reduction in HDL cholesterol levels among social drinkers who abstained from alcohol for a two-week period.[21] In women, light drinking (one drink or less a day) was associated with lower blood levels of bad cholesterol (LDL) and higher levels of good cholesterol (HDL).[22] A recently published article (Wakabayashi and Araki 2010) also demonstrated that serum HDL cholesterol was higher in drinkers than nondrinkers in all age-groups of men and women (twenty to sixty-nine), and the atherogenic index (risk of developing coronary heart disease), calculated by using serum total cholesterol and HDL cholesterol concentrations, was also lower in drinkers than nondrinkers in all age-groups of both men and women.[23]

In addition to increasing good cholesterol and reducing bad cholesterol, light to moderate consumption of alcohol also reduces the level of apolipoprotein-A (this lipoprotein, like LDL, increases the risk of coronary heart disease) and prevents clot formation, as well as reducing platelet aggregation.[24] Alcohol also diminishes thrombus formation on damaged walls of the coronary artery. This action of alcohol is due to its ability to inhibit Phospholipase A2, an enzyme that releases fatty acids.[25]

THE PROTECTIVE BENEFITS OF WINE
IN CARDIOVASCULAR HEALTH

Studies have indicated that the increased level of good cholesterol in blood may explain 50 percent of the protective effect of alcohol against cardiovascular disease, while the other 50 percent may be partly related to the inhibition of platelet aggregation, thus reducing blood clot formation in coronary arteries. It has been suggested that although alcohol can increase good cholesterol levels and inhibit platelet aggregation, the polyphenolic compounds found in abundance in red wine can reduce platelet activity via other mechanisms further than can alcohol. In addition, these polyphenolic compounds in red wine can also increase the level of vitamin E, an important antioxidant, thus providing further protection against various diseases. Therefore, it appears that red wine offers more protection against cardiovascular disease than other alcoholic beverages.[26] It has been postulated that resveratrol, a polyphenolic compound found abundantly in red wine but not in white wine, beer, or spirits, plays an important role as an antioxidant and inhibits platelet aggregation, which may explain the cardio protection received from consuming red wine.[27] A recently published article (Klatsky 2010) also suggests that wine, especially red wine, is more protective against coronary heart disease than beer or other liquors.[28]

> Drinking wine, especially red wine, may provide more protection against cardiovascular diseases than beer or other liquors.

THE CONSUMPTION OF ALCOHOL AND PREVENTING STROKE

Another beneficial effect of consuming alcohol in moderation is the dramatic reduction in the risk of having a stroke among both men and women regardless of age or ethnicity. The Copenhagen City Heart Study, with 13,329 eligible men and women ages forty-five to eighty-four (with a sixteen-year follow-up) showed that there was a U-shaped relation between intake of alcohol and risk of stroke. People who consumed low to moderate alcohol experienced the protective effect of alcohol against stroke, but heavy consumers of alcohol were more prone to stroke than moderate drinkers or nondrinkers. For moderate drinkers of wine, monthly drinking of alcohol reduced the risk of stroke by 17 percent, weekly drinking reduced the risk by 41 percent, and daily drinking reduced the risk by 30 percent. There was no association between risk of stroke and drinking beer or spirits.[29]

In the second examination of the Copenhagen City Heart Study, with 5,373 men and 6,723 women (with a sixteen-year follow-up), it was observed that at a high stress level, weekly total consumption of one to fourteen drinks compared to no consumption of alcohol was associated with a 43 percent lower risk of stroke in both men and women, but no clear association was observed between the risk of stroke and moderate consumption of alcohol in individuals who were at a lower stress level. In addition, this study also reported that only drinking beer or wine reduced the risk of stroke in individuals with high stress. It was suggested that alcohol may alter psychological responses to stress in addition to modifying physiological responses.[30]

The Northern Manhattan study, consisting of individuals ages forty and older (677 patients who had experienced a stroke were matched for gender, age, and ethnicity with 1,139 individuals in the community who had not), observed that moderate drinking of up to two drinks per day had a significantly protective effect against ischemic stroke. The protective effect of alcohol against stroke was detected in both younger and older groups of men and women in all ethnic groups (white, black, and Hispanic). However, this protective effect against stroke disappeared in heavy drinkers (seven or more drinks per day), and such chronic consumption of alcohol increased the risk of having strokes by approximately three times that of nondrinkers.[31] In a follow-up study, it was demonstrated that moderate drinkers (up to two drinks per day) had a 33 percent reduced risk of ischemic stroke (all ethnic groups, both men and women) compared to nondrinkers.[32] Ischemic stroke (cerebral infarction) is the death of an area of brain tissue due to blockage of an artery (most commonly a branch of one of the internal carotid arteries) that supplies blood to the brain. When consumed in moderate amounts, alcohol can prevent blood clot formation and fibrinolysis, which may protect from stroke, but in heavy drinkers, alcohol elevates blood pressure (a risk for stroke), may cause the rupture of arteries that deliver blood to the brain, and vasoconstriction (narrowing of blood vessels, which causes reduced blood flow), thus increasing the risk of stroke. In addition, at higher concentrations alcohol promotes blood clotting rather than preventing blood clotting, greatly increasing the risk of a stroke, because a blood clot in an artery may prevent blood flow to a certain part of the brain.[33]

MODERATE CONSUMPTION OF ALCOHOL AND REDUCING THE RISK OF DEVELOPING DIABETES

Diabetes mellitus, commonly referred to as diabetes, is a condition where a person has a high blood sugar level (more than 126 mg/dL after overnight fasting) either due to not producing enough insulin (type 1 diabetes, insulin dependent), or not utilizing insulin properly (type 2 diabetes, insulin resistant). Although either type of diabetes may develop at any age, usually the onset of type 1 diabetes occurs at an early age and requires a person to have a daily injection of insulin for maintaining normal glucose blood levels. Type 2 diabetes, which is more common and diagnosed later in life (thirty-five years or older), can be managed with lifestyle changes, diet control, and medication. The prevalence of diabetes for all age groups worldwide was estimated to be 2.8 percent in 2000 and projected to be 4.4 percent in 2030. The total number of people suffering from diabetes is projected to rise from 171 million in 2000 to 366 million in 2030. Most people with diabetes suffer from type 2 diabetes.[34]

Studies have shown that moderate consumption of alcohol reduces the risk of developing type 2 diabetes. Based on fifteen studies conducted in the United States, Finland, the Netherlands, Germany, the United Kingdom, and Japan with 369,862 men and women and an average follow-up of twelve years, light drinkers (less than half a drink per day or 6 gm of alcohol) had a 13 percent lower chance of developing type 2 diabetes, while moderate drinkers (half a drink to four drinks per day, 6–12 gm of alcohol per day) had a 30 percent lower risk of developing type 2 diabetes compared to nondrinkers. It made little difference whether an individual consumed beer, wine, or spirits, and it was best to consume alcohol frequently (such as daily or several times in a week) rather than occasionally. In contrast, heavy consumption of alcohol (more than three and a half drinks per day or 48 gm of alcohol per day) did not have any protective effect against developing type 2 diabetes, and these individuals were at a slightly higher risk (4 percent more) of developing type 2 diabetes than nondrinkers.[35]

The Finnish Twin Cohort Study followed 22,778 twins with different drinking patterns over the course of twenty years and found that moderate alcohol consumption (half a drink to two drinks [5–29.9 gm/day] for men and half to one and a half drinks [5–19.9 gm/day] for women) was associated with a lower risk of developing type 2 diabetes than light alcohol consumption (less than half a drink or less than 5gm/day). Overweight subjects (body mass index equal to or greater than 25.0 kg/m^2) showed more beneficial effects from moderate alcohol consumption, as risk of developing diabetes was 30 percent lower in overweight men and 40 percent lower in overweight women, than from no alcohol consumption. On the other hand, binge drinking and high alcohol consumption may increase the risk of type 2 diabetes in women, especially lean women, but affected men to a lesser extent.[36]

After reviewing twenty studies, Balinus et al. (2009) observed a U-shaped relationship between alcohol consumption and the risk of developing type 2 diabetes, where moderate alcohol consumption decreased the risk and heavy alcohol consumption increased the risk. Compared to lifetime abstainers of alcohol, those who drank an average of 22 gm of alcohol per day (one and a half drinks) had a 17 percent lower risk of developing diabetes. Women with the highest level of protection (40 percent lower risk) were those who consumed 24 gm of alcohol per day. Drinking became deleterious among men who consumed more than 60 gm of alcohol per day (four and a half drinks) and among women who consumed more than 50 gm of alcohol (almost four drinks) per day.[37]

Alcohol at lower levels decreases insulin resistance and thus may play a protective role against developing diabetes, but this effect is lost with higher alcohol consumption. In a twelve-year prospective study using nearly 47,000 men who were health care professionals, those who consumed one to two drinks per day (15–29 gm of alcohol) had a 36 percent lower incidence of diabetes compared to abstainers. In this study, consuming even less than one alcoholic drink five days a week provided the greatest protection, with the risk of diabetes reduced by 52 percent. In the Nurses' Health study, which followed 85,000 nurses, it was shown that consuming even less than one drink per day (10 gm of alcohol) reduced the risk of diabetes by 46 percent.

Insulin resistance is a key factor in developing type 2 diabetes. In one study of 883 individuals ages sixty-five and older, it was observed that individuals who consumed alcohol daily in moderation had significantly lower fasting glucose levels, and, after receiving a dose of 75 gm of glucose, they had a lower level of blood glucose compared to nondrinkers. Serum insulin levels were lower in drinkers compared to nondrinkers, indicating that drinkers had lower insulin resistance, because serum insulin levels are elevated in diabetics (cells do not properly take insulin from blood to use glucose as fuel). This phenomenon was observed in both diabetics and nondiabetics, indicating that a diabetic person may also get benefits from moderate alcohol consumption. For example, among diabetic drinkers, the mean fasting glucose (137.5 mg/dL) and the mean insulin (14.5 picomole per liter) were lower compared to diabetic nondrinkers (fasting glucose 150.6 mg/dL and insulin 31.2 picomole per liter). Hyperinsulinemia (high insulin level in serum) is associated with an increased risk of type 2 diabetes and obesity. The authors concluded that the abstainers with their relative hyperinsulinemia appeared to be more insulin resistant than daily moderate drinkers. The difference in insulin sensitivity may explain the lower prevalence of diabetes in drinkers.[38]

Shai et al. (2007) investigated the effect of daily consumption of alcohol on glycemic control (control of blood sugar) in patients with type 2 diabetes using 109 patients (forty-one to seventy-four years old) who had previously abstained from alcohol. The subjects were divided into two groups. One group received 150 mL of wine daily (one standard drink/14 gm of alcohol) and another group received nonalcoholic beer during dinner for three months. The fasting glucose was significantly reduced from an average value of 139.6 mg/dL initially to 118.0 mg/dL after three months in diabetics who consumed one drink during dinner for three months. In contrast, the mean fasting glucose value did not change in diabetic patients who abstained from alcohol during the three-month period of the study (136.7 mg/dL at the beginning to 138.6 at the end of the study). Participants in the alcohol group reported an improvement in the ability to fall asleep. Therefore, moderate alcohol consumption may help diabetic patients with glycemic control.[39]

MODERATE ALCOHOL CONSUMPTION FOR PREVENTING DEMENTIA AND ALZHEIMER'S DISEASE

Moderate alcohol consumption can dramatically reduce the risk of age-related dementia and developing Alzheimer's disease. A French study using 3,777 community residents ages sixty-five years or older demonstrated that the subjects who drank three to four glasses of alcoholic beverages (mostly wine) per day (318 subjects) had 82 percent lower risk of developing senile dementia and 75 percent lower risk of getting Alzheimer's disease compared to nondrinkers (971 subjects).[40] However, chronic abusers of alcohol are at a higher risk of developing memory loss, dementia, and lack of appropriate motor control due to alcohol-related brain damage. Younger people, especially underage drinkers, are also at higher risk of alcohol-related brain damage (see chapter 3).

MODERATE ALCOHOL CONSUMPTION AND REDUCED RISK OF CANCER

Moderate consumption of alcohol may reduce the risk of certain types of cancer. It has been suggested that moderate drinking facilitates the elimination of *Helicobacter pylori* (*H. pylori*), a bacteria found in the gut that causes chronic atrophic gastritis (CAG) and gastric cancer. Gastritis commonly refers to inflammation of the lining of the stomach, but the term is often used to cover a variety of symptoms, including stomach discomfort and a severe burning sensation. Gao et al. (2009), using 9,444 subjects ages fifty to seventy-four, observed that moderate drinkers (less than 60 gm of alcohol per week or four drinks per week) had 29 percent lower chance of developing CAG than nondrinkers. Both beer and wine drinking provided protection against CAG. In addition to facilitating elimination of *H. pylori*, other mechanisms may also contribute to reducing the risk of CAG in moderate drinkers.[41] In the California Men's Health Study using 84,170 men ages forty-five to sixty-nine, consumption of one or more drinks per day was associated with approximately 60 percent reduced lung cancer risk, including smokers. Even heavy smokers benefited from consuming red wine in moderation. No clear association was observed between moderate drinking and alcohol in individuals who consumed white wine, beer, or other liquors.[42]

Moderate consumption of red wine reduces the risk of lung cancer.

In another study, the author observed that although moderate consumption of wine (one drink or less per day) was associated with approximately 23 percent reduced risk of developing lung cancer, moderate consumption of beer (one or more per day) increases the risk of developing lung cancer by 23 percent in men but not in women.[43] Jiang et al. (2007) reported that people drinking beer and wine but not spirits (hard liquor) can reduce the risk of bladder cancer by up to 32 percent compared to nondrinkers.[44] Consumption of up to one drink per day reduced the risk of head and neck cancer in both men and women, but consuming more than three alcoholic beverages increased the risk of developing cancer.[45] In two Italian studies, the authors observed that moderate consumption of alcohol reduced the risk of developing renal cell carcinoma (kidney cancer) in both men and women.[46] However, chronic heavy drinkers are at increased risk of developing many types of cancers, especially cancer of the mouth (see chapter 5).

CAN MODERATE ALCOHOL CONSUMPTION PROLONG LIFE?

Because moderate consumption of alcohol can prevent many diseases, including the number one killer, cardiovascular disease, it is expected that moderate drinkers may live longer than lifetime abstainers of alcohol. Freiberg et al. (2009), using 10,576 African American and 105,610 Caucasian postmenopausal women and an eight-year follow-up, demonstrated that moderate drinking (one to less than seven drinks per week) was associated with lower mortality among both hypertensive and nonhypertensive Caucasian women, but among African American women only hypertensive women received benefits from moderate drinking. Even those who currently started drinking (versus lifetime drinkers) only one drink or more per month increased longevity among Caucasian hypertensive and nonhypertensive women, as well as among African American hypertensive women. Low mortality was also observed among the African American lifetime nondrinking women with normal blood pressure.[47] Klatsky et al. (1981) studied ten-year mortality in relation to alcohol in 8,060 subjects and observed that people who consumed two drinks or fewer daily fared best and had a 50 percent reduction in the mortality rate than nondrinkers. The heaviest drinkers (six or more drinks per day) had double the mortality rate of moderate drinkers, while people who drank three to five drinks per day had a similar mortality rate as nondrinkers. Therefore, consuming two or less drinks per day is the best practice.[48]

In the Physician's Health Study, which involved 22,071 U.S. male physicians between the ages of forty and eighty-four (with no history of myocardial infarction, stroke, or cancer) and a ten-year follow-up, the authors observed that men who consumed two to six drinks per week had the most favorable results (20–28 percent lower mortality rate than people who consumed one drink per week). In contrast, people who consumed more than two drinks per day had an approximately 50 percent chance of higher mortality than people who consumed just one drink per week.[49] A Chinese study also reported that consuming not more than two drinks per day was associated with a 19 percent reduction in mortality risk among Chinese men.[50]

It has been suggested that wine consumption increases longevity more than drinking beer or other liquors. Klatsky et al. (2003) collected data from 128,934 adults undergoing health evaluations in 1978–1985, with subsequent death ascertained by an automated linkage system with a twenty-year follow-up. The authors observed that wine drinking was associated with a lower mortality risk largely because of lower coronory disease risk. The authors concluded that those who drink any type of wine have a lower mortality risk than those drinking beer or other liquor.[51]

A nationwide survey based on 17,600 people in the United States revealed that those who currently drink are hospitalized less often than abstainers. Among men the possibility of one or more hospitalizations among current drinkers was 26 percent lower and in women 33 percent lower in current drinkers who consume alcohol in moderation as opposed to lifetime abstainers.[52] A study from the Netherlands reported that in the presence of stress, moderate drinkers are less likely to be absent from work than nondrinkers.[53] The nine-year Alameda County Study (1980) indicated that moderate consumption of alcohol was associated with the most favorable health scores, indicating that moderate drinkers in general enjoy better overall health quality than abstainers.[54] The authors of a study conducted in Copenhagen using 12,039 subjects reported that light to moderate wine drinking (one to two glasses of wine per day) was associated with good self-perceived health, whereas this was not the case with consumers of beer or spirits. However, heavy drinkers of any type of beverage (wine, beer, or spirits) had a higher prevalence of suboptimal health than nondrinkers.[55]

MODERATE ALCOHOL CONSUMPTION AND ARTHRITIS

Moderate alcohol consumption reduces the risk of developing rheumatoid arthritis. Results from two Scandinavian studies indicated that among moderate drinkers, the risk of rheumatoid arthritis was significantly reduced (40–50 percent). Smokers had a higher risk of developing rheumatoid arthritis. The authors advised that smokers should be advised to quit smoking in order to reduce the risk of developing arthritis, but moderate drinkers should not be discouraged from sensible alcohol consumption.[56] Moderate alcohol consumption not only reduces the risk of developing rheumatoid arthritis but also may slow the progression of the disease. Based on a study using 2,908 patients suffering from rheumatoid arthritis, Nissen et al. (2010) reported that occasional or daily consumption of alcohol reduces the progression of the disease based on radiological studies (X-rays). Best results were observed in men.[57] However, drinking beer, even one drink per day, increases the risk of developing gout in men. Individuals who drank spirits (even one drink a day) also had a somewhat increased risk of developing gout, although the risk was highest among beer drinkers. In contrast, moderate wine drinking did not increase the odds of developing gout.[58]

CAN MODERATE ALCOHOL CONSUMPTION PREVENT THE COMMON COLD?

Cohen et al. (1993) observed that smokers are at greater risk of developing the common cold than nonsmokers. Moderate alcohol consumption reduced the incidence of the common cold among nonsmokers but had no protective effect against the common cold in smokers.[59] In a large study using 4,272 faculty and the staff of five Spanish universities as subjects, the investigators observed that total alcohol intake from drinking beer and spirits had no protective effect against the common cold, where moderate wine consumption was associated with reduced risk of the common cold. When individuals consumed fourteen or more glasses of wine per week, the relative risk of developing the common cold was reduced by 40 percent compared to teetotalers. It was also observed that consumption of red wine provided superior protection against the common cold. The authors concluded that wine drinking, especially drinking red wine, may have a protective effect against the common cold.[60]

CONCLUSION

The Dietary Guideline for Americans has been published jointly every five years since 1980 by the Department of Health and Human Services and the Department of Agriculture. These guides serve as the basis for federal food and nutritional education programs. In the latest published guideline (2005), it was stated that consumption of alcohol can have a beneficial or a harmful effect on health depending on the amount consumed, age, gender, and other characteristics of the person. In 2002, approximately 55 percent of adults living in the United States were drinking alcohol, while the other 45 percent were abstainers. Fewer Americans drink today than fifty or a hundred years ago. Alcohol is beneficial only when consumed in moderation and reduces all causes of mortality at an intake of one to two drinks a day. The lowest coronary heart disease mortality also occurs at an intake of one to two drinks per day. In contrast, morbidity and mortality are highest among those drinking large amounts of alcohol. This guideline also defines moderate drinking as up to two drinks per day for men and up to one drink per day for women. The definition of moderation is not based on an average of alcohol consumption over several days but rather as the amount consumed every day. Consuming more than one drink per day for women and more than two drinks per day for men increases the risk of motor vehicle accidents and other injuries, high blood pressure, stroke, violence, and certain types of cancer. Alcohol must be avoided under certain circumstances, such as for those who plan to drive, operate machinery, or other activities requiring skill and attention. Pregnant women and women who plan to get pregnant should not drink at all. It appears that only middle-aged and older people receive benefits from moderate drinking, while benefits are few among younger people. Alcoholic drinks supply calories but few essential nutrients. Total caloric intake from one standard drink of various alcoholic beverages is listed in table 4.4. Although the consumption of one to two drinks per day is not associated with micronutrient deficiency or with overall dietary quality, heavy drinkers may be at risk of malnutrition if the calories derived from alcohol are substituted for those in nutritious food.[61]

Table 4.4. Calories in Selected Alcoholic Beverages

Alcoholic Drink	Serving Size	Total Calories
Regular beer	12 ounces	144
Light beer	12 ounces	108
White wine	5 ounces	100
Red wine	5 ounces	105
Sweet dessert wine	3 ounces	141
80 proof spirit (Gin, rum, whiskey, vodka)	1.5 ounces	96

Source: Dietary Guidelines for Americans, U.S. Department of Health and Human Resources, 2005, http://www.health.gov./dietaryguidelines/dga2005/document/default.htm.

NOTES

1. S. Renaud and J. M. de Lorgeril, "Wine, Alcohol, Platelets and the French Paradox for Coronary Heart Disease," *Lancet* 339, no. 8808 (June 1992): 1523–26.

2. A. M. Minino and R. J. Klein, "Health Mortality from Major Cardiovascular Diseases: United States, 2007," *Heath E-Stats*, National Center for Health Statistics, March 2010, Center for Disease Control and Prevention.

3. T. A. Gaziana, A. Bitton, S. Anand, S. Abrahams-Gessel, et al., "Growing Epidemic of Coronary Heart Disease in Low- and Middle-Income Countries," *Current Problems in Cardiology* 35, no. 2 (February 2010): 72–115.

4. Alcohol Alert, No. 45, October 1999, National Institute of Alcohol Abuse and Alcoholism, http://pubs.niaaa.nih.gov/publications/aa45.htm.

5. L. A. Friedman and A. W. Kimball, "Coronary Heart Disease Mortality and Alcohol Consumption in Framingham," *American Journal of Epidemiology* 124, no. 3 (September 1986): 481–89.

6. W. P. Castelli, "Diet, Smoking, and Alcohol: Influence on Coronary Heart Disease Risk," *American Journal of Kidney Disease* 16, no. 4, supplement 1 (October 1990): 41–46.

7. P. Boffetta and L. Garfinkel, "Alcohol Drinking and Mortality among Men Enrolled in an American Cancer Society Prospective Study," *Epidemiology* 1, no. 5 (September 1990): 342–48.

8. M. J. Thun, R. Peto, A. D. Lopez, and J. H. Monaco, "Alcohol Consumption and Mortality among Middle-Aged and Elderly U.S. Adults," *New England Journal of Medicine* 337, no. 24 (December1997): 1705–14.

9. M. Foerster, P. Marques-Vidal, G. Gmel, J. B. Daeppen, et al., "Alcohol Drinking and Cardiovascular Risk in a Population with High Mean Alcohol Consumption," *American Journal of Cardiology* 103, no. 3 (February 2009): 361–68.

10. H. D. Sesso, N. R. Cook, J. E. Buring, J. E. Manson, et al., "Alcohol Consumption and the Risk of Hypertension in Women and Men," *Hypertension* 51, no. 4 (April 2008): 1080–87.

11. H. D. Sesso, M. J. Stampfer, B. Rosner, C. H. Hennekens, et al., "Seven-Year Changes in Alcohol Consumption and Subsequent Risk of Cardiovascular Disease in Men," *Archives of Internal Medicine* 160, no. 17 (September 2000): 2605–12.

12. U. A. Ajani, J. M. Gaziana, P. A. Lotufo, C. H. Hennekens, et al., "Alcohol Consumption and Risk of Coronary Heart Disease by Diabetes Status," *Circulation* 102, no. 5 (August 2000): 500–505.

13. J. Tolstrup, M. K. Jensen, A. Tjonneland, K. Overvad, et al., "Prospective Study of Alcohol Drinking Patterns and Coronary Heart Disease in Women and Men," *British Medical Journal* 332, no. 7552 (May 2006): 1244–48.

14. K. J. Mukamal, M. Maclure, J. E. Muller, J. B. Sherwood, et al., "Prior Alcohol Consumption and Mortality Following Acute Myocardial Infarction," *Journal of the American Medical Association* 285, no. 15 (April 2001): 1965–70.

15. T. Brugger-Andersen, V. Ponitz, S. Snapinn, K. Dickstein, et al., "Moderate Alcohol Consumption Is Associated with Reduced Long-Term Cardiovascular Risk in Patients Following a Complicated Acute Myocardial Infarction," *International Journal of Cardiology* 133, no. 2 (April 2009): 229–32.

16. M. De Lorgeril, P. Salen, J. L. Martin, F. Boucher, et al., "Wine Drinking and Risks for Cardiovascular Complications after Recent Acute Myocardial Infarction," *Circulation* 106, no. 12 (September 2002): 1465–69.

17. C. L. Bryson, K. J. Mukamal, M. A. Mittleman, L. P. Fried, et al., "The Association of Alcohol Consumption and Incident Heart Failure: The Cardiovascular Health Study," *Journal of the American College of Cardiology* 48, no. 2 (July 2006): 305–11.

18. W. M. Snow, R. Murray, O. Ekuma, S. L. Tyas, et al., "Alcohol Use and Cardiovascular Health Outcomes: A Comparison across Age, Gender in the Winnipeg Health and Drinking Survey Cohort," *Age and Aging* 38, no. 2 (March 2009): 206–12.

19. H. D. Sesso, "Alcohol and Cardiovascular Health: Recent Findings," *American Journal of Cardiovascular Drugs* 1, no. 3 (March 2001): 167–72.

20. T. Gordon, N. Ernst, M. Fisher, and B. M. Rifkind, "Alcohol and High-Density Lipoprotein Cholesterol," *Circulation* 64, no. 3, part 2 (September 1981): 3:63–67.

21. S. B. Hulley and S. Gordon, "Alcohol and High-Density Lipoprotein Cholesterol: Casual Inference from Diverse Study Designs," *Circulation* 64, no. 3, part 2 (September 1981): 3:57–63.

22. I. Wakabayashi and Y. Araki, "Association of Alcohol Consumption with Blood Pressure and Serum Lipid in Japanese Female Smokers and Nonsmokers," *Gender Medicine* 6, no. 1 (April 2009): 290–99.

23. I. Wakabayashi and Y. Araki, "Influence of Gender and Age on Relationship between Alcohol Drinking and Atherosclerosis Risk Factor," *Alcoholism: Clinical and Experimental Research* 34, supplement 1 (February 2010): S54–60.

24. D. P. Agarwal, "Cardioprotective Effects of Light to Moderate Consumption of Alcohol: A Review of Putative Mechanisms," *Alcohol and Alcoholism* 37, no. 5 (September–October 2002): 409–15.

25. R. Rubin, "Effect of Ethanol on Platelet Function," *Alcoholism: Clinical and Experimental Research* 23, no. 6 (June 1999): 1114–18.

26. J. C. Ruf, "Alcohol, Wine and Platelet Function," *Biological Research* 37, no. 2 (February 2004): 209–15.

27. J. M. Wu, Z. R. Wang, T. C. Hsieh, J. L. Bruder, et al., "Mechanism of Cardio Protection by Resveratrol, a Phenolic Antioxidant Present in Red Wine," *International Journal of Molecular Medicine* 8, no. 1 (July 2001): 3–17.

28. A. L. Klatsky, "Alcohol and Cardiovascular Health," *Physiology and Behavior* 100, no. 1 (April 2010): 76–81.

29. T. Truelsen, M. Gronbaek, P. Schnohr, and G. Boyen, "Intake of Beer, Wine and Spirits and Risk of Stroke: The Copenhagen City Heart Study," *Stroke* 29, no. 12 (December 1998): 2467–72.

30. N. R. Nielsen, T. Truelsen, J. C. Barefoot, S. P. Johnsen, et al., "Is the Effect of Alcohol on Risk of Stroke Confined to Highly Stressed Persons?" *Neuroepidemiology* 25, no. 3 (March 2005): 105–13.

31. R. L. Sacco, M. Elkind, B. Boden-Albala, I. F. Lin, et al., "The Protective Effect of Moderate Alcohol Consumption on Ischemic Stroke," *Journal of the American Medical Association* 281, no. 1 (January 1999): 53–60.

32. M. S. Elkind, R. Sciacca, B. Boden-Albala, and T. Rundek, "Moderate Alcohol Consumption Reduces Risk of Ischemic Stroke: The Northern Manhattan Study," *Stroke* 37, no. 1 (January 2006): 13–19.

33. M. Hillbom and H. Numminen, "Alcohol and Stroke: Pathophysiologic Mechanisms," *Neuroepidemiology* 17, no. 6 (June 1998): 281–87.

34. S. Wild, G. Roglic, A. Green, R. Sicree, et al., "Global Prevalence of Diabetes," *Diabetes Care* 27, no. 5 (May 2004): 1047–53.

35. L. L. Koppes, J. M. Dekker, H. F. Hendriks, L. M. Bouter, et al., "Moderate Alcohol Consumption Lowers the Risk of Type 2 Diabetes: A Meta-analysis of Prospective Observational Studies," *Diabetes Care* 28, no. 3 (March 2005): 719–25.

36. S. W. Carrison, N. Hammar, V. Grill, and J. Kaprio, "Alcohol Consumption and the Incidence of Type 2 Diabetes: 20-Year Follow-Up of the Finnish Twin Cohort Study," *Diabetes Care* 26, no. 10 (October 2003): 2785–90.

37. D. O. Balinus, B. J. Taylor, H. Irving, M. Roereke, et al., "Alcohol as a Risk Factor for Type 2 Diabetes: A Systematic Review and Meta-analysis," *Diabetes Care* 32, no. 11 (November 2009): 2123–32.

38. P. V. Kenkre, R. D. Linderman, C. Lillian Yau, R. N. Baumgartner, et al., "Serum Insulin Concentrations in Daily Drinkers Compared with Abstainers in the New Mexico Elder Health Survey," *Journal of Gerontology Series A: Biological Sciences and Medical Sciences* 58, no. 10 (October 2003): M960–963.

39. I. Shai, J. Wainstein, I. Harman-Boehm, I. Raz, et al., "Glycemic Effects of Moderate Alcohol Intake among Patients with Type 2 Diabetes: A Multicenter Randomized Clinical Investigation," *Diabetes Care* 30, no. 12 (December 2007): 3011–16.

40. J. M. Orgogozo, J. F. Dartigues, S. Lafont, L. Letenneur, et al., "Wine Consumption and Dementia in the Elderly: A Prospective Study in the Bordeaux Area," *Revue Neurologique* (Paris) 153, no. 3 (April 1997): 185–92.

41. L. Gao, M. N. Weck, M. Stegmaier, D. Rothenbacher, et al., "Alcohol Consumption and Chronic Atrophic Gastritis: Population-Based Study among 9,444 Older Adults from Germany," *International Journal of Cancer* 125, no. 12 (December 2009): 2918–22.

42. C. Chao, J. M. Slezak, B. J. Caan, and V. P. Quinn, "Alcoholic Beverage Intake and Risk of Lung Cancer: The California Men's Health Study," *Cancer Epidemiology and Biomarkers Prevention* 17, no. 10 (October 2008): 2692–99.

43. C. Chao, "Association between Beer, Wine, and Liquor Consumption and Lung Cancer Risk: A Meta-analysis," *Cancer Epidemiology and Biomarkers Prevention* 16, no. 11 (October 2007): 2436–47.

44. X. Jiang, K. E. Castelao, V. K. Cortessis, R. K. Ross, et al., "Alcohol c and Risk of Bladder Cancer in Los Angeles County," *International Journal of Cancer* 121, no. 4 (August 2007): 839–45.

45. N. D. Freedman, A. Schatzkin, M. F. Leitzmann, M. F. Hollenbeck, et al., "Alcohol and Head and Neck Cancer Risk in a Prospective Study," *British Journal of Cancer* 96, no. 9 (May 2007): 1469–74.

46. C. Pelucchi, C. Galeone, M. Montella, J. Polesel, et al., "Alcohol Consumption and Renal Cell Cancer Risk in Two Italian Case-Control Studies," *Annals of Oncology* 19, no. 5 (May 2008): 1003–8.

47. M. S. Freiberg, Y. F. Chang, K. L. Kraemer, J. G. Robinon, et al., "Alcohol Consumption, Hypertension, and Total Mortality among Women," *American Journal of Hypertension* 22, no. 111 (November 2009): 1212–18.

48. A. L. Klatsky, G. D. Friedman, and A. B. Siegekaub, "Alcohol and Mortality: A Ten-Year Kaiser-Permanente Experience," *Annals of Internal Medicine* 95, no. 2 (August 1981): 139–45.

49. C. A. Camargo, C. H. Hennekens, J. M. Gaziano, R. J. Glynn, et al., "Prospective Study of Moderate Alcohol Consumption and Mortality in US Male Physicians," *Archives of Internal Medicine* 157, no. 1 (January 1997): 79–85.

50. L. C. De Groot and P. L. Zock, "Moderate Alcohol Intake and Mortality," *Nutritional Review* 596, no. 1, part 1 (January 1998): 25–26.

51. A. L. Klatsky, G. D. Friedman, M. A. Armstrong, and H. Kipp, "Wine, Liquor, Beer and Mortality," *American Journal of Epidemiology* 158, no. 6 (September 2003): 585–95.

52. M. P. Longnecker and B. MacMohon, "Association between Alcoholic Beverages Consumption and Hospitalization, 1983 National Health Interview Survey," *American Journal of Public Health* 78, no. 2 (February 1998): 1543–56.

53. R. M. Vasse, F. J. Nijhuis, and G. Kok, "Association between Work Stress, Alcohol Consumption and Sickness Absence," *Addiction* 93, no. 2 (February 1998): 231–41.

54. J. A. Wiley and T. C. Camacho, "Life-style and Future Health: Evidence from Alameda County Study," *Preventive Medicine* 9, no. 1 (January 1980): 1–21.

55. M. Gronbaek, E. L. Mortensen, K. Mygind, A. T. Andersen, et al., "Beer, Wine, Spirit and Subjective Health," *Journal of Epidemiology and Community Health* 53, no. 11 (November 1999): 731–24.

56. H. Kallberg, S. Jacobsen, C. Bengtsson, M. Pedersen, et al., "Alcohol Consumption Is Associated with Decreased Risk of Rheumatoid Arthritis: Results from Two Scandinavian Studies," *Annals of Rheumatoid Diseases* 68, no. 2 (February 2009): 222–27.

57. M. J. Nissen, C. Gabay, A. Scherer, and A. Finchk, "The Effect of Alcohol on Radiographic Progression in Rheumatoid Arthritis," *Arthritis and Rheumatology* 62, no. 5 (May 2010): 1265–72.

58. H. K. Choi, K. Atkinson, E. W. Karlson, W. Willett, et al., "Alcohol Intake and Risk of Incident Gout in Men: A Prospective Study," *Lancet* 363, no. 9417 (April 2004): 1277–81.

59. S. Cohen, D. A. Tyrell, M. A. Russell, N. J. Jarvis, et al., "Smoking, Alcohol Consumption and Susceptibility to the Common Cold," *American Journal of Public Health* 83, no. 9 (September 1993): 1277–83.

60. B. Takkouch, C. Regueira-Mendez, R. Garcia-Closas, A. Figueiras, et al., "Intake of Wine, Beer, and Spirits and the Risk of Clinical Common Cold," *American Journal of Epidemiology* 155, no. 9 (May 2002): 853–58.

61. Dietary Guidelines for Americans, 2005, Chapter 9: Alcohol, U.S. Department of Health and Human Resources, http://www.health.gov./dietaryguidelines/dga2005/document/default.htm.

5

Harmful Effects of Chronic Alcohol Consumption

Drinking in moderation has many health benefits, but all such positive effects quickly disappear in people who drink heavily or who are alcoholics. Although the majority of Americans drink sensibly, and per capita consumption of alcohol from all alcoholic beverages in 2007 was 2.31 gallons or 289 ounces (approximately twenty-four beers a year per person), according to the National Institute of Alcohol Abuse and Alcoholism (NIAAA), approximately 8 percent of Americans are alcohol dependent. The group Healthy People 2010 has set a national objective of reducing per capita consumption to no more than 1.96 gallons of alcohol,[1] because the average total societal cost due to alcohol abuse as a percentage of gross domestic product (GDP) in high-income countries, including the United States, is approximately 1 percent. This is a high toll for a single factor and an enormous burden on public health.[2] According to a report by Dr. Ting-Kai Li, the director of the NIAAA, in 2008, alcohol-related problems cost the United States an estimated $185 billion annually, with almost half the costs from lost productivity due to alcohol-related disabilities. In the United States more than 18 million people ages eighteen and older suffer from alcohol abuse or dependency and only 7 percent of these people receive any form of treatment. In addition, heavy drinkers who are not alcoholics but are at high risk for developing alcohol-related physical or mental damage are seldom identified. The highest prevalence of alcohol dependency in the United States is observed among younger people between the ages of eighteen and twenty-four.

The World Health Organization (WHO) lists alcohol as one of the leading causes of disability in the world.[3]

According to studies conducted by the Center for Disease Control (CDC), alcohol abuse kills approximately 75,000 Americans each year and shortens the life of alcoholics by an average of thirty years. In 2001, 34,833 Americans died from cirrhosis of the liver, a major complication of alcohol abuse, and another 40,933 died from car crashes and other alcohol-related fatalities. Men accounted for 72 percent of the deaths due to alcohol abuse and 6 percent were twenty-one years old or younger.[4] In 2005, liver cirrhosis was the twelfth leading cause of death in the United States, claiming 28,175 lives. Among all cirrhosis-related deaths, 45.9 percent were alcohol related.[5] California is the largest alcohol market in the United States, and Californians consumed almost 14 billion alcoholic drinks in 2005, which resulted in an estimated 9,439 deaths and 921,029 alcohol-related problems such as crime and injury. The economic burden was estimated to be $38.5 billion of which $5.4 billion was for medical and mental health spending, $25.3 billion due to loss of work, and another $7.8 billion in criminal justice spending.[6] In the United Kingdom, alcohol consumption was responsible for 31,000 deaths in 2005, and the National Health Services spent an estimated 3 billion pounds in 2005–2006 for treating alcohol-related illness and disability. Alcohol consumption was responsible for approximately 10 percent of disabilities (male: 15 percent; female: 4 percent).[7]

Many studies demonstrate the harmful effects of alcohol on a variety of organ systems, including the liver, heart, brain, immune system, endocrine system, and bones. Alcoholic liver disease and alcoholic liver cirrhosis take many lives every year worldwide. Major adverse effects of chronic alcohol consumption include:

Decreased life span
Increased risk of violent behavior and tendency for substance abuse
Alcoholic liver disease
Anxiety and mood disorder
Brain damage (see chapter 3)
Damage to heart
Increased risk of stroke
Damage to immune system
Damage to endocrine system, including both male and female reproductive systems
Bone damage
Increased risk of various cancers
Poor outcome of pregnancy (see chapter 10)

DEFINITION OF HEAVY CONSUMPTION
OF ALCOHOL AND RISKY DRINKING

The definition of moderate and heavy drinking has been discussed in chapter 2. Briefly, moderate drinking means consuming up to two alcoholic drinks per day for men, up to one alcoholic drink per day for women, and up to one drink per day for both men and women older than sixty-five. For all practical purposes, the NIAAA sets this threshold at no more than fourteen drinks per week for men (or more than four drinks per occasion) and no more than seven drinks per week for women (or more than three drinks per occasion). Individuals whose drinking exceeds these guidelines are at increased risk for adverse health effects. Hazardous drinking is defined as twenty-one or more drinks per week by men or more than seven drinks per occasion at least three times a week. For women, more than fourteen drinks per week or drinking more than five drinks in one occasion at least three times a week is considered hazardous drinking. Risky drinking is defined as the consumption of five or more drinks in a single occasion or day for men and four or more drinks for women. Risky drinking is also referred to as binge drinking.

There is a misconception that if the number of total drinks in a week does not exceed fourteen for men and seven drinks for women, then the drinking practice is safe. In reality, frequency of drinking is an important criterion for defining moderate drinking. It is wise not to consume more than one drink a day for both men and women because the beneficial effects of alcohol can be achieved from consuming as little as one to six drinks per week. Consuming seven drinks on Friday and seven drinks on Saturday and not drinking at all for the remainder of the week—thus consuming a total of fourteen drinks per week for a male—is risky behavior. Risky drinking or binge drinking, even practiced occasionally, is a dangerous behavior. For example, consuming five drinks within two hours would certainly elevate blood alcohol level over the legal limit of 0.08 percent in a lean and moderately built person, and if stopped by the police, a DWI charge would be extremely likely.

Risky drinking is also associated with violent behavior, mood swings, and behavior-related problems such as self-harm and injury, risky sexual practices and sexual victimization, spousal abuse, and risk of developing obesity. Consuming more than five drinks just once a month may increase the risk of developing dementia, and a study with Canadian adults ages eighteen to sixty-four found that having ever consumed more than one drink in a single day during the preceding year was associated with an increased risk of heart disease and hypertension among men and an increased risk of heart disease among women. Dawson et al. (2001), following 22,245 Americans, reported that 59.9 percent of drinkers never engaged in risky drinking behavior, 16.9 percent engaged in risky drinking less than once a month, about 9 percent did so one to three times a month, and a small minority of 3 percent did three to four times a week or nearly every day. Risky drinkers were younger and usually not married. Daily or nearly daily risky drinkers were more than seven times more likely to develop alcohol dependency compared to moderate drinkers. The odds of developing liver disease were also high in individuals who were involved in risky drinking just once or twice a week. Daily or near daily risky drinking was also associated with high odds of divorce, spousal abuse, and poor job performance. In addition, daily or near daily risky drinkers are also prone to drug abuse, drug dependence, and nicotine abuse.[8]

CHRONIC ABUSE OF ALCOHOL AND REDUCED LIFE SPAN

Although moderate drinking is associated with increased longevity, heavier drinking is associated with decreased longevity compared to abstainers. Heavy consumption of alcohol causing reduced longevity depends on two factors: frequency of drinking and number of drinks consumed in one occasion. As described in chapter 4, studies that demonstrated increased life span among moderate drinkers also established that heavy drinking reduces normal life span. Moderate drinking reduces the risk of heart disease, but excess alcohol consumption is toxic to the heart. Similarly, moderate drinking reduces the risk of stroke but heavy drinking increases the risk.

Even occasional heavy drinking may be detrimental to health. Dawson reported an increased risk of mortality among individuals who usually drink more than five drinks per occasion but who drank even less than once a month.[9] Irregular heavy drinking even once a month (five or more drinks per occasion) increases the risk of heart disease rather than protecting the heart as observed in moderate drinkers. The cardioprotective effect of moderate drinking also disappears when light to moderate drinking is mixed with occasional heavy drinking episodes.[10]

In a British study of 5,766 men ages thirty-five to sixty-four with a twenty-one-year follow-up, it was observed that consuming between fifteen to twenty-one standard drinks per week increases the risk of all causes of mortality compared to moderate drinkers (up to fourteen standard drinks per week) and nondrinkers by 34 percent, while drinking more than thirty-five standard drinks per week increases the risk by 49 percent. The authors further observed that men drinking thirty-five or more standard drinks per week had double the risk of stroke compared to nondrinkers. The authors concluded that in general the overall association between alcohol consumption and mortality is unfavorable for men drinking twenty-two standard alcoholic drinks per week or more.[11]

Using more than 43,000 participants and a fourteen-year follow-up (2,547 people died), Breslow and Graubard (2008) observed that men who consumed five or more drinks on a drinking day had a 30 percent higher risk of mortality from heart disease, a more than 50 percent higher risk of cancer, and a more than 40 percent of all-cause mortality compared to individuals who drank one drink on a drinking day. The risk of mortality was also increased to some extent with just two drinks per day or more for men. Women drinkers who consumed alcohol (two drinks or more in a session) more often than in moderation (one drink or less a day) also showed all-cause higher mortality than moderate drinkers. Among men both quantity and frequency of drinking were significantly associated with mortality from cardiovascular disease, cancer, and other causes, but among women the quantity of alcohol was more important, and women who drank more than in moderation showed a higher risk of mortality from cancer than from men.[12] The London-based Whitehall II Cohort Study, using 10,308 government employees between the ages of thirty-five and fifty-five with an eleven-year follow-up, also concluded that optimal drinking is one drink or less daily consumed once or twice a week. People who consumed alcohol twice a day or more had an increased risk of mortality compared to those drinking once or twice a week.[13]

Binge drinking is also dangerous. In one study (based on a population of 1,641 men who drank beer), the authors observed that the risk of death in men who drank six or more bottles of beer in one occasion was almost three times higher than those who consumed less than three bottles in one occasion.[14] Another study (Anda et al. 1988) based on 13,251 adults also reported that individuals who drank five or more drinks in one occasion were nearly twice as likely to die from injuries than people who drank fewer than five drinks in a single occasion. People drinking nine or more drinks in a single occasion were 3.3 times more likely to die from injuries than people consuming less than five drinks.[15]

Consuming five or more drinks in one occasion increases the risk of fatal injuries significantly compared to individuals who consume less than five drinks.

Other than increasing mortality from various diseases, alcohol abuse is associated with increased risk of suicide, accidents, and violent crimes.

Alcohol-related traffic accidents causing fatalities are discussed in chapter 6. Based on a survey of 31,953 school students, Schilling et al. (2009) observed that both drinking while depressed and episodic heavy drinking were associated with self-reported suicide attempts in adolescents.[16] Swahn et al. (2008) reported that in a high-risk school district in the United States, 35 percent of seventh graders reported alcohol use initiation at age thirteen or younger. Preteen alcohol users were more involved in violent behavior than nondrinkers. Early alcohol use was also associated with higher risk of suicide attempts among these adolescents.[17]

ALCOHOL ABUSE AND INCREASED RISK OF VIOLENT BEHAVIOR

Many investigators have reported a close link between violent behavior, homicide, and alcohol intoxication. Studies conducted on convicted murderers suggest that about half of them were under the heavy influence of alcohol at the time of the murder.[18] According to the latest report on alcohol and crime published by the U.S. Department of Justice, alcohol is involved in many violent crimes (table 5.1).

Alcohol may induce aggression and violent behavior by disrupting normal brain function when consumed in high doses. By impairing the normal information-processing capability of the brain, a person can misjudge a perceived threat and may react more aggressively than warranted. Serotonin, a neurotransmitter, is considered a behavioral inhibitor. Alcohol abuse may lead to decreased serotonin activity, causing aggressive behavior. High testosterone concentrations in criminals have been associated with violent crimes. Adolescents and young adults with

Table 5.1.   Involvement of Alcohol in Violent Crimes and Offenses in the United States

- On average each year 183,000 rapes and sexual assaults involve alcohol abuse by offenders.
- Approximately 197,000 robberies, 661,000 aggravated assaults, and nearly 1.7 million simple assaults are caused by heavy drinkers each year.
- Two-thirds of the victims attacked by a known individual (spouse or former spouse, boyfriend, or girlfriend) reported that alcohol was involved. In contrast, 31 percent of victimization by strangers is alcohol related.
- Approximately 118,000 family violences annually are alcohol related.
- Approximately 36 percent of convicted offenders abuse alcohol during committing the crime. Male offenders are more likely to be drinking than female offenders.
- Half of the convicted murderers in state prisons abused alcohol before committing the crime.

Source: "Alcohol and Crime," 1998 report by the U.S. Department of Justice, Bureau of Justice Statistics.

higher levels of testosterone compared to the general population are more often involved in heavy drinking and consequently violent behavior. Young men who exhibit antisocial behavior often "burn out" with older age due to decreased levels of testosterone and increased levels of serotonin. By modulating serotonin and testosterone concentration, alcohol may induce aggressive and violent behavior when consumed in excess.[19]

ALCOHOLIC LIVER DISEASE

The liver is one of the largest and most complex organs of the human body. It synthesizes important proteins vital for life, stores some nutrients, and breaks down (metabolizes) drugs and toxins, including alcohol, thus protecting the body from harmful effects. Although the liver has an amazing capacity for self-healing through regeneration, certain liver diseases, such as cirrhosis of the liver, are irreversible and may even cause death. Alcohol-induced liver disease can be classified under three categories: (1) fatty liver; (2) alcoholic hepatitis; and (3) liver cirrhosis.

Heavy drinking for as little as a few days may produce fatty changes in the liver (steatosis), which can be reversed after abstinence. However, drinking heavily for a longer period may cause severer alcohol-related liver injuries, such as alcoholic hepatitis and cirrhosis of the liver. The diagnosis of alcoholic hepatitis is a serious medical condition because approximately 70 percent of such patients may progress to liver cirrhosis, a major cause of death worldwide. However, if a patient with alcoholic hepatitis practices complete abstinence, this condition may be reversible.

> In general, women are more susceptible to alcoholic liver disease than are men.

Drinking in moderation has no ill effects on the liver. One drink or less a day for both men and women is safe, and all the health benefits of alcohol can be enjoyed from consumption of such a moderate amount of alcohol, but heavy drinkers are susceptible to alcoholic liver disease. Although fatty liver may develop in approximately 90 percent of alcoholics, only 10–35 percent of them develop alcoholic hepatitis, while 10–20 percent of them develop liver cirrhosis. In the United States it is estimated that more than 2 million people are suffering from alcohol-related liver diseases. Liver cirrhosis is the seventh-leading cause of death among young and middle-aged adults and approximately 10,000 to 24,000 deaths from liver cirrhosis annually may be attributable to alcohol abuse.[20] The risk of developing alcoholic hepatitis and liver cirrhosis depends on several factors:

Amount of alcohol consumed per day
Length of heavy drinking
Gender
Ethnicity and genetic predisposition
Nutritional status and obesity
Type of alcoholic beverage consumed
Family history of alcohol abuse
Presence of hepatitis C

The amount of alcohol consumed is a determining factor in developing alcoholic hepatitis and liver cirrhosis. In one report (Bellentani and Tribelli 2001) the authors commented that cirrhosis of the liver does not develop below a lifetime ingestion of 100 kg of alcohol (one standard drink is approximately 14 gm of alcohol; therefore, this would be a lifetime consumption of 7,143 drinks). This amount corresponds to an average of five drinks a day for about four years. The authors also commented that consuming alcohol with food lowers the risk of developing cirrhosis of the liver compared to consuming alcohol on an empty stomach.[21]

Although only a small percentage of alcoholics develop alcoholic hepatitis and liver cirrhosis, other alcohol-related liver damage occurs at a much lower intake of alcohol. In general, it is considered that the threshold of alcohol-induced liver toxicity is 40 gm of alcohol per day (approximately three drinks a day) for men and 30 gm (more than just two drinks) or more of alcohol a day for women. But in one report (Bellentani et al. 1997) the authors concluded—based on a study of 6,917 subjects—that risk of any alcohol-induced liver damage (noncirrhotic liver damage) may have a threshold of just 30 gm or more of alcohol consumption (a little more than two standard drinks) per day for both men and women, and the risk increases with increasing daily consumption. Drinking outside mealtime and drinking multiple different alcoholic beverages increased alcohol-induced liver damage.[22]

However, another study (Walsh and Alexander 2000) indicated that above a threshold of seven to thirteen drinks per week for women and fourteen to twenty-seven drinks per week for men, there is a risk of developing some alcohol-related liver problems. In general women are more sensitive than men to the toxic effects of alcohol. One of the reasons is that women break down alcohol more slowly than do men due to genetic differences. In addition, toxic metabolites of alcohol tend to accumulate more in women than in men. Consumption of coffee may protect men against alcohol-induced liver damage, but no such data is currently available for women.[23] It has also been postulated that heavy drinkers of spirits are more susceptible to alcoholic liver damage than wine drinkers.

Although fatty liver is common in heavy drinkers, those who develop alcoholic hepatitis, liver cirrhosis, and other severe alcohol-related liver diseases have usually been abusing alcohol for more than a decade. Daily alcohol consumption of three to six drinks for men and two to three drinks for women over a period of twelve years would most likely cause alcoholic liver diseases. However, lower amount of alcohol consumption may cause alcoholic liver disease in certain ethnic populations. One Chinese study (Lu et al. 2004) using 1,300 alcohol drinkers indicated that the risk threshold was only 20 gm of alcohol daily (one and a half drinks) for five years, with a greater risk when alcohol is consumed on an empty stomach, especially with hard liquor (spirits). In addition, obese people showed more morbidity from alcohol-related liver diseases.[24]

Hepatitis C is a liver disease caused by *Hepatitis C virus*. This virus can be spread by sharing needles or other equipment for injecting illicit drugs and also through sexual contact with infected partners. It has been estimated that approximately 4 million Americans are infected with hepatitis C, and between 10,000 and 12,000 die annually. Hepatitis C infection is common among alcohol abusers, and this infection may even accelerate alcohol-related liver diseases, including cirrhosis of the liver and liver cancer. How much alcohol consumption is safe for a person with hepatitis C has not been clearly established. In one study (Hezode et al. 2003) the authors observed that moderate alcohol consumption of 31–50 gm per day for men (two and a half drinks to three and a half drinks) and 21–50 gm per day for women (one and a half drinks to three and a half drinks) could adversely affect the progression of liver damage.[25] Anyone with a confirmed hepatitis C infection must consult with his or her physician before drinking any alcoholic beverages.

DIAGNOSIS AND TREATMENT
OF ALCOHOLIC LIVER DISEASES

Common symptoms of alcoholic hepatitis are weakness, weight loss, nausea, vomiting, diarrhea, pain in the upper abdomen, and jaundice. Laboratory findings include increased levels of liver-specific enzymes in the blood, and increased levels of bilirubin may correlate with the severity of the disease. Serum bilirubin over 15 mg/dL (100 milliliters of serum) indicates a severe case of liver damage. In general, lab tests show that the liver enzyme aspartate aminotransferase (AST) is more elevated than alanine aminotransferase (ALT). Prothrombin time is usually prolonged and the albumin level in the blood is usually reduced. Viral hepatitis can also cause similar laboratory findings, and negative tests for hepatitis combined with a prolonged history of heavy drinking may confirm the diagnosis of alcoholic liver damage.

Hepatitis C and concurrent alcohol abuse could cause more severe liver damage and a poor prognosis. Liver biopsy may or may not be performed depending on the physical examination of the patient and laboratory test results. However, liver biopsy may be helpful to rule out non-alcohol-related liver damage. In figure 5.1, representative liver biopsies of fatty liver, alcohol hepatitis, and alcoholic liver cirrhosis are shown. Patients with severe liver cirrhosis have poor survival rates, and 50 percent may die within thirty days after diagnosis of the disease, but people with a diagnosis of alcoholic hepatitis have a much better prognosis, with only 15 percent mortality within thirty days.

The severity of alcoholic liver disease can be estimated by using the following formula:

Risk factor = 4.6 × (prothrombin time prolongation in seconds) + serum bilirubin (mg/dL)

A value higher than 32 indicates severe disease.

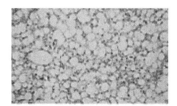

Fatty Liver

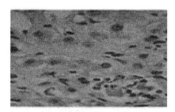

Alcoholic Hepatitis

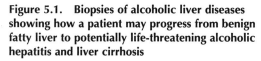

Figure 5.1.   Biopsies of alcoholic liver diseases showing how a patient may progress from benign fatty liver to potentially life-threatening alcoholic hepatitis and liver cirrhosis

Source: L. S. Marsano et al., "Diagnosis and Treatment of Alcoholic Liver Disease and Its Complications," *Alcohol Research and Health* 27, no. 3 (2003): 247–56. A publication of the National Institute of Alcohol Abuse and Alcoholism. Information in the public domain.

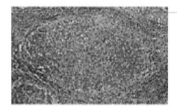

Cirrhosis

Liver transplant is the replacement of a severely diseased liver (usually in a patient suffering from end-stage liver disease), which can no longer perform the physiological functions required for sustaining life, with a healthy liver, usually from a deceased donor. Live liver transplant, where a living person donates a portion of liver to another person, is usually performed in children. The first such surgery was performed in 1989 when a child received a segment of his mother's liver.

The most commonly used liver transplant technique is orthotopic transplantation, where the damaged liver is removed and then the new liver is placed at the same anatomic spot. The mathematical formula widely used to assess the need for liver transplant in patients with severe end-stage liver disease is called the MELD score (model for end-stage liver disease), which is based on natural logarithm (ln) values of bilirubin, creatinine, and international normalization ratio (INR), indicating the coagulation status of blood.

MELD score = 3.8 (ln bilirubin, mg/dL) + 11.2 (ln INR) + 9.6 (ln creatinine mg/dL) + 6.4

A value of 6 or less indicates a good prognosis, while a score higher than 26 indicates fatalities in ninety days for about 90 percent of patients after diagnosis.

Treatment of alcoholic liver diseases includes lifestyle modification and practicing complete abstinence. Alcoholic hepatitis can often be reversed if complete abstinence is practiced, and even patients who have progressive liver cirrhosis can benefit from practicing abstinence. Other therapies include nutritional supplementation and medications, such as pentoxifylline or steroids. Liver transplantation may greatly increase the chance of survival in some patients (table 5.2).

Table 5.2.   Therapy for Alcoholic Liver Disease

Treatment	Comments
Alcohol abstinence	Survival is greatly increased in patients with liver cirrhosis and alcoholic liver disease.
Nutritional supplements	Many alcoholics get almost half of their daily calories from alcohol and experience severe vitamin and nutritional deficiencies including thiamine deficiency.
Pentoxifylline	May be beneficial in some patients
Prednisone	May be beneficial in some patients
Antioxidant therapy	Therapy with antioxidant including vitamin E
Liver transplant	Patient must be alcohol free for a specified time prior to transplant. This is a very effective way of treating alcoholic liver cirrhosis with about 70 percent survival after five years. In contrast, patients with severe forms of alcoholic liver disease, including cirrhosis, may die in days or months.

Mechanism of Liver Damage by Alcohol

The mechanism for alcohol-induced liver disease is complex. While in moderate drinkers alcohol is mostly metabolized by alcohol dehydrogenase in the liver, in alcoholics CYP2E1, a member of the cytochrome P-450 drug-metabolizing family of enzymes in the liver, becomes activated. In this process free oxygen radicals are generated, causing oxidative damage to liver cells. In addition, acetaldehyde—a toxic product of alcohol metabolism if not removed quickly by further metabolism—may cause liver toxicity. In alcoholics, the tremendous burden of alcohol on the liver for metabolism causes both acetaldehyde and nicotinamide adenine dinucleotide hydrogen (NADH) to accumulate, leading to oxidative stress to the liver and increased production of fatty acid. Metabolism of fatty acid is also impaired, causing fatty acid buildup, which is eventually turned into fat (triglycerides) by the liver. Fatty liver with more alcohol consumption may proceed to liver cirrhosis.

Another mechanism of liver damage by alcohol is the excess cytokine production by Kupffer cells of the liver due to the release of bacterial endotoxin in the blood by the action of excess alcohol on bacteria present in the gut. Excess cytokine can stimulate the inflammatory process, causing further liver damage. The mechanism of liver damage by alcohol is schematically presented in figure 5.2.

HEAVY ALCOHOL CONSUMPTION, DEPRESSION, AND BRAIN DAMAGE

Although alcohol can cause relaxation and mild euphoria with moderate consumption, these pleasurable effects of alcohol are reversed when blood alcohol levels go above 100 mg/dL (0.1 percent). Alcohol has more damaging effects on the adolescent brain than the adult brain. The onset of drinking at an early age (thirteen or earlier) has devastating effects on the brain as well as on the life of the person, and such effects follow the person throughout his or her life. Early onset of drinking is also linked to a greater risk of alcohol dependence in adult life. Although thiamine deficiency is one of the major factors involved in alcohol-related brain damage, both alcohol and its toxic metabolite acetaldehyde have direct toxic effects on neurons (brain cells). Please see chapter 3 for an in-depth discussion on this topic.

HEAVY ALCOHOL CONSUMPTION AND RISK OF HEART DISEASE AND STROKE

As discussed in chapter 4, if consumed in moderation, alcohol can reduce the risk of heart disease and stroke, but if consumed chronically in excess,

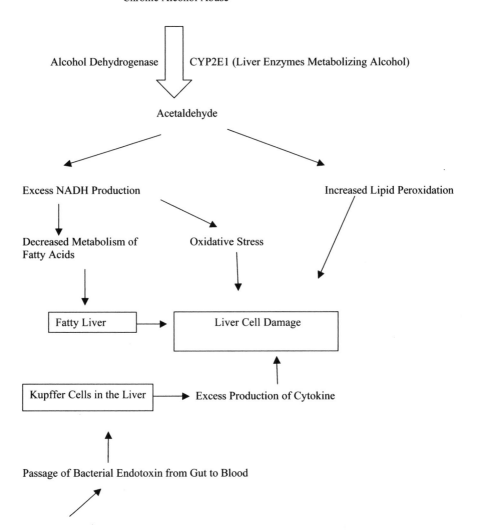

Figure 5.2.   Mechanism of alcohol-induced liver damage

it increases the risk of both heart disease and stroke. Drinking more than three drinks per day (any type of alcoholic beverage) may be harmful to the heart. Chronic alcohol abuse for several years may result in the following serious medical conditions:[26]

- Alcoholic cardiomyopathy and heart failure
- Systematic hypertension (high blood pressure)

- Heart rhythm disturbances
- Hemorrhagic stroke

Alcoholics who consume 90 gm or more of alcohol per day (seven to eight drinks) for five years are at risk of developing alcoholic cardiomyopathy, and if they continue drinking alcohol, cardiomyopathy may proceed to heart failure, a potentially fatal medical condition. This distinct form of heart failure (congestive heart failure) is responsible for 21–36 percent of all cases of nonischemic heart failure. Without complete abstinence, 50 percent of these patients will die from heart failure within four years of diagnosis.[27]

A stroke occurs when the blood supply in a particular part of the brain is interrupted or decreased, depriving brain cells from the supply of glucose (fuel for brain cells), oxygen, and essential nutrients. Within a few minutes brain cells start dying, and if not treated soon, the stroke may lead to severe brain damage, paralysis, or even death. Fortunately, there are many excellent options for treating stroke today if the patient receives prompt medical attention. Today fewer Americans die from stroke than thirty or forty years ago. Controlling high blood pressure, abstinence from tobacco, and lowering cholesterol can all reduce the risk of stroke. *Hemorrhage* means "bleeding" and a hemorrhagic stroke occurs when a blood vessel in the brain ruptures, causing interruption in the blood flow to a part of the brain. A blood vessel may rupture from high blood pressure or a weak spot in the blood vessel wall (aneurysm). Heavy drinking increases the risk of stroke, but particularly the risk of hemorrhagic stroke. Ikehara et al. (2009) observed that the risk of hemorrhagic stroke increases in an individual drinking 300 gm or more of alcohol weekly (twenty-one or more drinks).[28]

HEAVY ALCOHOL CONSUMPTION AND DAMAGE TO THE IMMUNE SYSTEM

Alcohol abuse is associated with increased risk of bacterial infections and opportunistic infections (including viral infections). The increased risk of infection in alcohol abusers is due to the impairment of the immune system by alcohol. Exposure to alcohol can result in reduced cytokine production. Mast cells are important immune cells that are widely distributed in tissues that are in contact with the external environment, such as skin and the mucosa of the lung and the gastrointestinal tract. Mast cells produce a variety of compounds, including cytokines, histamine, eicosanoid, and TNF-α (tumor narcosis factor-alpha), that play important roles in the defense against bacteria and parasites. Therefore, mast cells are considered the first line of defense against invading bacteria and parasites. Alcohol reduces the viability of mast cells and may cause cell death. Alcohol-induced reduction of the viability of mast cells could contribute to the impaired immune system function associated with alcohol abuse.[29] Alcohol also accelerates disease progression in patients with HIV infection because of immunosuppression. In one study using 231 patients with HIV infection who were undergoing antiretroviral therapy, Baum et al. (2010) observed that even consumption of two or more drinks daily can cause a serious decline in CD4+ cell count (higher CD4+ counts indicates good response to therapy).[30]

> Even two drinks a day may have serious consequences in the progression of HIV infection.

Adult respiratory distress syndrome (ARDS) is a severe form of lung injury. Approximately 200,000 individuals develop ARDS in the United States each year, and nearly 50 percent of these patients have a history of alcohol abuse. The mortality from ARDS is high (more than 40 percent) and for alcohol abusers approximately 65 percent. In ARDS survivors, alcohol abuse was also associated with a longer stay under ventilation in intensive care units. Alcohol impairs immune function and decreases the level of pulmonary antioxidants and thus may cause ARDS.[31]

ALCOHOL ABUSE AND DAMAGE TO THE ENDOCRINE, REPRODUCTIVE, AND SKELETAL SYSTEMS

Hormones are chemical messengers that control and coordinate the function of tissues and organs. Each hormone is secreted from a particular gland and distributed throughout the body to carry out its physiological function. The hypothalamus, located deep within the brain, is the control center for most of the body's hormonal system. The hypothalamus, the pituitary gland (also located in the brain), and the adrenal glands (located on the kidneys) function together as a well-coordinated unit, controlling the hormonal balance of the body. The hypothalamus secretes corticotrophin-releasing factor, which through complex mechanisms stimulates the adrenal glands to secrete glucocorticoid hormones, which influence carbohydrate, lipid, protein, and nucleic acid metabolism, and play a vital role in the cardiovascular system, bone development, and immune function.

The major circulating glucocorticoid hormone in humans is cortisol. Alcohol abuse may lead to a disease known as pseudo–Cushing's syndrome, indistinguishable from Cushing's syndrome, characterized by excess production of cortisol, which causes high blood pressure, muscle weakness, diabetes, obesity, and a variety of other physical disturbances. Diminished sexual function in alcoholic men has been described for many years. Administration of alcohol in healthy young male volunteers causes diminished levels of testosterone. Even drinking three or more drinks a day may cause significant problems in women, including delayed ovulation or failure to ovulate and menstrual problems, but such problems do not affect women who consume two or fewer drinks a day. This may be related to alcohol-induced estrogen levels in women. Alcoholic women often experience reproductive problems. However, these problems may resolve when a woman practices abstinence from alcohol. To form healthy bone calcium, phosphorus and the active form of vitamin D is essential. Chronic consumption of alcohol may reduce bone mass through a complex process of inhibition of the hormonal balance needed for bone growth, including testosterone in men, which is diminished in alcoholics. Alcohol abuse may also interfere with pancreatic secretion of insulin, causing diabetes.[32]

ALCOHOL ABUSE AND
INCREASED RISK OF VARIOUS CANCERS

Although moderate drinking reduces the risk of certain cancers (see chapter 4), chronic abuse of alcohol increases cancer risk. Cancer kills an estimated 526,000 Americans annually, and ranks second only to heart disease. Cancers of the lung, large bowel, and breast are most common in the United States, and approximately 2 to 4 percent of all cancer cases may be linked to alcohol abuse. Epidemiological research has demonstrated a dose-dependent relationship between consumption of alcohol and certain types of cancers; as alcohol consumption increases, so does the risk of cancer. The strongest link was found between alcohol abuse and cancer of the mouth, pharynx, larynx, and esophagus. An estimated 75 percent of all esophageal cancers are attributable to chronic alcohol abuse, while nearly 50 percent of cancers of the mouth, pharynx, and larynx are associated with chronic heavy consumption of alcohol. Prolonged drinking may result in alcoholic liver disease and cirrhosis of the liver, and such diseases can progress to liver carcinoma (liver cancer). There are weak links between alcohol abuse and cancer of the colon, stomach, lung, and pancreatic cancer.[33] Disease of the pancreas (pancreatitis) and gallstones are common among alcohol abusers. In alcoholics, endotoxin may be released from gut bacteria and trigger progression of acute pancreatitis into chronic pancreatitis. Chronic pancreatitis may lead to pancreatic cancer.[34] Pancreatic cancer is related to a high mortality rate.

Moderate alcohol consumption and the risk of breast cancer is debatable because there are conflicting reports in the medical literature. One Spanish study of 762 women between the ages of eighteen and seventy-five showed that even one drink a day may increase the risk of breast cancer, and one and a half drinks or more per day results in a 70 percent higher chance of developing breast cancer than nondrinkers.[35] In contrast, another study reported that women who consumed 10 to 12 gm of wine per day (one glass of wine) had a lower risk of developing breast cancer compared to nondrinkers. However, the risk of breast cancer increases in women who drink more than one drink per day.[36] Nagata et al. (based on a review of eleven reports on the association between alcohol consumption and the risk of breast cancer) concluded that epidemiological evidence of the link between alcohol consumption and the risk of developing breast cancer remains insufficient.[37]

In general, studies have shown that heavy drinking of more than 46–69 gm of alcohol per day (three and half drinks to five drinks) contributes to the total cancer risk, especially among men who drink heavily.[38] Various factors may contribute to the development of alcohol-related cancer, including the action of acetaldehyde, the toxic metabolite of alcohol. The main liver enzymes involved in alcohol and acetaldehyde metabolism are alcohol dehydrogenase and acetaldehyde dehydrogenase, which are encoded by various genes. Because some of these genes demonstrate polymorphism (a variant that may control enzymatic activities), in certain individuals, lower activity of acetaldehyde dehydrogenase may lead to an accumulation of toxic acetaldehyde in the blood. Acetaldehyde is carcinogenic (cancer-promoting) and can react with DNA to form cancer-promoting compounds. In addition, the generation of reactive oxygen free radicals when alcohol is metabolized by CYP2E1 liver enzyme can also damage DNA, thus promoting cancer.[39]

ALCOHOL ADDICTION AND GENES

Research on alcohol addiction has indicated that genetics play some role in the development of alcohol abuse, and it is not just the influence of environment alone. Based on large well- characterized studies involving twins, it has been established that alcoholism is a moderately inherited psychiatric disorder, with children of alcoholic parents more prone to alcohol abuse. The variation of gene coding that determines the activities of alcohol-metabolizing enzymes and genes that code for receptors or transmitters of neurochemical pathways for action of alcohol on the brain influence individuals' response and susceptibility to alcohol consumption.

Based on genetic variation, the liver enzymes alcohol dehydrogenase (ADH) and acetaldehyde dehydrogenase (ALDH) can accelerate or slow down the metabolism of alcohol. Acetaldehyde dehydrogenase exits in two major forms, ALDH1 and ALDH2. Although both forms can convert toxic acetaldehyde into acetate (which eventually breaks down into carbon dioxide and water), ALDH2 is the major enzyme responsible for the transformation of toxic acetaldehyde metabolite of alcohol. For both ADH and ALDH enzymes, genetically determined variants (also called isoforms) exist in their different levels of activity. People carrying different ADH and ALDH isoforms metabolize alcohol at different rates. ADH and ALDH isoforms arise from a natural variation (polymorphism) in the structures of the genes that code these enzymes. Two alcohol dehydrogenase genes (ADH2 and ADH3) on chromosome 4 and one acetaldehyde dehydrogenase gene (ALDH2) on chromosome 12 are known to exhibit polymorphism, thus controlling the activities of both enzymes. The frequency of these polymorphisms differs in different ethnic groups.

One of the best understood polymorphisms of alcohol-metabolizing enzymes is associated with the ALDH2 enzyme. One ALDH2 isoform, known as ALDH2*2, which is found in approximately 40 percent of people of Far East Asian descent but rarely in Caucasians, is partially inactive because of a specific mutation in the gene encoding this enzyme. In people carrying the ALDH2*2 enzyme, even moderate alcohol consumption results in acetaldehyde accumulation in the blood, because acetaldehyde is only slowly removed from the blood due to the less active form of the enzyme. An elevated acetaldehyde level after drinking may lead to unwanted reactions toward alcohol, such as flushing, nausea, and rapid heartbeat, and thus deter people from drinking.

The high prevalence of alcohol abuse and alcohol dependence among American Indians may also be mediated partly by genetic factors. Wall et al. (2003) reported that American Indians who consumed more alcohol and were alcohol dependent had different polymorphism in the ADH gene than non-alcohol-dependent subjects. This genetic difference in alcohol dehydrogenase enzyme may be linked to alcohol dependence in some American Indians.[40] Interestingly, in some Asians genetic polymorphism of acetaldehyde dehydrogenase enzyme may protect them from alcohol abuse, while genetic polymorphism of alcohol dehydrogenase may make some American Indians more prone to alcohol dependence.

Addiction to alcohol and drugs is related to brain function, and individuals who are addicted to alcohol may also be addicted to illicit drug abuse. Research indicates that genes affecting the activity of the neurotransmitter serotonin and gamma-aminobutyric acid (GABA) are likely candidates to be involved in the genetic mechanism of alcohol dependence. In one study, the authors (Herman et al. 2003) found that Caucasian college students with a particular variant of the serotonin transporter gene (short variant S of the serotonin transporter promoter polymorphism) consumed more alcohol per occasion, drank more often to get drunk, and also engaged in binge drinking more often than students with another variant of the gene. A higher frequency of S homozygotes (both parents contribute S variant, the other variant is long variant) is associated with adult alcoholics who exhibited an increased frequency of binge drinking.[41] Stacey et al. (2009) commented that heritability estimates for alcoholism range from 50 to 60 percent, pointing out the importance of both genetic and environmental factors in its etiology. Corticotropin-releasing factor, glutamatergic and opioidergic systems, and the genes regulating them may all play a role in the genetics of alcoholism.[42]

ALCOHOL REHABILITATION

Alcohol addiction is an illness that can be cured with proper treatment. The most widely used definitions for alcohol use disorders are those determined by the editions of the *Diagnostic and Statistical Manual of Mental Disorders* (*DSM-IV*) of the American Psychiatric Association and the *International Classification of Disease* (*ICD-10*) of the World Health Organization (WHO). Alcoholism treatments, as well as research studies on alcohol (including epidemiological studies), all rely on these definitions. Currently *DSM-IV* and *ICD-10* criteria are widely used to determine alcohol dependence.

Alcoholism can be classified under two broad categories based on the research of C. Robert Cloninger:

- *Type 1.* Less severe form with later onset of alcohol-related problems, and the problems are more psychological than physical dependence on alcohol. Children of type 1 alcoholism tend to develop type 1 alcoholism in the later part of their lives but under strong environmental influence may become type 2 alcoholics.
- *Type 2.* More severe form of alcoholism found most commonly in men. The onset of alcohol dependence starts at an earlier age, and these individuals show compulsive alcohol-seeking behavior and are disruptive socially when drinking. Children of type 2 alcoholics tend to be type 2 alcoholics, regardless of environment. Although originally considered male limited, later research indicated that type 2 alcoholism may also be found in females.[43]

More than 700,000 Americans receive alcoholism treatment in a given day. Self-help groups are the most commonly used source of help for people suffering from alcohol-related problems. Alcoholics Anonymous (AA), one of the most widely used self-help groups, outlines twelve consecutive steps that an alcohol-dependent person is encouraged to follow to achieve continuous sobriety. There are also psychosocial treatments available for an alcohol-dependent person. These therapies include Motivational Enhancement Therapy, Couples Therapy, Cognitive Behavioral Therapy, and Motivational Interviewing. In addition, drug therapy can be initiated if necessary to combat withdrawal symptoms from alcohol abuse.[44]

Currently there are three Federal Drug Administration (FDA)–approved medications for treating alcohol dependence. The oldest one, disulfiram (Antabuse), interferes with metabolism of alcohol by blocking the action of acetaldehyde dehydrogenase enzyme, resulting in the accumulation of acetaldehyde. Therefore, a person undergoing alcohol rehabilitation experiences unpleasant reactions, such as flushing, nausea, and palpitation, if he or she drinks alcohol. Therefore, disulfiram deters a person from drinking. This drug is given orally once a day. Naltrexone, another drug used in treating alcohol dependence, blocks opiate receptors that are involved in the rewarding effects of drinking alcohol. It is available in oral form (Depade, ReVia) to be taken once a day or in extended release form (Vivitrol), which is given by injection once a month. Because a person no longer gets the pleasurable effect from drinking, this medication acts as a deterrent. The third FDA-approved drug for treating alcoholism is acamprosate (Campral), which acts on gamma-aminobutyric acid (GABA) and glutamate neurotransmitter symptoms, and reduces symptoms of protracted alcohol abstinence, including insomnia, anxiety, restlessness, and dysphoria (unpleasant and uncomfortable mood). This medication is given orally three times a day. Although not FDA-approved for treating alcohol dependence, the anticonvulsant drug topiramate and several new antidepressant agents, such as fluoxetine and ondansetron, have been shown to increase abstinence rates and decrease drinking among alcohol-dependent people.[45]

CONCLUSION

All beneficial effects of alcohol disappear if it is not consumed in moderation. Interestingly, if consumed in moderation, alcohol reduces the risk of heart disease, stroke, certain types of cancer, and even Alzheimer's disease, but if consumed in excess instead increases the risk of developing the same diseases. Moderate drinkers enjoy longer life, while alcohol abuse shortens life. Chronic alcohol abuse for a longer period of time may cause alcoholic hepatitis and even liver cirrhosis, which are potentially fatal medical conditions. Alcoholism is part genetically controlled and part environmentally controlled. Fortunately, alcohol dependence is an illness, and intervention and treatment can return an alcohol-dependent person to a normal life again.

NOTES

1. R. LaValle, G. D. Williams, and H. Ti, "Apparent Per Capita Alcohol Consumption: National, State, Regional Trends, 1977–2007," Surveillance Report #87, National Institute on Alcohol Abuse and Alcoholism, September 2009.

2. S. Mohapatra, J. Patra, S. Popova, A. Duhig, et al., "Social Cost of Heavy Drinking and Alcohol Dependence in High-Income Countries," *International Journal of Public Health* 55, no. 3 (June 2010): 149–57.

3. National Institute of Alcohol Abuse and Alcoholism (NIAAA): FY 2009 Presidents' Budget Request for NIAAA, Directors' Statement before the House Subcommittee on Labor, HHS Appropriations, March 5, 2008, presented by Ting-Kai Li, M.D., http://www.niaaa.nih.gov/AboutNIAAA/CongressionalInformation/Testimony/statement.html.

4. "Alcohol Linked to 75,000 U.S. Deaths a Year," Msnbc.com news update, June 25, 2005 (no author listed), http://www.msnbc.msn.com/id/6089353.

5. Y. H. Yoon and H. Yi, "Liver Cirrhosis Mortality in the United States, 1970–2005," Surveillance Report #83, National Institute on Alcohol Abuse and Alcoholism, August 2008.

6. S. M. Rosen, T. R. Miller, and M. Simon, "The Cost of Alcohol in California," *Alcoholism: Clinical and Experimental Research* 32, no. 11 (November 2008): 1925–36.

7. R. Balakrishnan, S. Allender, P. Scarborough, P. Webster, et al., "The Burden of Alcohol-Related Ill Health in the United Kingdom," *Journal of Public Health* (Oxford) 31, no. 3 (September 2009): 366–73.

8. D. A. Dawson, T. K. Li, and B. Grant, "A Prospective Study of Risk Drinking: At Risk of What?" *Drug and Alcohol Dependence* 95, no. 1 (May 2008): 62–72.

9. D. A. Dawson, "Alcohol and Mortality from External Causes," *Journal of Studies on Alcohol and Drugs* 62, no. 6 (November 2001): 790–97.

10. M. Roerecke and J. Rehm, "Irregular Heavy Drinking Occasions and Risk of Ischemic Heart Disease: A Systematic Review and Meta-analysis," *American Journal of Epidemiology* 171, no. 6 (March 2010): 633–44.

11. C. L. Hart, G. D. Smith, D. J. Hole, and V. M. Hawthorne, "Alcohol Consumption and Mortality from All Causes, Coronary Heart Disease, and Stroke: Results from a Prospective Cohort Study of Scottish Men with 21 Years of Follow-Up," *British Medical Journal* 318, no. 7200 (July 1999): 1725–29.

12. R. A. Breslow and B. I. Graubard, "Prospective Study of Alcohol Consumption in the United States: Quantity, Frequency and Cause of Cause-Specific Mortality," *Alcoholism: Clinical and Experimental Research* 32, no. 3 (March 2008): 513–21.

13. A. Britton and M. Marmot, "Different Measures of Alcohol Consumption and Risk of Coronary Heart Disease and All-Cause Mortality: 11-Year Follow-Up of the Whitehall II Cohort Study," *Addiction* 99, no. 1 (January 2004): 109–16.

14. J. Kauhanen, G. A. Kaplan, D. E. Goldberg, and J. T. Salonen, "Beer Binging and Mortality: Results from Kuopio Ischemic Heart Disease Risk Factor Study; a Prospective Population-Based Study," *British Medical Journal* 315, no. 4 (October 1997): 846–51.

15. R. F. Anda, D. F. Williamson, and P. L. Remington, "Alcohol and Fatal Injuries among U.S. Adults: Findings from the NHANES I Epidemiologic Follow-Up Study," *Journal of the American Medical Association* 260, no. 17 (November 1988): 2529–32.

16. E. A. Schilling, R. H. Aseltine, J. L. Glanovsky, A. James, et al., "Adolescent Alcohol Use, Suicidal Indention and Suicide Attempts," *Journal of Adolescent Health* 44, no. 4 (April 2009): 335–41.

17. M. H. Swahn, R. M. Bossarte, and E. E. Sullivent III, "Age of Alcohol Use Initiation, Suicidal Behavior, and Peer and Dating Violence Victimization and Perception among High-Risk Seventh Grade Adolescents," *Pediatrics* 121, no. 2 (February 2008): 297–305.

18. T. Z. Palijan, D. Kovacevic, S. Radeljak, M. Kovac, et al., "Forensic Aspects of Alcohol Abuse and Homicide," *Collegium Anthropologium* 33, no. 3 (September 2009): 893–97.

19. "Alcohol, Violence, and Aggression," Alcohol Alert No. 38, National Institute on Alcohol Abuse and Alcoholism, October 1997, http://pubs.niaaa.nih.gov/publications/aa38thm.

20. S. F. DeBarkey, F. S. Stinson, B. F. Grant, and M. C. Dufour, "Liver Cirrhosis Mortality in the United States, 1970–1993," Surveillance Report #41, National Institute of Alcohol Abuse and Alcoholism, 1996.

21. S. Bellentani and C. Tribelli, "Spectrum of Liver Disease in General Population: Lessons from Dionysos Study," *Journal of Hepatology* 35 (2001): 531–37.

22. S. Bellentani, G. Saccoccio, G. Costa, C. Tribelli, et al., "Drinking Habits as Cofactors of Risk for Alcohol Induced Liver Damage: The Dionysos Study Group," *Gut* 42, no. 6 (December 1997): 845–50.

23. K. Walsh and G. Alexander, "Alcoholic Liver Disease," *Postgraduate Medicine* 281 (2000): 280–86.

24. X. Lu, J. Y. Luo, M. Tao, et al., "Risk Factors for Alcoholic Liver Disease in China," *World Journal of Gastroenterology* 10 (2004): 2423–26.

25. C. Hezode, I. Lonjon, F. Roudot-Thorval, J. M. Pawlotsky, et al., "Impact of Moderate Alcohol Consumption on Histological Activity and Fibrosis in Patients with Chronic Hepatitis C, and Specific Influence of Steatosis: A Prospective Study," *Alimentary Pharmacology and Therapeutics* 17, no. 8 (April 2003): 1031–37.

26. A. L. Klatsky, "Alcohol and Cardiovascular Health," *Physiological Behavior* 100, no. 1 (April 2010): 76–81.

27. I. Laonigro, M. Correale, M. Di Biase, and E. Altomare, "Alcohol Abuse and Heart Failure," *European Journal of Heart Failure* 11, no. 5 (May 2009): 453–62.

28. S. Ikehara, H. Iso, K. Yamagishi, and S. Yamamoto, "Alcohol Consumption, Social Support and Risk of Stroke and Coronary Heart Disease among Japanese Men: The JPHC Study," *Alcoholism: Clinical and Experimental Research* 33, no. 6 (June 2009): 1025–32.

29. K. Numi, K. Methuen, T. Maki, K. A. Lindstedt, P. T. Kovanen, et al., "Ethanol Induces Apoptosis in Human Mast Cells," *Life Sciences* 85, nos. 19–20 (November 2009): 678–84.

30. M. K. Baum, C. Rafie, C. Lai, S. Sales, et al. "Alcohol Use Accelerates HIV Disease Progression," *AIDS Research and Human Retroviruses* 26, no. 5 (May 2010): 511–18.

31. D. M. Boe, R. W. Vandivier, E. L. Burnham, and M. Moss, "Alcohol Abuse and Pulmonary Disease," *Journal of Leukocytes Biology* 76, no. 5 (November 2009): 1097–1104.

32. N. Emanuele and M. A. Emanuele, "Alcohol Alters Critical Hormonal Balance," *Alcohol Health and Research World* 21, no. 1 (1997): 53–64.

33. "Alcohol and Cancer," Alcohol Alert No. 21, PH 345 (July 1993), National Institute of Alcohol Abuse and Alcoholism.

34. M. Apte, R. Pirola, and J. Wilson, "New Insights into Alcoholic Pancreatitis and Pancreatic Cancer," *Journal of Gastroenterology and Hepatology* 24, no. 3, supplement 3 (October 2009): S351–56.

35. J. M. Martin-Moreno, P. Boyle, L. Gorgojo, W. C. Willett, et al., "Alcoholic Beverage Consumption and Risk of Breast Cancer in Spain," *Cancer Causes and Control* 4, no. 4 (July 1993): 345–53.

36. F. Bessaoud and J. P. Daures, "Pattern of Alcohol (Especially Wine) Consumption and Breast Cancer Risk: A Case-Controlled Study among a Population in Southern France," *Annals of Epidemiology* 18, no. 6 (June 2008): 467–75.

37. C. Nagata, T. Mizoue, K. Tanaka, I. Tsuji, et al., "Alcohol Drinking and Breast Cancer Risk: An Evaluation Based on a Systematic Review of Epidemiological Evidence among the Japanese Population," *Japanese Journal of Clinical Oncology* 37, no. 8 (August 2007): 568–74.

38. M. Inoue, K. Wakai, C. Nagata, T. Mizoue, et al., "Alcohol Drinking and Total Cancer Risk: An Evaluation Based on a Systematic Review of Epidemiological Evidence among the Japanese Population," *Japanese Journal of Clinical Oncology* 37, no. 9 (September 2007): 692–700.

39. H. K. Seitz and P. Becker, "Alcohol Metabolism and Cancer Risk," *Alcohol Research and Health* 30, no. 1 (January 2007): 44–47.

40. T. L. Wall, L. G. Carr, and C. L. Ehlers, "Protective Association of Genetic Variation in Alcohol Dehydrogenase with Alcohol Dependence in Native American Mission Indians," *American Journal of Psychiatry* 160, no. 1 (January 2003): 41–46.

41. A. I. Herman, J. W. Philbeck, N. L. Vasilopoulos, and P. B. Depertrillo, "Serotonin Transporter Promoter Polymorphism and Differences in Alcohol Consumption Behavior in a College Student Population," *Alcohol and Alcoholism* 38, no. 5 (September–October 2003): 446–49.

42. D. Stacey, T. K. Clarke, and G. Schumann, "The Genetics of Alcoholism," *Current Psychiatry Report* 11, no. 5 (October 2009): 364–69.

43. A. Magnusson, M. Goransson, and M. Heilig, "Early Onset Alcohol Dependence with High Density of Family History is Not 'Male Limited,'" *Alcohol* 44, no. 2 (March 2010): 131–39.

44. "New Advances in Alcoholism Treatment," Alcohol Alert No. 49 (October 2000), National Institute on Alcohol and Alcoholism.

45. J. C. Garbutt, "The State of Pharmacotherapy for the Treatment of Alcohol Dependence," *Journal of Substance Abuse and Treatment* 36, no. 1 (January 2009): S15–23.

6

DWI and Alcohol Testing

Breath Analyzer versus Blood Alcohol

Drinking and driving do not mix at all. "Driving while impaired" (DWI) and "driving under the influence" (DUI) are used interchangeably to describe impaired drivers. In chapter 2, detailed guidelines have been provided regarding consumption of alcohol and estimated blood alcohol levels based on gender and body weight. The objective of this chapter is to reinforce the philosophy of drinking sensibly and drinking in moderation.

Injury from motor vehicle crashes is the leading cause of death in the United States among people ages one to thirty-four and approximately 40 percent of all traffic-related deaths involve alcohol. According to the statistics released by the National Highway Traffic Safety Administration, there were 16,694 deaths and 258,000 injuries from alcohol-related motor vehicle crashes in 2004. The estimated annual economic cost of alcohol-related crashes is $51 billion.[1]

Although injuries from alcohol-related crashes have declined over the past two decades due to implementation of legal blood alcohol limits and strict enforcement of DWI laws, alcohol-related fatalities from traffic accidents remained relatively stable in the last decade. In 2003 there were 17,041 alcohol-related fatalities in the United States that were attributed in part to repeat DWI offenders.[2] In 2007, nearly 13,000 alcohol-impaired people were killed in driving accidents, and, as in 2003, many alcohol-impaired drivers involved in fatal crashes were previously arrested for driving while intoxicated. In 2007, drivers with a blood alcohol level exceeding the legal limit (0.08 percent or above) in fatal crashes were eight times more likely to have a prior DWI conviction compared to drivers with no alcohol in their blood.

According to the U.S. Department of Transportation and the National Highway Traffic Safety Administration (NHTSA) reports, 1.46 million drivers were arrested in the United States in 2006 for driving under the influence of alcohol or narcotics.[3] In 2008, 11,733 people were killed in driving crashes caused by alcohol impairment, accounting for one-third (32 percent) of all traffic-related deaths in the United States. Of the 216 child passengers ages fourteen and younger who died in driving crashes caused by alcohol/drug impairment in 2008, 99 were riding in the vehicle with an alcohol-impaired driver.

Although the number of deaths due to alcohol-related traffic crashes was reduced from 2007 to 2008, alcohol-related crashes remained a major cause of traffic fatalities. In 2008, 1.4 million drivers were arrested for driving under the influence of alcohol or narcotics.[4] However, one report (Quinlan et al. 2005) estimated that the number of alcohol-impaired drivers in the United States was 159 million annually based on surveys of self-reported episodes of alcohol-impaired driving.[5] Therefore, DWI arrests represent only 1 percent of all drivers on the road who are driving after consuming alcohol.

> Despite continued efforts from law enforcement, deaths caused by alcohol-impaired driving take an enormous toll in the United States: approximately one person every forty minutes or thirty-two people a day.

Incidents of alcohol-impaired driving increase during holidays such as Christmas and New Year's. On average, from 2001 to 2005, about 40 percent of all fatalities during the Christmas and New Year's holidays in the United States have occurred in crashes where at least one of the involved drivers was impaired due to consumption of alcohol. Compare that to approximately 28 percent of all fatalities during the rest of December and 31 percent during the entire year being alcohol related. During 2001–2005, the average number of fatalities per day during New Year's was fifty-four and during Christmas was forty-five, and both numbers were significantly higher than the average fatality rate of thirty-three per day during the rest of December.[6]

In general, alcohol involvement in fatal crashes in 2007 was more than three times higher at night (6 PM to 6 AM) than during the day (6 AM to 6 PM), with 62 percent of crashes involving alcohol at night versus 19 percent of crashes involving alcohol during the day. Alcohol involvement in fatal crashes was also higher (54 percent) on the weekend compared to weekdays (35 percent). In addition, nearly one in four drivers (23 percent) of a personal vehicle and more than one in four motorcyclists (27 percent) involved in fatal crashes were intoxicated with a blood alcohol level of 0.08 percent or higher. The drivers between twenty-one and thirty-two years of age had the highest proportion of drivers with blood alcohol levels over the legal limit, followed by drivers between twenty-five and thirty-four. Elderly drivers (seventy-five or older) showed the smallest percentage (only 4 percent) of driving over the legal limit. Interestingly, only 1 percent of drivers of commercial vehicles (heavy trucks) had blood alcohol concentrations over the legal limit.[7]

One of the major problems of alcohol-impaired driving is the habit of binge drinking, which is defined as consuming more than five drinks in one episode by a man or four or more drinks by a woman (see chapter 2). Based on a survey of 14,085 adults, Naimi et al. (2009) reported that overall 11.9 percent of binge drinkers drove during or within two hours of their most recent binge episode. Those drinking in licensed establishments (bars, clubs, or restaurants) consumed an average of 8.1 drinks, and 25.7 percent of them consumed more than ten drinks.[8] These episodes are considered heavy drinking and certainly cause serious impairment in a driver.

Consuming two standard drinks by a man and one standard drink by a woman in one episode is considered moderate drinking, and after such moderate consumption of alcohol driving is safe within an hour, because blood alcohol level would be well below the legal limit of driving. A man weighing 175 pounds or more can safely consume three standard drinks with food and wait for at least two hours before driving. A woman weighing 125 pounds or more can safely consume two standard drinks with food and wait for two hours before driving. Binge drinking may produce a blood alcohol level that is two to three times higher than the legal limit for driving, and if the driver is stopped by the police, it would certainly result in a DWI charge.

The legal drinking age in the United States is twenty-one, and there is a sizable amount of literature on the effect of minimum drinking age restrictions on teenage drunk driving. The effect of lowering the minimum drinking age, as has been proposed in Vermont, could lead to sizable increases in teenage involvement in fatal accidents due to the evasion of local alcohol restrictions.[9] In addition to the legal drinking age of twenty-one, most states have a zero-tolerance policy for underage drinking. The role of age (youth and driving inexperience) and alcohol as major risk factors for traffic accidents has been firmly established by numerous studies over the last fifty years. Some investigators have hypothesized that there is a synergistic effect in which young drivers with less experience and a greater tendency to take risks are more adversely affected at lower blood alcohol concentrations compared to older, more experienced drivers. Peck et al. (2008) demonstrated that positive blood alcohol in drivers younger than twenty-one is associated with a higher relative crash risk than would be predicted from the added effect of blood alcohol level and age. In addition, crash-avoidance skills of young drivers are adversely affected by alcohol. These results support a zero-tolerance policy for blood alcohol level laws for minors.[10]

Parents and other adults also have the responsibility of influencing the attitude of younger drivers about drinking. A study by Leadbeater et al. (2008) found that young drivers' risk behaviors were associated independently with their own experiences of riding with adults and peers who drove while under the influence of drugs and/or alcohol. The authors concluded that prevention efforts for youth drinking and driving should be expanded to include the adults and peers who are role models for new drivers, and that awareness should be raised concerning their own responsibility of not drinking and driving for their own personal safety and the safety of others.[11] Social host laws for minors aim to reduce alcohol consumption by imposing liability on adults who host parties. These laws have an impact on reducing alcohol-related traffic accidents. One study reported that among those who were eighteen to twenty, social host liability for minors reduced the drunken driving rate by 9 percent.[12]

In addition to fatalities from traffic accidents, alcohol-related traffic accidents and injuries are a major public health and public safety concern. Rosen et al. (2008) reported that alcohol consumption in California led to an estimated 9,439 deaths and 921,029 cases of alcohol-related problems, such as crime and injury, in 2005.[13] Alcohol intoxication may confound the initial assessment of trauma patients, even minimally injured patients, resulting in more diagnostic and therapeutic procedures, thus increasing the cost of care. The Uniform Policy Provision Law, which permits insurance providers to deny coverage for medical treatment due to alcohol-related injuries, exists in many states. In one report (O'Keefe et al. 2009), the authors demonstrated that of the patients admitted to the emergency room with similar injuries, those individuals with a positive blood alcohol level required more procedures, such as intubation, cauterization, and so on, at an average cost of $1,833 more than similar patients with no alcohol in their blood. In addition, a significant amount of trauma center costs are primarily attributable to alcohol use by patients.[14]

Fortunately, alcohol-related traffic fatalities are on the decline thanks to tough DWI implementation, public education, and other prevention programs. Mothers Against Drunk Driving (MADD), which was established in 1980, is considered one of the most successful public health citizen advocacy organizations in the United States. This group has been given credit for changing the attitude of Americans regarding drinking and driving. Alcohol-related traffic deaths in the United States declined from an estimated 30,000 in 1980 to 16,694 in 2004, partly due to the public's understanding of the perils of alcohol-impaired driving.[15]

LEGAL BLOOD ALCOHOL POLICY IN THE UNITED STATES AND OTHER COUNTRIES

If you are stopped by the police on suspicion that you are driving while under the influence of alcohol or drugs, the officer first conducts a field sobriety test and, based on his or her judgment, may ask you to take a breath alcohol test, submit a urine specimen for drug testing, or give a blood specimen for alcohol testing. If you have a choice, always agree to submit to a blood alcohol test. The blood is drawn in a detention center or a health care facility, and the blood alcohol test is more accurate than the breath alcohol test. However, depending on the state and county, you may not have the option of a blood alcohol test and will need to agree to a breath alcohol test.

The officer may or may not carry an evidentiary breath analyzer where the results produced by such analyzers can be admitted to a court of law as evidence. If the officer uses a breath analyzer for screening purposes, you may have to go to a police station where breath analysis is performed by a qualified person using an evidentiary breath analyzer. For this purpose, an officer may observe you for fifteen minutes and then ask you to blow into a disposable mouthpiece for five to ten seconds, and when enough exhaled air is collected, the instrument usually produces a buzzing noise. Before performing the test, the officer may perform a blank test to ensure the instrument is working properly. Then a second test may be performed to ensure validity of the test results, and, based on the results, you may be charged with DWI and your driver's license may be taken.

Usually you have the right to go for an administrative hearing to get your license back prior to trial. If you are found guilty and have a very high blood alcohol level, such as 0.15 percent or 0.2 percent, you may need to put an ignition lock device in your car at your own expense. This ignition lock device does not allow you to start a car if you have any alcohol in your blood (usually 0.02 percent or 0.01 percent). The best policy is to have a designated driver or drink in moderation so that your blood alcohol is half of the legal limit for driving (see later in this chapter for details). Many states also have open container laws where it is illegal to have an open bottle of an alcoholic beverage in the car, regardless of whether the driver or the passenger is drinking while the car is in motion.

Since 2002, the legal limit for driving in the United States in all states is 0.08 percent blood alcohol concentration (BAC), which is equivalent to 80 mg of ethyl alcohol in 100 mL of blood. This is more conveniently expressed as 80 mg/dL. Although DWI conviction is based on BAC, a BAC at or over the legal limit can be established by indirect means, such as by using a breath analyzer, which indirectly estimates blood alcohol by measuring alcohol concentration in the exhaled air. License suspension or revocation traditionally takes place after a DWI conviction. Under a procedure called "Administrative License Suspension," the license may be taken before a conviction if a driver fails or refuses to take a breath analyzer test or a similar test to determine the blood alcohol level.

Justification of 0.08 percent BAC Limit

The legal limit for blood alcohol is the amount of alcohol in the whole blood that is drawn directly from an individual by puncturing a vein on the arm. Whole blood alcohol is also commonly referred to as legal blood alcohol. Sometimes the alcohol level is not determined in a laboratory directly on the whole blood but may be determined in serum or plasma. When a whole blood specimen is drawn, after clotting, the blood cells settle at the bottom, leaving a yellowish liquid at the top, which is the water component of blood, or serum. If an anticoagulant is used, such as heparin, citrate, or ethylenediaminetetraacetic acid (EDTA) in the blood collection tube, upon centrifugation the aqueous (water) part of the blood is separated from the blood cells; the aqueous layer is called plasma. If an anticoagulant is not used in the blood collection tube, the serum can also be separated from the cellular components by centrifugation. Alcohol determined in serum or plasma is higher than whole blood alcohol. Therefore, it is important to establish how the alcohol level was determined in the blood (whole blood versus serum) during a DWI trial (this is covered more thoroughly later in this chapter). For our purposes here, BAC represents alcohol content in whole blood (legal blood).

Scientific research has indicated that drivers with a BAC between 0.05 and 0.08 percent are twice as likely to have accidents as drivers with no alcohol in their blood. Drivers with BAC from 0.1 percent to 0.14 percent are ten times more likely to have accidents than nondrinkers. There is a general agreement that BAC of about 0.05 percent results in some impairment of the ability to drive. Initially the legal BAC in the United States was 0.1 percent, but it was lowered to 0.08 percent in 1998 when President Clinton directed the secretary of transportation to work with Congress, state agencies, and other concerned safety groups to promote the adoption of 0.08 percent BAC nationwide.

In 1998, as part of the Transportation Equity Act for the 21st Century (TEA-21), a new federal program was created to encourage states to adopt 0.08 percent BAC as the legal limit of driving. Fourteen independent studies in the United States indicated that lowering the legal limit of BAC from 0.1 percent to 0.08 percent has resulted in a 5 to 16 percent reduction in alcohol-related crashes, fatalities, or injuries. Legal BAC is 0.05 percent in numerous countries, and several studies indicate that lowering BAC from 0.08 percent to 0.05 percent also reduces alcohol-related fatalities to some extent.[16]

Legal Limit of Blood Alcohol in Various Countries

The United States, Mexico, and some other countries have a legal BAC of 0.08 percent, but several countries in the world have a zero-tolerance policy of blood alcohol, meaning it is illegal to drive with any detectable alcohol in the blood. In addition, several countries in the world have a 0.02 percent and 0.03 percent BAC limit, while others have a limit of 0.05 percent BAC for driving (table 6.1). In fact, to my knowledge, 0.08 percent BAC is the highest acceptable legal limit for driving in any country, and in this light, a 0.08 percent limit of BAC as the legal limit of driving in the United States can be considered very fair and generous.

Table 6.1.   Legal Limits for Driving in Various Countries in the World by Blood Alcohol Concentration (BAC) Percentage

Blood Alcohol Concentration (BAC) %	Countries
0.08	United States, Mexico, United Kingdom, New Zealand, Ireland, Malta
0.05	Austria, Belgium, Bulgaria, Costa Rica, Denmark, Finland, Greece, Hong Kong, Israel, Peru, Portugal, Serbia, Spain, Switzerland, Thailand, Turkey
0.03	India, Japan, Russia
0.02	China, Poland, Norway, Sweden, Estonia
Zero tolerance	Saudi Arabia, United Arab Emirates, Brazil, Bangladesh, Hungary, Czech Republic

A BAC of 0.08 percent is the highest acceptable legal limit for driving in a few countries in the world, including the United States. Many
countries have a 0.05 percent BAC as the highest legal limit for driving.

DIFFERENT BIOLOGICAL MATRICES OF MEASURING ALCOHOL

For medical purposes, such as in the emergency room, alcohol is usually
measured in serum or plasma and is referred to as "medical alcohol."
Legal blood alcohol may be measured in whole blood or in serum/
plasma. Although medical alcohol may be used in the prosecution of a
DWI trial at the discretion of the judge, there are some differences between medical and legal alcohol. Breath alcohol measurement is usually
performed by police officers in a suspected impaired driver. In addition, alcohol can be measured in the urine, but determination of alcohol
levels in urine specimens is less common than blood alcohol testing
or breath alcohol analysis. Alcohol determination in a urine specimen
may be employed in a workplace alcohol and drug testing program (see
chapter 9).

Alcohol level can also be determined in saliva, also called "oral fluid."
In general, alcohol concentration in saliva is slightly higher than in blood.
In a study of forty-eight male volunteers, researchers demonstrated that
saliva/blood alcohol ratio was 1.082. The saliva/blood alcohol ratio was
remarkably constant throughout the absorption, distribution, and elimination of alcohol from the body, and the saliva alcohol level also reached
zero when the blood alcohol level was undetectable. Because saliva alcohol reflects blood alcohol level, saliva alcohol can be used as supportive
evidence in legal cases involving alcohol intoxication.[17]

Nevertheless, saliva alcohol measurement is less common than breath
alcohol measurement or blood alcohol measurement in determining intoxication in a suspected individual. In addition, saliva alcohol measurement is rarely used in medical settings despite commercial availability of
saliva-collecting devices and analytical methods for measuring alcohol
concentration in a saliva specimen. Interestingly, in many European
countries saliva drug testing is employed to identify a driver suspected
of driving under the influence of illicit drugs, and there are established
guidelines for cutoff levels of various drugs in saliva specimens. However, saliva testing of alcohol is rarely performed to identify a driver driving under the influence of alcohol.

Drug testing in hair specimens is gaining popularity and is used in legal
settings. Drugs stay in hair much longer than in urine. However, alcohol

is a small molecule that is readily soluble in water and is not deposited in hair. Metabolites of alcohol, such as ethyl sulfate and ethyl glucuronide, are trapped in hair and can be analyzed to determine whether an individual is abusing alcohol (see chapter 7 for more detail).

Breath Alcohol Analysis

A very small amount of alcohol is found in human breath. Only air in the deepest portion of the lung, known as alveolar sacs, comes in contact with the alcohol found in blood, and there is equilibrium between the alcohol level in the exhaled air and blood alcohol. The estimated ratio between breath alcohol and blood alcohol is 2100:1, and this ratio is utilized in various breath alcohol analyzers to calculate blood alcohol level based on the concentration of ethanol in exhaled air. This process is based on Henry's law, which states that the ratio between alcohol in blood and alcohol in deep lung air is constant. After measuring the concentration of alcohol in the exhaled air, the microprocessor of the instrument automatically converts the value to a calculated blood alcohol level.

Breath alcohol analysis was first developed in the 1950s, at a time when the understanding of pulmonary physiology was limited. Over the past fifty years, the research has revealed that the mechanism by which air in breath comes into contact with alcohol in the lungs is very complex. Alcohol is exchanged with the airway via diffusion from the bronchial tubes. Therefore, depending on the breathing pattern, variation in breath alcohol content may occur.[18] Because of this complex mechanism of exchange of alcohol from blood to exhaled air and individual variation in the ratio of alcohol between breath and blood, as well as interferences, legal challenges can be made at a court of law if breath alcohol value is just above the cutoff of the legal limit. In contrast, blood alcohol levels are more difficult to challenge during DWI defense because they are subject to no interferences if measured by using gas chromatography (GC), even if the value is just above the legal limit for driving.

Blood alcohol measurement is a direct measurement and there are established guidelines for assessing degree of impairment of an individual based on BAC and drinking history. In contrast, breath alcohol measurement is an indirect measurement but is considered a reasonable estimate of blood alcohol using a noninvasive technique with an assumption that an exhaled breath sample accurately reflects the alveolar air alcohol concentration, which is assumed to be in equilibrium with blood in pulmonary circulation. Despite considerable research in this field, forensic toxicologists still have only a very basic understanding of the physiological basis of breath alcohol analysis and associated limitations.[19]

How Breath Analyzers Work

The earliest developed breath analyzer was based on a chemical principle in which exhaled air was allowed to pass through a cocktail of chemicals containing sulfuric acid, potassium dichromate, silver nitrate, and water. Silver nitrate acts as a chemical catalyst in the reaction (a catalyst remains unchanged after a chemical reaction) where alcohol in the presence of sulfuric acid (sulfuric acid absorbs alcohol from air and also provides an acidic medium for facilitating the reaction) turns orange potassium dichromate solution into green due to the conversion of potassium dichromate into chromium sulfate, which is green in color. The intensity of the green color can be used to estimate the amount of alcohol in the exhaled air. Captain Robert Borkenstein of the Indiana State Police used this chemical principle to develop breath analyzers in 1954, and some breath alcohol analyzers still use this principle today.[20] In general, breath alcohol analyzers work on any of the following mechanisms:

- Analyzers that utilize color change due to a chemical reaction to determine alcohol level
- Analyzers based on detecting ethanol in breath based on infrared spectroscopy
- Analyzers based on fuel cell technology
- Analyzers based on mixed technology (infrared and fuel cell) and other techniques.

Breath analyzers can be further classified into screening devices and evidentiary breath analyzers. Screen breath analyzers can be used by a police officer for screening a suspected alcohol-impaired driver, but for the purpose of prosecution, a result obtained by an evidentiary breath analyzer approved by the U.S. Department of Transportation (DOT) must be used. Evidentiary breath analyzers are more expensive and more accurate, and results obtained correlate well with blood alcohol values. In addition, to ensure proper function of such analyzers, regular calibration against known alcohol standards are performed, and other preventive maintenances are carried out at regular intervals. Breath analyzers, which are small pocket-sized devices, are also available for consumers. These devices are helpful to determine an individual's alcohol level before driving so that a person may decide not to drive after a party; or if you think your teenager is drinking, the breath analyzer result can be used to verify your suspicion.

Breathalyzer (Analyzers Based on Color Change Due to a Chemical Reaction with Alcohol)

Breathalyzer is the oldest technology of breath alcohol analyzer and is based on the principle of color change of potassium dichromate solution in the presence of alcohol (as described earlier) and then analysis by using spectroscopy after a specified time to ensure complete reaction. The analyzer contains two vials of a chemical cocktail. After a subject exhales into the device, the air is passed through one vial, and if alcohol is present in the exhale, a color change occurs. A system of photocells connected to a meter to measure color change associated with the chemical reaction by comparing the response from the second vial (where no air is passed through) produces an electrical signal proportional to the color change in the reaction vial. This electrical signal can move the meter (more alcohol, more signal and a higher reading), and alcohol level in the subject can be determined. Breathalyzer was the brand name originally developed and marketed by Smith and Wesson, and the company then sold that brand to a German company called Draeger. The old Breathalyzer 900 model was replaced by newer versions, such as model 1100, but this technology is subject to interferences from a variety of substances, and because of that, other companies have focused on developing more robust technology for breath alcohol analysis.

Analyzers Based on Infrared Spectroscopy

There are several evidentiary breath alcohol analyzers that are based on the principle of infrared spectroscopy (IR spectroscopy) for quantitative determination of alcohol (ethanol) in exhaled air. The Intoxilyzer was originally developed by Omicron in Palo Alto, California, and later sold to CMI, Inc., in Owensboro, Kentucky. The earlier models were 4011A and 4011S, and then the Intoxilyzer 5000 was developed, which is used as an evidentiary breath alcohol analyzer, and, more recently, the Intoxilyzer 8000 model was introduced, which is now commercially available. Many states use this analyzer as their evidentiary breath analyzer. In addition to Intoxilyzer, DataMaster cdm (National Patent Analytical System, Mansfield, Ohio), which is also used in many states as the evidentiary breath alcohol analyzer, is based on IR spectrum technology.

The IR spectrum of a specimen is produced by passing a beam of infrared light through the specimen and then recording the transmitted light. A spectrum is formed when a particular wavelength of infrared light is absorbed by the specimen. This takes place when the frequency of the IR is the same as the frequency of a particular chemical bond in the molecule, absorption occurs, and the chemical bond vibrates due to the absorption of the energy. If a compound has multiple different bonds, absorption at multiple wavelengths should be observed.

In a more advanced version of IR spectroscopy, Fourier Transform IR spectroscopy, the instrument can measure all wavelengths at once and then perform a very complex technique of background correction to produce the IR spectrum. IR spectrum is like a picture of the molecule, indicating different chemical bonds that join various atoms together to produce the molecule, but it is unable to show atomic structures because energy is not sufficient to excite electrons in an atom. Infrared has less energy than the visible region of the electromagnetic spectra, and wavelengths of infrared are much longer than the wavelengths of the electromagnetic spectra we see visually (light and color). The infrared beam used for obtaining IR spectra of various organic compounds has a wavelength range between 1,500 to 16,000 nm (1.5 to 15 microns).

Alcohol breath analyzers that operate on the IR spectroscopic principle utilize the "Lambert-Beer Law," which states that the amount of electromagnetic radiation absorbed depends on the concentration of the active component that absorbs in that particular wavelength. Therefore, the amount of infrared radiation absorbed is proportional to the concentration of the alcohol in the breath; when more alcohol is present, more absorption of the infrared radiation is absorbed.

The newer version of Intoxilyzer (Intoxilyzer 5000) uses a five-wavelength filter at 3.36, 3.4, 3.47, 3.52, and 3.8 microns and can thus differentiate between ethanol and common interferences in exhaled air, such as acetone, acetaldehyde, and toluene. The 3.4 micron wavelength is used to detect alcohol, the 3.47 wavelengths identify interfering substances, and the 3.8 micron is used as the reference wavelength. The latest model, Intoxilyzer 8000, uses a pulsed IR source instead of a moving wavelength filter, and uses a dual wavelength for measuring alcohol (3.4 and 9.36 micron) in the breath. It also has more advanced computer technology to accurately provide alcohol level results. Razatos et al. (2005) evaluated the performance of both Intoxilyzer 5000 and 8000 by comparing results obtained by these instruments and direct analysis of alcohol using blood from the same subjects. Based on analysis of 700 specimens, both analyzers demonstrated good comparison with direct blood alcohol determinations. Based on their study, Intoxilyzer 8000 was approved as an evidentiary breath alcohol analyzer in the state of New Mexico.[21]

However, another report (Hardings et al. 1990) based on comparison of blood alcohol determined directly and blood alcohol determination based on breath alcohol analysis using 395 pairs of specimens indicated that in general, the Intoxylizer 5000 reported values 10 mg/dL less than blood alcohol most of the time, and in only 2 percent of the cases reported an alcohol value that was higher than the true blood alcohol level determined directly. The range of blood alcohol values determined directly ranged from zero to 338 mg/dL, while blood alcohol level estimates based on the Intoxylizer 5000 ranged from zero to 320 mg/dL.[22]

DataMaster cdm, an evidentiary breath analyzer widely used by police officers in many states, is also based on the principle of IR spectra, where alcohol is detected using two different wavelengths (3.37 and 3.44 microns). Kechagias et al. (1999) compared blood alcohol values with values obtained by a breath alcohol analyzer (DataMaster) in patients suffering from gastroesophageal reflux disease (GERD) and concluded that breath alcohol analyzers can overestimate true blood alcohol value due to the eruption of alcohol from the stomach to the mouth from gastric reflux.[23]

Analyzers Based on Fuel Cell Technology

There are several different brands of evidentiary breath alcohol analyzers that are based on the principle of fuel cell technology, such as Alcotest Models 6510, 6810, 7410, and so on (National Draeger, Durango, Colorado), and Alco-Sensor III and IV (Intoximeters, Inc., St. Louis, Missouri), which are evidentiary breath analyzers. The fuel cell is a porous disk coated with platinum oxide (also called platinum black) on both sides. The porous layer is impregnated with an acidic solution containing various salts (electrolytes) so that charged particles such as hydrogen ions can travel through that medium. In addition, both sides of the disk containing platinum oxide are connected through a platinum wire. The manufacturer mounts this fuel cell in a case along with the entire assembly so that when a person blows into the disposable mouthpiece, the air can travel through the fuel cell. If any alcohol is present in the exhaled air, then the alcohol is converted into acetic acid, hydrogen ion, and electrons on the top surface by the platinum oxide. Then hydrogen ions travel to the bottom surface (also containing platinum oxide) and are converted into water by combining with oxygen present in the air. In this process, electrons are removed from the platinum oxide. Because there is an electron excess on the top surface and electron deficit on the bottom surface, electrons flow from one surface to another, generating an electric current (the electric current is the flow of electrons through the wire) that flows through the platinum wire, with the intensity of the current being proportional to the amount of alcohol present in the exhaled air. The microprocessor of the instrument then converts that current to equivalent blood alcohol.

Some evidentiary breath analyzers are based on both fuel cell and infrared spectroscopy technology, giving them good sensitivity and specificity to analyze alcohol on breath. Various models of the Intox EC/IRl desktop evidentiary alcohol breath analyzers, also manufactured by Intoximeters, Inc., combine reliable fuel cell analysis with real-time analytical advantages of infrared technology.

Interferences in Measuring Alcohol Using Various Breath Analyzers

As mentioned before, blood alcohol determination is more accurate than breath alcohol analysis because substances with structural similarity with ethanol (alcohol) may be falsely identified as alcohol. This phenomenon, where a compound is falsely identified as the target compound, is called "interference," and the substance that causes this false identification is called an "interfering substance." Because false identification of another compound as alcohol has grave legal consequences, readers should be aware of such problems. If you think you are wrongly accused of DWI based on a false reading from an evidentiary breath analyzer, please contact an experienced DWI attorney in your area. There are legal books on the market that discuss this topic in detail, and an attorney specializing in DWI defense is very familiar with this situation. In general, if the breath analyzer results (based on two readings after fifteen minutes with each reading correlating very well) are just above the 0.08 percent level, it is possible that an interfering substance may have skewed the results. However, research indicates that when alcohol levels are significantly above the legal limit (such as two to three times higher), the effect of interfering substances may be insignificant. Again: do not drink and drive.

Partition Ratio

Unlike blood alcohol determination, which is a direct measurement of the alcohol level in a blood specimen, a breath alcohol analyzer uses a 2100:1 partition ratio between the breath alcohol level and the blood alcohol level based on Henry's law to calculate blood alcohol from breath alcohol. It is assumed that 2,100 mL of breath contains the same amount of alcohol as 1 mL blood, therefore 210,000 mL (210 liters) of breath contains the same amount of alcohol as 100 mL (1dL) of blood. Therefore, if the breath measures 80 mg of alcohol in 210 liters of breath, it is translated to 80 mg of alcohol in 100 mL of blood or 0.08 percent blood alcohol.

Although this ratio of 2100:1 is a very conservative estimate and valid for most people, variation from this partition ratio has also been reported in medical journals. Jones and Anderson (2003) reported that the average ratio between breath and blood alcohol levels was 2448:1, but varied widely, between 1836:1 and 4082:1. The median value (midpoint in the distribution) was 2351:1. Therefore, for an individual with a ratio below 2100:1, a breath alcohol analyzer would overestimate blood alcohol level, and for an individual with a breath-to-blood alcohol ratio greater than 2100:1, a breath alcohol analyzer would underestimate the true blood alcohol level. The authors concluded that breath test results obtained with the Intoxilyzer 5000S model were generally lower than the blood alcohol level, which gives an advantage to a suspect who provides breath compared to blood in cases close to a legal cutoff alcohol level of 0.08 percent.[24]

Mouthwash, Acetone, Propyl Alcohol, and Methanol

Sometimes a driver stopped by the police may use mouthwash to hide any alcoholic breath. Because most mouthwash contains alcohol, use of a mouthwash prior to taking a breath alcohol analysis may cause a falsely elevated alcohol result. However, residual alcohol evaporates from the mouth rapidly, and this is the reason for waiting for fifteen minutes in a police station under supervision so that the suspect cannot take anything by his or her mouth during the waiting period. Fessler et al. (2008) studied the effect of alcohol-based substances such as mouthwash, cough mixture, and breath spray just prior to breath alcohol measurement using the Draeger evidentiary portable breath alcohol analyzer with twenty-five volunteers and concluded that a fifteen-minute waiting period is necessary to ensure that there is no residual alcohol in the mouth following using mouthwash and other alcohol-containing products. Otherwise mouth alcohol interference in breath alcohol analysis may occur.[25]

Drinking an energy drink while driving a car is not against the law, but some energy drinks contain very low levels of alcohol. When volunteers drank various energy drinks, eleven out of twenty-seven drinks gave positive results using evidentiary breath analyzers when testing was done just after drinking. However, after a fifteen-minute waiting period, all breath alcohol analysis reports were negative. The authors concluded that a fifteen-minute waiting period eliminates the possibility of testing false positive after consuming an energy drink with a low alcohol content.[26]

Laakso et al. (2004) studied the effect of various volatile solvents for potential interference with breath alcohol analysis using the Draeger 7110 evidentiary breath analyzer and concluded that acetone, methyl ethyl ketone, methyl isobutyl ketone, ethyl acetate, and diethyl ether do not influence breath alcohol measurement significantly, but propyl alcohol and isopropyl alcohol have a significant effect on breath alcohol measurement.[27] Isopropyl alcohol is rubbing alcohol. If an individual abuses isopropyl alcohol, the person may produce a false positive ethanol result using an evidentiary breath analyzer. Jones and Rossner (2007) described a case where a fifty-nine-year-old man undergoing a weight-loss program using a ketogenic diet attempted to drive a car that was fitted with an alcohol ignition interlock device, and the vehicle would not start. Because he had completely stopped drinking, he was surprised and upset. Ketogenic diets used for treating obesity and controlling seizures in some epileptic children are high in fat, very low in carbohydrate, and have adequate protein. The goal of the diet is to burn fat to get energy rather than getting it from glucose, which is formed by carbohydrate metabolism. However, in this case, consuming the ketogenic diet led to a stage called ketonemia, where concentrations of acetone, acetoacetic acid, and beta hydroxybutyric acid are high. This high amount of acetone may be found in exhaled air. The interlock device in the car determines alcohol by an electrochemical oxidation method, and acetone does not interfere with the process. However, acetone is known to be converted into isopropyl alcohol by the action of liver alcohol dehydrogenase, and isopropyl alcohol can be falsely identified as alcohol (ethanol) by the ignition interlock device. In addition, methanol and propanol can also be falsely identified as alcohol. The authors concluded that side effects of ketogenic diets need further evaluation by authorities, especially for people involved in safety-sensitive positions, such as airline pilots and bus drivers who are subjected to much tougher alcohol tolerance policies.[28]

Methanol poisoning is dangerous because it may cause death or blindness (see chapter 12 for more detail), but drinking methanol is not against the law. A recent article reported the case of a forty-seven-year-old man who was found at a public park and acting intoxicated (methanol poisoning may cause intoxication). A breath analyzer (Intoxilyzer 5000EN) measured 288 mg of alcohol in 210 liters of breath, which was translated to 288 mg/dL blood alcohol or 0.28 percent blood alcohol (legal limit is 0.08 percent blood alcohol). In the emergency room, the patient admitted he drank gas line antifreeze, which contains 99 percent methanol. The patient was subsequently treated and survived, but this case indicates that methanol poisoning can be mistaken by a breath analyzer as alcohol poisoning.[29]

In another report (Caldwell and Kim 1997) the authors showed that toluene, xylene, methanol, and isopropyl alcohol in exhaled air can be mistakenly identified as breath alcohol by the Intoxilyzer 5000 evidentiary breath alcohol analyzer.[30] Although exposure to toluene or xylene may occur in certain workers in the chemical industry, taking proper protective measures to control such exposure would eliminate any possibility of being wrongly charged with DWI following an analysis by an evidentiary breath analyzer. A small amount of methanol is produced after eating certain foods high in pectin (see chapter 12), but again, the small amount of methanol found in the exhaled air has a negligible effect on breath alcohol analysis. A small amount of ethanol is also produced during normal human metabolism, but the amount is negligible and would not interfere with a breath alcohol measurement.

BLOOD ALCOHOL MEASUREMENT

Legal limit for driving is based on whole blood alcohol content in most states. Blood alcohol can be determined in whole blood or can be determined in serum or plasma, which is obtained after separating the aqueous part of the blood from various blood cells. The red color of the blood is due to the presence of hemoglobin and serum, while plasma has a yellowish appearance due to the absence of sufficient hemoglobin. A small amount of hemoglobin, called plasma-free hemoglobin, may be found in plasma but is not sufficient to produce a red color. Because alcohol is readily soluble in water, serum or plasma alcohol content is approximately 15–20 percent higher than whole blood alcohol content. Therefore, serum or plasma alcohol must be converted to a whole blood value by multiplying it by a correction factor. Serum and plasma alcohol content are virtually identical. In one report (Winek and Carfagna 1987), the authors found that the average ratio of ethanol in serum versus plasma is 1, while the ratio varied only slightly from 0.98 to 1.04 among different individuals. The serum to whole blood alcohol ratio is 1.12, which is identical to plasma to whole blood alcohol ratio.[31]

In general, a whole blood alcohol level is determined using gas chromatography in a crime or forensic laboratory, while serum or plasma blood alcohol is determined in a hospital laboratory, either by an enzymatic method or by using gas chromatography. In one study (Barnhill et al. 2007), using 212 consecutive patients admitted to a hospital trauma center, serum was analyzed for ethanol using an enzymatic method, while whole blood was analyzed using gas chromatography in a forensic toxicology laboratory. The authors observed that serum to whole blood alcohol ratio was dependent on alcohol concentration, but the average value was 1.12 up to an alcohol concentration of 300 mg/dL (0.3 percent) and may be as high as 1.18. Therefore, a serum blood alcohol of 90 mg/dL (0.09 percent) corresponds to a whole blood alcohol level of 80 mg/dL (0.08 percent).[32]

Rainey (1993) reported that the ratio between serum and whole blood alcohol ranged from 0.88 to 1.59, but the median was 1.15. Therefore, dividing the serum alcohol value by 1.15 would calculate the whole blood alcohol concentration. The serum to whole blood alcohol ratio was independent of serum alcohol concentration and hematocrit.[33] Hematocrit is a measure of the proportion of volume in blood occupied by red blood cells (erythrocytes) and is approximately 46 percent in men and 38 percent in women.

Gas Chromatography–Based Methods

Gas chromatography is a complex analytical technique capable of analyzing volatile substances in a mixture. In forensic toxicology laboratories, whole blood alcohol is always analyzed by a gas chromatographic method. Gas chromatography can also be used for quantitative estimation of serum of plasma alcohol. In gas chromatography, the stationary phase is a high boiling point liquid coated on a tube with a thin internal bore (gas chromatography column), and the mobile phase is an inert gas such as helium. A small sample (usually a few microliters) is drawn into a syringe, and then the needle of the syringe is placed on a hot injector and the specimen is injected into the gas chromatograph. The injection chamber is kept at a higher temperature than the column, and all components of the mixture are volatilized at the injector chamber. Then these compounds are swept by a stream of inert carrier gas through the heated column, and as these compounds pass through the column, they go back and forth between the carrier gas and the high boiling liquid coating of the column. More volatile compounds (lower boiling point) have more affinity for carrier gas and elute from the column before high volatile components. Thus, the complex mixture can be separated into individual compounds.

As soon as a compound in the mixture comes out of the column, it passes through a detector. When the detector sees a compound, it sends an electrical signal to the recorder, which recodes each compound as it comes out of the column as a function of the time it takes to elute from the column. Each compound thus has a specific time for which it is retained in the column, and this time is called the retention time.

For a particular instrument and a particular set of conditions, this retention time is specific for a compound, and in gas chromatographic determination of alcohol, the compound is identified based on the retention time. In order to measure the amount of alcohol (ethanol) in the specimen, a fixed amount of another compound with a similar structure to alcohol, for example, 1,2-butanediol, is added to the specimen prior to analysis. Then the concentration of alcohol in the specimen can be determined by comparing the response of the detector when alcohol eluted from the column (peak area of ethanol) to the peak area of 1,2-butanediol, which elutes from the column after alcohol. This is possible because concentration of 1,2-butanediol in the specimen is known.

A common technique applied to the analysis of blood alcohol using gas chromatography is called headspace gas chromatography. In this process blood is mixed with the internal standard and a solution containing various salts that make alcohol less soluble in blood and then placed in a sealed sample vial. Then the vial is heated, and in this process the alcohol and the internal standard is vaporized and an equilibrium is reached between alcohol in the air space above the liquid level (vapor phase) and blood. Then the air in the space above the liquid, which is also called headspace, is drawn into a syringe and then injected into the gas chromatograph.

There are many published methods of analysis of alcohol using gas chromatography. One advantage of gas chromatography is that alcohol (ethyl alcohol) along with similar compounds such as methanol, propyl alcohol, isopropyl alcohol, and acetone can be analyzed simultaneously. Another advantage of having a gas chromatograph in the laboratory is that ethylene glycol can also be analyzed using this equipment.

On the other hand, an enzymatic method for analysis of alcohol (ethyl alcohol) cannot be used to measure similar compounds, although there is an enzymatic method available for analysis of ethylene glycol. Because methanol, isopropyl alcohol, and ethylene glycol poisoning also occur, especially during winter months, many university hospital–based toxicology laboratories utilize a gas chromatographic method for analysis of alcohol, which is capable of simultaneously analyzing similar compounds. Such laboratories usually use a serum or plasma specimen for such analysis.

Smith (1984) reported determination of various alcohols and acetone in human serum using capillary gas chromatography, using propanol as the internal standard. In a 2 mL centrifuge tube containing 200 μl of serum, 200 μl of internal standard solution (containing propanol in deionized water), 200 μl of sodium tungstate (200 mmol/L), and 200 μl of copper sulfate (200 mmol/L) solution were added. After mixing and centrifuging to precipitate serum proteins, 1 μl of supernatant was injected into the gas chromatography column. Helium was used as the carrier gas, and both injector and detector (flame ionization detector) temperature was 280°C. The column temperature was maintained at 35°C. After the injection, methanol eluted at 2.06 minutes followed by alcohol (ethanol), acetone, and isopropyl alcohol (fig. 6.1).[34]

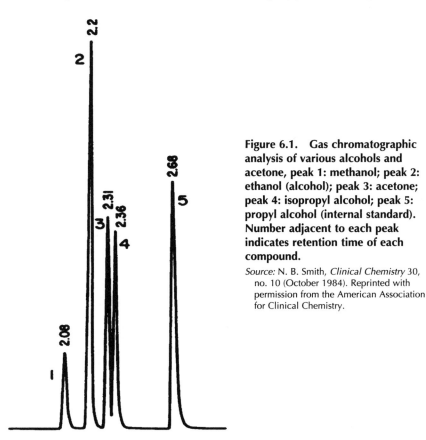

Figure 6.1. Gas chromatographic analysis of various alcohols and acetone, peak 1: methanol; peak 2: ethanol (alcohol); peak 3: acetone; peak 4: isopropyl alcohol; peak 5: propyl alcohol (internal standard). Number adjacent to each peak indicates retention time of each compound.

Source: N. B. Smith, *Clinical Chemistry* 30, no. 10 (October 1984). Reprinted with permission from the American Association for Clinical Chemistry.

Enzymatic Methods

In hospital laboratories, alcohol (ethyl alcohol) is also analyzed using enzymatic methods and automated analyzers. There are several different automated analyzers available from various diagnostic companies that are capable of analyzing alcohol in serum or plasma. Enzyme-based automated methods are generally not applicable for analysis of whole blood, although modified methods are available for analysis of alcohol in urine specimens. Commonly used automated analyzers in hospital laboratories include Dimension Vista Platform and ADVIA Platform (Siemens Diagnostics), Vitros Platform (Johnson and Johnson), and SYNCHRON LX20 analyzers (Beckman Corporation) to name a few.

Enzymatic automated analysis of alcohol is based on the principle of conversion of alcohol to acetaldehyde by alcohol dehydrogenase, and in this process nicotinamide adenine diphosphate (NAD) is converted into NADH (which is NAD plus one hydrogen atom). NAD has no absorption at ultraviolet light at 340 nm wavelength, while NADH absorbs at 340 nm. Therefore, an absorption peak is absorbed when alcohol is converted into acetaldehyde because NAD is also converted into NADH. The intensity of the peak is proportional to the amount of alcohol present in the specimen. If no alcohol is present, no peak is absorbed. Usually methanol, isopropyl alcohol, ethylene glycol, and acetone have negligible effect on alcohol determination using enzymatic methods, but propanol, if present, may cause 15–20 percent cross-reactivity with alcohol assay. Although isopropyl alcohol, which is used as rubbing alcohol, is common in the household, propanol is used in much less frequency in household products. Moreover, if 100 mg/dL of propanol is present in serum, the maximum false positive alcohol level would be 20 mg/dL (0.02 percent) and would not cause any serious problem in interpreting legal blood alcohol.

However, interference of lactate dehydrogenase and lactate in the enzymatic method of alcohol determination is significant and may cause misinterpretation of alcohol value over legal limit in a patient suffering from lactic acidosis (where high concentrations of lactate and lactate dehydrogenase are observed in blood), a serious medical condition requiring treatment in an emergency room. In addition, enzymatic alcohol assay is unsuitable for determination of alcohol in postmortem blood because of high concentrations of lactate dehydrogenase (LDH) and lactate; only gas chromatography can be used for measuring alcohol in postmortem blood. In one report (Thompson et al. 1984), the authors observed 690 mg/dL (0.69 percent) of alcohol in serum using an enzymatic method for alcohol in a patient, but the gas chromatography did not show any alcohol in the serum. This patient had end-stage renal disease and received a kidney transplant, and at the time when blood was drawn, she had severe metabolic acidosis and was admitted to the hospital. Her LDH concentration was 27,000 units/L and her lactate concentration was 15.0 mmol/L. However, the authors observed no apparent alcohol level in any specimen containing normal levels of LDH and lactate.[35]

End-stage liver disease, liver transplant (biliary atresia), Duchene muscular dystrophy, and chronic myelogenous leukemia may also lead to high LDH and lactate in living patients, which may cause false positive ethanol readings by immunoassays. Nine et al. (1995) observed a correlation between increasing lactate and LDH concentration and false positive ethanol results. This interference was most noticeable with the EMIT assay (enzyme multiplied immunoassay technique, Syva, San Jose, California) for alcohol and less remarkable with Abbott (Abbott Laboratories, Abbott Park, Illinois) and Roche (Roche Diagnostics, Indianapolis, Indiana) assays. With EMIT assay, false positive ethanol started at an LDH activity of 682 U/L and lactate concentration of 14 mmol/L.[36] Lactate concentrations also tend to increase in trauma patients. Dunne et al. (2005) reported that 27 percent (3536) of 13,102 patients they studied had positive alcohol screen (mean alcohol: 141mg/dL, range: 10 mg/dL–508 mg/dL).[37]

In contrast, Winek et al. (2004) compared alcohol concentration obtained by an enzyme assay (Dimension Analyzer, Siemens Diagnostics, Deerfield, Illinois) and gas chromatography in trauma patients and observed no false positives by immunoassays. Alcohol concentrations obtained by immunoassays correlated well with GC values, and, only in six specimens (out of twenty-seven), the difference between GC and immunoassay values exceeded 10 percent, and the highest difference was 22 percent. The authors concluded that immunoassay methods can be used in hospital laboratories for determination of alcohol concentrations in trauma patients.[38]

In my experience, false positive alcohol measured by an enzyme assay in an individual with high lactate and LDH is only expected in severely ill patients and should not be a concern in terms of being wrongly accused of DWI. Powers and Dean (2009) described a case where a driver, a thirty-three-year-old man, was involved in a single motor vehicle collision (hitting a tree). He was transferred to a local hospital emergency room where blood was drawn for various tests, including blood alcohol. The serum alcohol level was 200 mg/dL (0.2 percent), which was more than twice the legal limit, indicating that the driver was intoxicated during the accident. Blood tests also revealed that the patient experienced a certain degree of trauma following the accident because his liver enzymes were elevated due to some liver damage. Amylase and lipase levels were also elevated. During criminal prosecution of DWI, hospital alcohol results were admitted as evidence by the court. Although lactate and LDH were not measured in this patient, based on other blood tests, it was estimated

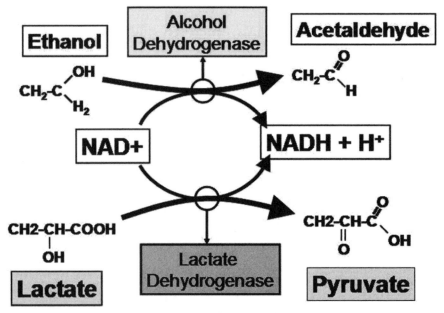

Figure 6.2. Chemical transformation (oxidation) of lactate to pyruvate and ethanol (alcohol) to acetaldehyde and generation of NADH from NAD. In the absence of alcohol, lactate can be transformed to pyruvate by lactate dehydrogenase (LDH), and in this process excess NAD can be converted into NADH thus providing a false alcohol measurement. However, both lactate and pyruvate must be present in very high amounts to cause this interference. Reprinted with permission from *The Journal of Analytical Toxicology* (Preston).

that both lactate and LDH were not elevated sufficiently to interfere with the enzymatic alcohol determination in this case. Both lactate and LDH must be present in very high amounts to cause this interference, and lactate alone cannot cause this interference. Lactate must be converted into pyruvate catalyzed by lactate dehydrogenase enzyme in order for NAD to be transformed to NADH. The mechanism of this interference is explained in figure 6.2.[39]

FORENSIC VERSUS MEDICAL ALCOHOL

Forensic or "legal" blood refers to the sample of blood the police obtain pursuant to their investigation of DWI. When blood is drawn for determination of forensic alcohol, a chain of custody is maintained where there is always a written record of all personnel who had possession of the sample until the time of analysis. The name of the analyst is also recorded in the chain of custody. Because of this chain of custody, integrity of the specimen is guaranteed, and there is no possibility of misidentification of the specimen. Moreover, most forensic toxicology laboratories determine whole blood alcohol using a specific and sensitive gas chromatographic technique. Therefore, a forensic alcohol level over the legal limit is difficult to challenge in a court of law unless a loophole can be discovered in the chain of custody process during the trial.

Medical blood refers to a blood sample that was either voluntarily given or involuntarily taken by medical personnel in the course of providing medical treatment to the patient. For an injured DWI suspect who is transferred to an emergency room of a local hospital, and who is incapable of providing a breath sample, a blood sample given for medical treatment purposes may be subpoenaed or obtained pursuant to a search warrant and used against him or her in his or her criminal DWI trial with the approval of the judge. The legal standard of causation is usually the same when requesting medical blood as it is for forensic blood alcohol level, but a medical alcohol may be challenged in court if a chain of custody is not maintained and alcohol analysis is conducted by an enzymatic method rather than a chromatographic technique. However, maintaining a chain of custody may be practiced in a hospital if a police officer brings in a suspect injured in a drunk-driving accident. Modern enzymatic alcohol assays are very robust and correlate well with the gas chromatographic methods, the gold standard for alcohol determination.

Both forensic and medical alcohol determination is subject to a precision issue. Precision means percent variation expected if alcohol level is measured by the same method multiple times. For example, one determination of alcohol may be 80 mg/dL and analysis of the same specimen by the same instrument could be 78 mg/dL or 82 mg/dL. Most gas chromatographic methods and enzymatic alcohol determination methods have variability less than 5 percent, but depending on an individual case, a maximum allowance of 10 percent may be granted. For example, if the whole blood alcohol level is 84 mg/dL, a defense lawyer could argue that the true value may be between 76 and 92 mg/dL, and if the level was determined by another person, it could well be below 80 mg/dL, the legal limit.

However, if an alcohol value is measured twice (as we do in our hospital for any emergency room patients involved in a motor vehicle crash) and both values are over the legal limit, the defendant may be out of luck. Therefore, both medical and legal alcohol value can be challenged in a court if the value is just above 80 mg/dL limit for whole blood or 90 mg/dL for serum or plasma. Higher blood alcohol values are difficult to challenge. In a report by Chang et al. (2001) the conviction rate of trauma patients involved in motor vehicle crashes was high based on alcohol levels determined in the author's hospital. Of 213 intoxicated drivers studied, 172 were followed up by law enforcement personnel, and 156 were arrested and charged with DWI. Out of 156 individuals arrested, 135 individuals (93.8 percent) were convicted for DWI.[40]

EXTRAPOLATION OF ALCOHOL VALUE AT COURT

Reliable information about the elimination rate of alcohol from the body is often needed in forensic science and legal medicine when alcohol-related crimes, such as alcohol-impaired driving or alcohol-related crimes, are being investigated. The courts usually want to know the defendant's blood alcohol level at the time of the accident based on a blood alcohol level determined several hours later. After drinking on an empty stomach, the elimination rate of alcohol from the human body falls within the range of 10–15 mg/dL per hour. In other words, blood alcohol level declines 0.010 to 0.015 percent per hour. If alcohol is consumed with food, elimination rate tends to be 15–20 mg/dL per hour (0.015 to 0.02 percent per hour).

In general, women tend to eliminate alcohol slower than do men. In moderate drinkers the elimination rate of 15 mg/dL per hour (0.015 percent per hour) is used by many expert witnesses to extrapolate blood alcohol level during testimony. Alcoholics may eliminate alcohol faster than moderate drinkers.[41] Therefore, a defendant's blood alcohol may be 75 mg/dL (0.075 percent) two hours after an accident, which is below the legal limit, but prosecution may argue in court that two hours prior to the time of the accident the blood alcohol level was 75 + 2 × 15 = 105 mg/dL, a value above the legal limit of driving.

Therefore, the best policy is to not drink and drive, and if drinking, exercise caution. In chapter 2, I provided detailed information on how blood alcohol levels are related to a number of drinks based on body weight and gender. Always try to limit your drinking to one drink per hour, and do not consume more than two standard drinks in two hours if you are a man with no genetic defect for alcohol metabolism and weigh at least 140 pounds or more. For a woman who weighs 120 pounds or more, consuming one drink in a two-hour period prior to driving is safe, and the blood alcohol level would be significantly below the legal limit of driving. Always consume alcohol with food and be careful when you order a margarita or a specially prepared drink, because one drink may be equivalent to two or three standard drinks as far as alcohol content is concerned (see chapter 2).

CONCLUSION

As emphasized in this chapter, drinking and driving do not mix well. If you plan to drink on a night out, find a designated driver or hire a cab for your ride home. If you drink, drink in moderation. Information provided in this chapter should make you familiar with current laws and blood alcohol determinations. Law enforcement agencies, prosecutors, and expert witnesses exercise extreme care to ensure that an innocent person is not charged with a DWI. My experience is that doubts are always given in favor of defendants in borderline cases. However, despite tough enforcement of DWI laws in all states, fatalities from motor vehicle crashes due to alcohol-impaired drivers claim many lives each year and are major public safety concerns. Do not drink and drive so that you can enjoy a happy and prosperous life.

NOTES

1. N. T. Flowers, T. S. Naimi, R. D. Brewer, R. W. Elder, et al., "Patterns of Alcohol Consumption and Alcohol-Impaired Driving in the United States," *Alcoholism: Clinical and Experimental Research* 32, no. 4 (April 2008): 639–44.

2. T. H. Nochajski and P. R. Stasiewicz, "Relapse to Driving under the Influence (DUI): A Review," *Clinical Psychology Review* 26, no. 2 (March 2006): 179–95.

3. "Ignition Interlocks: What You Need to Know," Department of Transportation (U.S.), National Highway Traffic Safety Administration (NHTSA), National Highway Traffic Safety Administration Report, November 2009, www.nhtsa. gov/staticfiles/nti/impaired_driving/pdf/811246.pdf.

4. "Traffic Safety Facts 2008: Alcohol-Impaired Driving," Department of Transportation (U.S.), National Highway Traffic Safety Administration (NHTSA), Washington, D.C., 2009. Available at http://www-nrd.nhtsa.dot.gov/Pubs/811155. PDF.

5. K. P. Quinlan, R. D. Brewer, P. Siegal, D. A. Sleet, et al., "Alcohol-Impaired Driving among U.S. Adults, 1993–2002," *American Journal of Preventive Medicine* 28, no. 4 (May 2005): 346–50.

6. "Traffic Safety Facts: Fatalities Related to Alcohol-Impaired Driving during the Christmas and New Year's Day Holiday Periods," NHTSA Report Number DOT HS 810 870, December 2007, available on the NHTSA website, http://www. nhtsa.gov.

7. J. C. Fell, A. S. Toppetts, and R. B. Voas, "Fatal Traffic Crashes Involving Drinking Drivers: What Have We Learned?" *Annual Proceedings of the Association for Advancement of Automobile Research* 53 (2009): 63–76.

8. T. S. Naimi, D. E. Nelson, and R. D. Brewer, "Driving after Binge Drinking," *American Journal of Preventive Medicine* 37, no. 4 (October 2009): 314–20.

9. M. F. Lovenheim and J. Slemrod, "The Fatal Toll of Driving to Drink: The Effect of Minimum Legal Drinking Age Evasion on Traffic Fatalities," *Journal of Health Economics* 29, 1 (January 2010): 62–77.

10. R. C. Peck, M. A. Gebers, R. B. Voas, and E. Romano, "The Relationship between Blood Alcohol Concentration (BAC), Age and Crash Risk," *Journal of Safety Research* 39, no. 3 (March 2008): 311–19.

11. B. J. Leadbeater, K. Foran, and A. Grove-White, "How Much Can You Drink Before Driving? The Influence of Riding with Impaired Adults and Peers on the Driving Behaviors of Urban and Rural Youth," *Addiction* 103, no. 4 (April 2008): 629–37.

12. A. K. Dills, "Social Host Liability for Minors and Underage Drunk-Driving Accidents," *Journal of Health Economics*, January 15, 2010 (e-publication before print).

13. S. M. Rosen, T. R. Miller, and M. Simon, "The Cost of Alcohol in California," *Alcohol Clinical and Experimental Research* 32, no. 11 (November 2008): 1925–36.

14. T. O'Keefe, S. Shafi, J. L. Sperry, and L. M. Gentiello, "The Implications of Alcohol Intoxication and the Uniform Policy Provision Law on Trauma Centers: A National Trauma Data Bank Analysis of Minimally Injured Patients," *Journal of Trauma* 66, no. 2 (February 2009): 495–98.

15. J. C. Fell and R. B. Voas, "Mothers Against Drunk Driving (MADD): The First 25 Years," *Traffic Injury Prevention* 7, no. 3 (September 2006): 195–212.

16. J. C. Fell and R. B. Voas, "The Effectiveness of Reducing Illegal Blood Alcohol Concentration (BAC) Limits for Driving: Evidence for Lowering the Limit to 0.05 BAC," *Journal of Safety Research* 37, no. 3 (March 2006): 233–43.

17. A. W. Jones, "Distribution of Ethanol between Saliva and Blood in Man," *Clinical and Experimental Pharmacology and Physiology* 6, no. 1 (January–February 1979): 53–59.

18. M. P. Hlastala, "The Alcohol Breath Test: A Review," *Journal of Applied Physiology* 84, no. 2 (February 1998): 401–8.

19. M. Hlastala, "Paradigm Shift for the Alcohol Breath Test," *Journal of Forensic Sciences* 55, no. 2 (March 2010): 451–56.

20. DataMaster Operator Information Manual Review, October 2000, Washington State Patrol, http://www.breathtest.wsp.wa.gov.

21. G. Razatos, R. Luthi, and S. Kerrigan, "Evaluation of a Portable Evidentiary Breath Alcohol Analyzer," *Forensic Sciences International* 153, no. 1 (October 2005): 17–21.

22. P. M. Hardings, R. H. Laessing, and P. H. Field, "Field Performance of the Intoxilyzer 5000: A Comparison of Blood and Breath Alcohol Results in Wisconsin Drivers," *Journal of Forensic Sciences* 35, no. 5 (September 1990): 1022–28.

23. S. Kechagias, K. A. Jonsson, T. Franzen, L. Anderson, et al., "Reliability of Breath Alcohol Analysis in Individuals with Gastroesophageal Reflux Disease," *Journal of Forensic Sciences* 44, no. 4 (July 1999): 814–18.

24. A. W. Jones and L. Anderson, "Comparison of Ethanol Concentrations in Venous Blood and End-Expired Breath during a Controlled Drinking Study," *Forensic Sciences International* 132, no. 1 (March 2003): 18–25.

25. C. C. Fessler, F. A. Tulleners, D. G. Howitt, and J. R. Richards, "Determination of Mouth Alcohol Using the Dräger Evidential Portable Alcohol System," *Science and Justice: Journal of the Forensic Science Society* 48, no. 1 (March 2008): 16–23.

26. B. Lutmer, C. Zurfluh, and C. Long, "Potential Effect of Alcohol Content in Energy Drinks on Breath Alcohol Testing," *Journal of Analytical Toxicology* 33, no. 3 (April 2009): 167–69.

27. O. Laakso, T. Pennanen, K. Himberg, T. Kuitunen, et al., "Effect of Eight Solvents on Ethanol Analysis by Dräger 7110 Evidentiary Breath Analyzer," *Journal of Forensic Sciences* 49, no. 5 (September 2004): 1113–16.

28. A. W. Jones and S. Rossner, "False Positive Breath Alcohol Test after a Ketogenic Diet," *International Journal of Obesity* (London) 31, no. 3 (March 2007): 559–61.

29. E. M. Caravati and K. T. Anderson, "Breath Alcohol Analyzer Mistakes Methanol Poisoning for Alcohol Intoxication," *Annals of Emergency Medicine* 55, no. 2 (February 2010): 198–200.

30. J. P. Caldwell and N. D. Kim, "The Response of the Intoxilyzer 5000 to Five Potential Interfering Substances," *Journal of Forensic Sciences* 42, no. 6 (November 1997): 1080–87.

31. C. L. Winek and M. Carfagna, "Comparison of Plasma, Serum, and Whole Blood Ethanol Concentration," *Journal of Analytical Toxicology* 11, no. 6 (November 1987): 267–68.

32. M. T. Barnhill Jr., D. Herbert, and D. J. Wells Jr., "Comparison of Hospital Laboratory Serum Alcohol Levels Obtained by an Enzymatic Method with Whole Blood Levels Forensically Determined by Gas Chromatography," *Journal of Analytical Toxicology* 31, no. 1 (January–February 2007): 23–30.

33. P. Rainey, "Relation between Serum and Whole Blood Ethanol Concentrations," *Clinical Chemistry* 39, no. 11 (November 1993): 2288–92.

34. N. B. Smith, "Determination of Volatile Alcohols and Acetone in Serum by Non-polar Capillary Gas Chromatography after Direct Sample Injection," *Clinical Chemistry* 30, no. 10 (October 1984): 1672–74.

35. W. T. Thompson, D. Malhotra, D. P. Schammel, W. Blackwell, et al., "False Positive Ethanol in Clinical and Postmortem Sera by Enzymatic Assay: Elimination of Interference by Measuring Alcohol in Protein-Free Ultrafiltrate," *Clinical Chemistry* 40, no. 8 (August 1994): 1594–95.

36. J. Nine, M. Moraca, A. Virji, and K. Rao, "Serum Ethanol Determination: Comparison of Lactate and Lactate Dehydrogenase Interference in Three Enzymatic Assays," *Journal of Analytical Toxicology* 19, no. 3 (May–June 1995): 192–96.

37. J. R. Dunne, J. K. Tracy, T. M. Scalea, and L. Napolitano, "Lactate and Base Deficit in Trauma: Does Alcohol or Drug Use Impair Predictive Accuracy?" *Journal of Trauma* 58, no. 5 (May 2005): 959–66.

38. C. L. Winek, W. W. Wahba, R. Windisch, and C. L. Winek, "Serum Alcohol Concentrations in Trauma Patients Determined by Immunoassays Versus Gas Chromatography," *Forensic Sciences International* 139, no. 1 (January 2004): 1–3.

39. R. H. Powers and D. E. Dean, "Evaluation of Potential Lactate/Lactate Dehydrogenase Interference with an Enzymatic Alcohol Analysis," *Journal of Analytical Toxicology* 33, no. 5 (October 2009): 561–63.

40. S. Chang, J. G. Cushman, and M. D. Pasquale, "The Injured Intoxicated Driver: Analysis of the Conviction Process," *Journal of Trauma* 51, no. 3 (September 2001): 551–56.

41. A. W. Jones, "Evidence-Based Survey of the Elimination Rates of Ethanol from Blood with Applications in Forensic Cases," *Forensic Sciences International* 200, nos. 1–3 (July 2010): 1–20.

7

Biomarkers of Alcohol Abuse

One of the consequences of moderate ethanol ingestion is a reduced risk of cardiovascular events (heart disease) with the consumption of alcoholic products that contain specific flavonoids. This was first observed in conjunction with mild to moderate wine consumption, hence the term "French Paradox."[1] In order to get the health benefits of alcohol, one must practice moderate drinking. Although many alcoholics often have remarkably "clean" arteries at autopsy, chronic excessive ethanol ingestion leads to hyperlipidemia (high lipids or fats in the blood), and such fats tend to deposit in the liver, causing fatty livers and eventually cirrhosis of the liver, which can be fatal. Negative effects of heavy alcohol consumption include liver cirrhosis, esophageal cancer, pancreatitis, and epilepsy. Alcohol also plays a role in traffic accidents, violent crimes, sexual assaults, domestic violence, and child abuse.

It is estimated that about 5 percent of the general population drinks heavily and about 10 percent of the general population has alcohol-related medical problems. From 2001 to 2005, there were approximately 79,000 deaths per year attributed to excessive alcohol use. In fact, alcohol abuse is the third lifestyle-related cause of death in the United States each year.[2] The consumer expenditure on alcohol in the United States in 1999 was roughly $116.2 billion, and $22.5 billion was attributed to underage drinking. It has also been estimated that roughly 50 percent of underage people (twelve to twenty years old) drink alcohol and approximately 30.4 percent of adults in the United States drink more than two drinks a day, which is considered excessive alcohol consumption.[3] Heavy alcohol consumption causes serious public health issues that not only affect individuals and their families but society as a whole. Prevention of alcohol abuse is an important concern from both a medical and social point of view. The biomarkers of alcohol abuse are the latest techniques available to health care professionals to identify alcohol abusers and also to monitor individuals undergoing alcohol rehabilitation.

THE BIOMARKERS OF ALCOHOL ABUSE

A biological molecule found in blood, tissue, or body fluids that is a sign of an abnormal process or condition can be broadly termed a "biomarker." These markers can be used for diagnosis of a condition or a disease. Alternatively, biomarkers can also be used to measure the success of a particular therapy. Biomarkers are also called "molecular markers" or "signature molecules." In general, in the absence of a disease or a condition, concentration of a biomarker is very low, but when a condition develops further, the concentration may be increased significantly, thus indicating an abnormal condition or disease. For example, normal concentration of prostate specific antigen (PSA) in blood is less than 4 nanogram/milliliter (4 ng/mL), but in the event of prostate cancer, this value increases significantly over 4 ng/mL. In one report (Anai et al. 2007), the authors concluded that a PSA value higher than 30 ng/mL is an almost certain predictor of the presence of prostate cancer.[4]

Alcohol can usually be detected in blood several hours to less than a day after consumption of the last drink. Alcohol is metabolized by the liver, and alcohol concentration in blood is reduced by approximately 0.015 percent (15 mg/dL) per hour. For example, if a blood alcohol level is 0.08 percent (80 mg/dL, the legal limit of driving), 0.08 divided by 0.015 hours or 5.3 hours would be needed for the blood alcohol level to become zero. If more alcohol is consumed, then more time is needed for blood alcohol to return to the zero value (table 7.1).

Table 7.1. Number of Hours Needed for Blood Alcohol Concentration (BAC) to Become Zero

Percentage of Blood Alcohol Concentration (BAC)	Time Needed to Reach Zero Blood Alcohol Concentration (BAC)
0.2 (200 mg/dL)	13.3 hours
0.15 (150 mg/dL)	10 hours
0.12 (120 mg/dL)	8 hours
0.1 (100 mg/dL)	6.6 hours
0.08 (80 mg/dL)	5.3 hours
0.05 (50 mg/dL)	3.3 hours
0.03 (30 mg/dL)	2 hours

The determination of blood alcohol is not a good way to screen people who are at higher risk of alcohol abuse. In one report (Alkan et al. 2001), the authors described a case where a drunken person had fallen from the window of his girlfriend's apartment and died. This person's parents appealed to the public prosecutor that their child did not fall down but was murdered by his girlfriend. During the trial, the victim's autopsy revealed no blood alcohol—in contrast to his girlfriend's statement—and there was a reasonable doubt that the girlfriend was the murderer. However, later in the trial, the reason for detection of no alcohol in the autopsy was revealed, indicating that blood alcohol detection has many limitations in criminal cases.[5] Blood alcohol level cannot discriminate between acute and long-term alcohol consumption and risky behavior. The detection time frame of blood alcohol is very limited (from a few hours to twelve hours in most cases) and cannot detect a hangover stage.

Biomarkers for alcohol use have many advantages over the determination of blood alcohol level. First, biomarkers can stay elevated for a considerably longer period of time than blood alcohol. Although biomarkers are often used as screens for diagnosis of alcohol abuse or dependence, strictly speaking, alcohol biomarkers are reflections of the physiological response of the body to heavy alcohol consumption and have diagnostic value. Biomarkers can be broadly classified into two categories: slate markers and trait markers. Slate markers are valuable in addressing questions, such as evidence of recent alcohol intake versus chronic alcohol consumption, alcohol abuse versus moderate drinking, and whether there is any evidence of organ damage related to drinking. Trait markers can address broad questions, such as whether an individual has a genetic makeup that may make that individual more susceptible to alcohol abuse or alcoholic liver disease. In clinical practice physicians more often order tests that measure slate markers of alcohol, and in this chapter only slate markers of alcohol will be discussed. Many trait markers of alcohol abuse are in developmental and extensive research stages and not commonly measured in hospital laboratories. The slate markers of alcohol include:

Liver enzymes
Mean corpuscular volume (MCV)
Carbohydrate-deficient transferrin
Serum and urine hexosaminidase
Sialic acid
Acetaldehyde-protein adducts
Ethyl glucuronide and ethyl sulfate
Fatty acid ethyl ester

CLINICAL APPLICATION OF ALCOHOL BIOMARKERS

Alcohol biomarkers are primarily used for screening patients for possible alcohol abuse, mainly in primary care facilities. In addition, alcohol biomarkers are also useful in identifying pregnant women who may be abusing alcohol, because fetal alcohol syndrome is a totally preventable disorder. Alcohol biomarkers are also used in emergency room settings, psychiatric clinics, and internal medicine settings, because self-reporting of alcohol use is not always accurate, as some patients are reluctant to admit a problem with alcohol. The addition of biomarkers may help identify individuals who need treatment for alcohol abuse. The major clinical utilities of using biomarkers of alcohol use include

1. Identifying patients needing intervention for alcohol abuse
2. Physiological response to alcohol abuse and whether a medical problem exists related to heavy alcohol consumption
3. Monitoring patients undergoing alcohol rehabilitation and identifying any relapse of alcohol use
4. Outcome measures in studies evaluating new medication or behavior modification for intervening in alcohol abuse problems
5. Guiding patients in a positive manner to change their lifestyles and drinking habits
6. Documenting abstinence

Monitoring alcohol biomarkers is very helpful in motivating patients to change their habit of consuming alcohol. Giving feedback on elevations of biomarkers and reviewing their decline levels with the patient provides objective evidence of the patient's treatment success, personal needs, and the benefits of reducing alcohol consumption. Relapse is unfortunately common in alcohol detoxification programs, and identifying such relapse in a patient at an early stage using biomarkers is clinically very useful. In addition, alcohol biomarkers are very useful in documenting abstinence in these special populations: individuals younger than twenty-one, especially in the military; adolescents on probation for alcohol use or possession; individuals with previous alcohol-related problems who have custody of their children with the stipulation that they must practice abstinence; motorists with DWI convictions who must document abstinence in order to get their driving privilege back; medical professionals; pilots; and others who need to document abstinence from drinking due to previous alcohol-related problems and any other individuals where required by the law or company policy.

SCREENING ALCOHOL-RELATED HEALTH PROBLEMS IN PRIMARY CARE SETTINGS

Primary health care settings are ideal for screening patients for alcohol-related health problems because a majority of the population visits primary care physicians for routine annual checkups or seeks treatment for chronic conditions at least on a yearly basis. In addition, advice by the primary care physician regarding behavior modification in order not to consume excessive alcohol is usually well received by patients. The National Institute on Alcohol Abuse and Alcoholism recommends that all adult primary care patients be screened for alcohol use, because valid and reliable screening tools are available. Despite these guidelines, only 55–65 percent of physicians routinely ask their patients about alcohol use and only 35 percent screen patients during their annual visit. Together with self-reporting, alcohol screening tools, and using biomarkers of alcohol abuse, a reliable and accurate estimation of alcohol consumption by a patient can be reached, and intervention can be done by the primary care physician if needed. Unfortunately, there has been little translation of alcohol biomarker research into practical guidelines for primary care physicians. Many primary care physicians say that they will use alcohol biomarkers more often in their clinical practice if practical guidelines are readily available, and if they have additional knowledge regarding clinical use of such biomarkers.[6]

APPLICATION OF ALCOHOL BIOMARKERS IN OTHER MEDICAL AND SURGICAL SETTINGS

The utilization of alcohol biomarkers as disease risk indicators in specialty medical and surgical settings has many advantages and is a welcome trend, because heavy alcohol consumption may cause or aggravate many medical conditions, including hypertension, stroke, heart disease, liver disease, pancreatitis, and various types of cancer. Heavy alcohol consumption also significantly contributes to complications in trauma and surgical patients. Approximately one-fifth of patients seen in clinical practice have some alcohol use disorders, ranging from hazardous alcohol consumption to alcohol dependence. Early intervention for alcohol-related disorders is highly desirable because a variety of effective therapeutic options exist to treat such disorders, including behavior modification, prophylactic stress management, and therapy for alcohol-related complications and detoxification.

Between 16 and 39 percent of trauma victims have positive blood alcohol concentrations, but 11–45 percent of trauma patients may suffer from alcohol-related disorders, even though they have negative blood alcohol on admission. Therefore, blood alcohol determination is a poor measure of establishing whether a trauma patient is also suffering from alcohol-related disorders or not, and under such circumstances, an alcohol biomarker, such as carbohydrate-deficient transferrin, is very useful in detecting alcohol-related disorders in trauma patients.

Hypertension is the leading cause of stroke and heart disease, and heavy drinking (more than three drinks a day) increases blood pressure in both normal and hypertensive patients. In addition, excessive drinking is associated with uncontrolled treatment-resistant hypertension. There is a correlation between serum gamma-glutamyl transferase and carbohydrate-deficient transferrin, and these alcohol biomarkers can be successfully employed to diagnose patients with alcohol-related disorders who are also suffering from uncontrolled hypertension. A considerable amount of research indicates that alcohol screening and brief intervention can improve clinical outcome in patients and is also very effective in reducing medical costs.[7]

INDIRECT VERSUS DIRECT SLATE BIOMARKERS OF ALCOHOL

Traditional slate biomarkers of alcohol use are indirect biomarkers, which are elevated in a person consuming moderate to heavy amounts of alcohol. These biomarkers are elevated due to the toxicity of alcohol on a particular organ. For example, liver enzymes, such as gamma-glutamyl transferase (GGT), alanine aminotransferase (ALT), and aspartate aminotransferase (AST), are elevated after heavy alcohol consumption because alcohol has toxic effects on the liver. Mean corpuscular volume (MCV) as well as the first FDA-approved biomarker of alcohol abuse, carbohydrate-deficient transferrin, are also indirect markers. Serum and urine hexosaminidase and sialic acid are also indirect biomarkers of alcohol abuse. Alcohol metabolites such as ethyl glucuronide, ethyl sulfate, or biomolecules derived from the interaction of alcohol with other molecules, such as fatty acid ethyl ester and phosphatidyl ethanol, are direct biomarkers of alcohol consumption (table 7.2).

Liver Enzymes as Alcohol Biomarkers

Liver enzymes are elevated in individuals consuming excessive amounts of alcohol because alcohol has a direct toxic effect on the liver. Alanine transaminase (ALT) and aspartate transaminase (AST) are found inside liver cells (hepatocytes), and small amounts of these enzyme activities are detected in the serum of healthy individuals. However, in the case of liver injury, these

Table 7.2. Various Markers for Alcohol Abuse

Marker	Type of Slate Marker	Comment
Gamma-glutamyltransferase (GGT)	Indirect	Associated with heavy drinking; value returns to normal 2–6 weeks after abstinence. Not a specific marker and may be elevated in some diseases.
Alanine amino transferase (ALT)/ Aspartate amino transferase (AST)	Indirect	Also elevated in alcoholics but less sensitive than GGT. Not a specific marker and may be elevated in some diseases.
Mean corpuscular volume (MCV)	Indirect	Associated with heavy drinking but not a specific marker and may be elevated in certain types of anemia.
Carbohydrate-deficient transferrin	Indirect	More specific marker than MCV and liver enzymes (GGT, ALT, and AST) but more difficult to measure in blood. Value returns to normal 2–4 weeks after abstinence.
Serum and urine hexosaminidase	Indirect	Specific marker for heavy alcohol use (60 gm or more per day). Value returns to normal 7–10 days after abstinence. This is a complex test not readily available in small hospital laboratories.
Sialic acid	Indirect	Specific marker for heavy alcohol use, but it is a specialized test not readily available to small hospital laboratories. Value returns to normal after 7–10 days of abstinence.
Acetaldehyde-protein adducts	Direct	Distinguishes heavy drinkers from social drinkers and nondrinkers but amounts found in blood or urine are very small and difficult to measure.
Ethyl glucuronide and ethyl sulfate	Direct	Specific markers for alcohol abuse and can differentiate between heavy drinkers and social drinkers. Can be measured in blood or hair, but method of determination is complex.
Fatty acid ethyl ester	Direct	Specific markers for alcohol abuse and can differentiate between heavy drinkers and social drinkers. Can be measured in blood or hair, but method of determination is complex.

enzymes can be increased three- to tenfold from their normal expected values (ALT: 10–40 units/L, ALT: 5–40 units/L). Alkaline phosphatase (ALP), another enzyme found in the cell lining of the biliary ducts of liver, is also elevated during liver injury but may not be significantly elevated after heavy alcohol consumption. Gamma-glutamyl transferase (GGT) is also another marker of liver injury, and this enzyme is also elevated in people drinking alcohol.

Out of all liver enzymes, GGT is considered the most sensitive biomarker for alcohol consumption. GGT levels are elevated following heavy alcohol consumption, and with complete abstinence the level returns to normal within two to six weeks. GGT is elevated in response to alcohol consumption due to accelerated release from damaged liver cells. GGT levels are also high in patients suffering from severe alcoholic liver disease. However, GGT is elevated in individuals who consume high amounts of alcohol on a regular basis rather than individuals who consume high amounts of alcohol sporadically.

GGT may also be somewhat elevated in moderate drinkers compared to nondrinkers. In one report (Alatalo et al. 2009), the authors studied GGT along with ALT, AST, ferritin (a protein that binds iron), and albumin (major protein found in human blood) levels in 133 heavy drinkers (mean alcohol consumption 110 gm per day; approximately eight drinks per day as each standard drink contains 14 gm of alcohol), 1,504 moderate drinkers (less than 40 gm of alcohol per day or approximately three drinks or less a day), and 685 nondrinkers (abstainers). The heavy drinkers in this study were admitted for alcohol detoxification. The authors reported that GGT had the highest incidence of elevated levels in heavy drinkers compared to moderate drinkers and abstainers, followed by AST and ALT, where albumin was elevated in approximately 20 percent of heavy drinkers only.

Interestingly, significant differences between GGT and ALT levels were also observed between moderate drinkers and abstainers in the male population, but no such difference was observed in females. For example, average GGT levels in male heavy drinkers was 193 units per liter compared to 34 units per liter in moderate drinkers and 26 units per liter in abstainers. Similarly, the average AST value in heavy male drinkers was 65 units per liter compared to 26 units per liter in moderate drinkers and 25 units per liter in abstainers. Mean ALT value in heavy drinkers was 71 units per liter compared to 29 units per liter in moderate drinkers and 26 units per liter in abstainers.[8] This publication also demonstrates that GGT is a more sensitive marker than other liver enzymes (AST and ALT) for heavy alcohol consumption.

One limitation of GGT as a biomarker of alcohol is that it may also be elevated in a person taking a barbiturate, in nonalcoholic liver diseases, cardiovascular disease, individuals with high lipids, and obese individuals. Several epidemiological studies have indicated that there is an association between elevated GGT values and increased risk for cardiovascular disease, type 2 diabetes (diabetes that can be controlled without taking insulin shots), chronic kidney disease, and cancer, and these elevations in GGT levels are not associated with alcohol consumption.[9]

Mean Corpuscular Volume (MCV) as a Biomarker for Alcohol

Alcohol and its metabolites (breakdown products of alcohol produced by liver enzymes) have toxic effects on human red blood cells (erythrocytes). During a blood test, mean corpuscular volume or mean cell volume of erythrocytes (MCV) is calculated from the hematocrit (ratio of the volume of red cells to the volume of whole blood) and red cell counts. The normal range of MCV is 86–98 femtoliter (fl). A femtoliter is one quadrillionth of a liter (10^{-15} liter), an extremely small volume indicating the volume of an average erythrocyte. Excessive alcohol consumption is known to increase MCV, a pathogenic process known as macrocytosis (enlarged erythrocytes). If both GGT and MCV are elevated, it is likely that regular heavy alcohol consumption is the cause, because an erythrocyte remains in circulation 120 days on average; it takes MCV about three months to return to a normal level after abstinence.

Koivisto et al. (2006) studied MCV and other parameters in 105 alcoholics with a wide range of alcohol consumption (40 gm to 500 gm of ethanol per day or three to forty drinks per day), 62 moderate drinkers (less than 40 gm a day or three or less drinks a day), and 24 abstainers, and reported that the upper limit of MCV in moderate drinkers was 98 fl (range 82–98 fl), while the upper limit of abstainers was 96 fl (range 82–96). In contrast, in heavy consumers of alcohol, MCV can be as high as 104 fl. The increase in MCV due to alcohol consumption is due to the penetration of alcohol into erythrocytes, with this altering the erythrocyte membrane and affecting its stability. In addition, high concentration of acetaldehyde, the first metabolite of alcohol, is also detected in high amounts in erythrocytes of alcoholics. Acetaldehyde can increase erythrocyte volume by forming adducts with various components on the cell membrane, including proteins.[10]

Carbohydrate-Deficient Transferrin as an Alcohol Biomarker

Transferrin is a protein that is responsible for transporting iron in the blood from the intestine to bone marrow, so that iron can be incorporated into hemoglobin during the formation of red blood cells, also known as erythrocytes. Transferrin consists of 679 amino acids and is also a glycoprotein, meaning that the carbohydrate is an integral part of the transferrin structure, representing approximately 6 percent of the transferrin molecule. Carbohydrate is an organic compound that consists of carbon, hydrogen, and oxygen, and can be expressed as $C_m(H_2O)_n$, and glucose is a simple carbohydrate, expressed as $C_6H_{12}O_6$. Another common name for carbohydrate is saccharide. Glucose is a monosaccharide (a simple sugar that cannot be broken down further), while sucrose, or common cane sugar (table sugar), is a disaccharide (contains two monosaccharide molecules and can be broken down into two simple sugar molecules: glucose and fructose). Starch is a polysaccharide. Sialic acid, an integral component of transferrin, is a monosaccharide. So in a broader sense, sialic acid can also be termed as a carbohydrate.

Transferrin is found in blood in several different molecular forms called isoforms. These molecular forms differ in the number of their carbohydrate groups (sialic acid and other carbohydrate residues) and carry different electrical charges. The major form of transferrin is tetrasialotransferrin, which has four sialic acid moieties attached to the molecule and represents approximately 80 percent of all transferrin molecules in a healthy individual. Other transferrin molecules found in blood may have more (5–8 sialic acid moieties) or less (0–3 sialic acid moieties) carbohydrate.

Acetaldehyde formed from alcohol by the liver enzyme aldehyde dehydrogenase is known to interfere with the incorporation of sialic acid moiety to transferrin, resulting in the formation of transferrin molecules with zero, one, or two sialic acid moieties attached to the final molecules. In addition, these isoforms of transferrin may also have reduced carbohydrate residue. Chronic excess alcohol consumption (approximately 60 gm or more alcohol per day or five or more drinks per day) for one to two weeks causes an increase in transferrin molecules in blood with only two sialic acid moieties (disialotransferrin) attached to the final molecule with an accompanying lesser increase in the concentration of monosialotransferrin (one sialic acid) or asialotransferrin (no sialic acid). Because sialic acid is a carbohydrate and usually four sialic acid moieties or more are found in transferrin, collectively disialotransferrin, monosialotransferrin, and asialotransferrin are called carbohydrate-deficient transferrin.

Trisialotransferrin (three sialic acid moieties) is generally thought not to increase in response to heavy alcohol consumption. In the clinical laboratory, various forms of transferrin can be measured by separating them based on their electrical charges, using a complex technique known as capillary zone electrophoresis. Carbohydrate-deficient transferrin can also be measured in a clinical laboratory by other complex analytical techniques, such as high-performance liquid chromatography and N-Latex Direct carbohydrate-deficient transferrin immunoassay. The first developed assays for measuring carbohydrate-deficient transferrin were based on ion exchange chromatography to separate disialotransferrin, and carbohydrate-deficient transferrin value was expressed as units/liter.

Later other assays were developed, and currently carbohydrate-deficient transferrin in blood is reported as the percentage of total transferrin in blood. For example, in the automated immunoassay for transferrin (N-Latex Direct carbohydrate-deficient transferrin immunoassay), a specific monoclonal antibody that recognizes disialotransferrin, monosialotransferrin, and asialotransferrin is used in combination with a simultaneous assay for total transferrin, and the values are expressed as the percentage of carbohydrate-deficient transferrin.[11] Usually in heavy users of alcohol, the value of carbohydrate-deficient transferrin is above 2 percent of total transferrin.[12] In another report (Sorvajärvi et al. 1996), the authors stated that in alcohol abusers (consuming more than 80 gm of alcohol per day), the mean concentration of carbohydrate-deficient transferrin is 29.2 units/liter compared to the mean value of 19.0 units/liter observed in controls. In addition, the mean percentage of carbohydrate-deficient transferrin was 2.2 percent in alcohol abusers compared to 0.1 percent in controls (nondrinkers and social drinkers).[13] The advantage of knowing the percentage of carbohydrate-deficient transferrin is that it automatically corrects any fluctuations in transferrin levels not related to alcohol abuse.

It is generally assumed that at least 60 gm of alcohol per day for a man and at least 40 gm of alcohol per day for a woman for at least a week is needed for carbohydrate-deficient transferrin percentage in blood to rise above the cutoff reference value. Individuals who consume more alcohol than the level stated here (this is equivalent to heavy alcohol consumption) may have alcohol dependence (alcoholics), and these individuals also have a higher percentage of carbohydrate-deficient transferrin in their blood. A report by Rosalki (2004) stated that 50 percent of heavy drinkers and 80 percent of alcoholics demonstrated elevated carbohydrate-deficient transferrin levels in blood.

However, carbohydrate-deficient transferrin has less sensitivity for identifying female heavy drinkers than for identifying male heavy drinkers. This marker is also more sensitive for identifying older individuals who are heavy drinkers compared to younger individuals. Because some alcohol abusers show a higher percentage of carbohydrate-deficient transferrin but normal GGT and vice versa, combining both markers is ideal to identify individuals who abuse alcohol. After complete abstinence, carbohydrate-deficient transferrin returns to normal levels within two weeks.

There are ethnic variations in carbohydrate-deficient transferrin, as values are more elevated in alcoholic Puerto Ricans than alcoholic Blacks and alcoholic Caucasians but not when abstinent. Pregnant women, women using oral contraceptives, and patients suffering from iron-deficient anemia may also have higher percentages of carbohydrate-deficient transferrin. In addition, such increase may also be observed in people with hypertension, smokers, and in obese people.[14]

Whitfield et al. (2008) reported that carbohydrate-deficient transferrin increased in men who consumed more than seven drinks per week, and such increases were more significant with the number of drinks consumed per week. For women, however, a maximum value of the percentage of carbohydrate-deficient transferrin was reached with twenty-nine to thirty-five drinks per week, and then the value did not change significantly in women who drank more than that amount. Again, the authors used 2 percent as the cutoff concentration for the percentage of carbohydrate-deficient transferrin. The authors further stated that the percentage of carbohydrate-deficient transferrin is a poor marker for alcohol abuse in both men and women who are obese, and is also less useful in nonsmokers than smokers.[15]

Golka and Wiese (2004) commented that carbohydrate-deficient transferrin is a superior biomarker than conventional biomarkers such as GGT and MCV, but combining all these parameters may provide superior diagnostic value in identifying patients who are abusing alcohol, because mechanisms of elevation of these three biomarkers are different from one another. In addition, carbohydrate-deficient transferrin determinations are particularly useful to identify patients with chronic alcohol dependence and relapse after withdrawal, license reapplication after suspension for driving with blood alcohol exceeding the legal limit, and patients treated for galactosemia, as well as for identifying patients suffering from a genetic disorder called carbohydrate-deficient glycoprotein syndrome. The carbohydrate-deficient transferrin value is not usually affected by medications except in immunosuppressant patients who may show low carbohydrate-deficient transferrin values. The authors also stressed that carbohydrate-deficient transferrin values appear less elevated in women than men.[16]

Serum and Urine beta-Hexosaminidase as Alcohol Biomarkers

Hexosaminidase, also known as N-acetyl glucosaminidase, is a lysosomal enzyme (lysosome is a spherical organelle, a small structure with the cell that contains certain enzymes that can break down food) found in most body tissues, especially in the kidneys where the concentrations are even higher than other tissues. This enzyme breaks down carbohydrates and gangliosides. Gangliosides are complex lipids, also known as glycosphingolipids, that are found in cell membranes, particularly in nerve cells, and play an important role in cell-to-cell communication. The hexosaminidase molecule is composed of two units, alpha and beta, and both units are composed of amino acids (polypeptides), and variations of the arrangements of these chains result in various molecular forms of hexosaminidase known as isoforms. The hexosaminidase S is composed of two alpha chains, while hexosaminidase B, I, and P are composed of two beta chains. Hexosaminidase A is composed of one alpha and one beta chain. Isoforms B, I, and P are heat stable and collectively called beta-hexosaminidase, while isoforms A and S are heat labile.

The heat stable form of beta-hexosaminidase is elevated after heavy consumption of alcohol because lysosomes (small spherical structures inside the cell) are damaged, and subsequently enzymes are released in blood. Beta-hexosaminidase activity is also found in elevated concentration in urine. Total serum beta-hexosaminidase activity, particularly beta-hexosaminidase B isoform (beta-Hex B) activity, as well as total urinary beta-hexosaminidase activity, is increased in alcoholics compared to moderate drinkers and nondrinkers. Wehr et al. (1991) reported increased activity of serum and urinary beta-hexosaminidase after drinking more than 60 gm of alcohol daily (five or more drinks) for at least ten consecutive days.[17] The blood beta-hexosaminidase activity returns to normal usually after abstinence for seven to ten days, while it may take up to four weeks for urine beta-hexosaminidase activity to return to normal values. Serum beta-hexosaminidase B activity as a percentage of total hexosaminidase activity, expressed as the percentage of beta-Hex B, is also a very sensitive marker for alcohol abuse.

Stowell et al. (1997) compared carbohydrate-deficient transferrin and beta-hexosaminidase activity along with liver enzymes and MCV in alcoholic patients and compared the values obtained in moderate and nondrinking subjects. The total beta-hexosaminidase activity was in general 2.5 times higher in alcoholics compared to moderate drinkers, and this increase was mainly due to a fivefold increase in the activity of B isoform. The average beta-hexosaminidase activity in alcoholics was 49.6 units/liter compared to 19.4 units/liter in moderate drinkers. However, the average concentration of B isoform was 28.4 units/liter in alcoholics compared to 5.7 units/liter in moderate drinkers. Therefore, the percentage of beta-Hex B was 52.4 percent in alcoholics and 29.0 percent in moderate drinkers. The mean carbohydrate-deficient transferrin activity was 60.2 units/liter in alcoholics and 16.9 units/liter in moderated drinkers (cutoff concentration was 20 units/liter). Specimens from alcoholics were collected during admission to the authors' hospital for alcohol detoxification. The authors concluded that the serum percent of Hex B is a very sensitive and specific marker for detecting people who drink more than 60 gm of alcohol per day on a regular basis and is slightly more sensitive to carbohydrate-deficient albumin as a biomarker for alcohol. Beta-hexosaminidase activity can be measured by using inexpensive reagents and a spectrophotometer or a fluorometer.[18]

In another report Kärkkäinen (1990), using thirty-two alcoholic men admitted to the detoxification center for treatment for seven days and twenty-seven nondrinkers, demonstrated that total serum hexosaminidase activities were increased in 68.8 percent of alcoholics on admission while urine total beta-hexosaminidase activities were increased in 81.3 percent of patients compared to nondrinkers. Following a week of abstinence, serum and urine total beta-hexosaminidase activities were increased in 37.5 percent and 71.9 percent patients, respectively. These results indicate that urine beta-hexosaminidase activity may be a more sensitive marker of heavy alcohol consumption compared to serum beta-hexosaminidase activity.[19] Although beta-hexosaminidase activities are increased after heavy consumption of alcohol for at least ten days, a paper published in 2008 indicated that binge drinking (heavy consumption of alcohol in one occasion, see chapter 2 for more detail) may also significantly increase both serum and urine activities of beta-hexosaminidase. In this study, eight binge drinkers (reported binge drinking event one to two times a month) who abstained from consuming alcohol and drugs for ten days, in one occasion drank 120–160 gm of alcohol along with light meals and fruit juices between 7 PM and 1 AM while staying at home under supervision. Blood, urine, and saliva specimens were collected from these subjects 12 hours prior to drinking and also 36 and 108 hours after finishing drinking. The total beta-hexosaminidase activity in serum increased from a mean value of 33.0 prior to drinking to 50.0, 108 hours after drinking. At 36 hours significant increases in beta-hexosaminidase activities were also observed in saliva and urine. The authors concluded that binge drinking in one occasion may also increase beta-hexosaminidase activities in serum, urine, and saliva.[20]

Other than heavy alcohol consumption, elevated serum hexosaminidase activity may occur in patients with severe liver disease (such as cirrhosis of liver), hypertension, diabetes, after heart attack, thyrotoxicosis (a disorder causing very high thyroid hormones levels in the body, which may be life-threatening), and pregnancy.[21]

Sialic Acid as an Alcohol Biomarker

Sialic acids are a family of thirty-six naturally occurring acetylated derivatives of neuraminic acid, which are found in carbohydrate chains of glycoprotein (proteins with carbohydrate moieties) in biological fluids such as blood and cell membranes. The most abundant sialic acid is N-acetylneuraminic acid. These compounds play important roles in cell-to-cell communication or serve as a recognition site on the cell surface. Total sialic acid in blood can be measured after breaking down conjugated sialic acid (hydrolysis) using either a strong acid or an enzyme and then quantitation of total sialic acid by an analytical method such as high performance liquid chromatography. There are also immunoassays for estimating sialic acid in blood. In one study (Sillanaukee et al. 1999), the authors reported that total sialic acid level in the blood of female social drinkers (less than 30 gm of alcohol per week) and male social drinkers (less than 50 gm of alcohol per week) were 40–79 mg/100 mL and 42 to 97 mg/100 mL, respectively. In contrast, the total sialic acid content in female alcoholics (more than 800 gm of alcohol per week) varied from

62 to 132 mg/100 mL, while the sialic acid content of male alcoholics (more than 1000 gm of alcohol per week) varied from 62 to 158 mg/100 mL. The authors measured the total sialic acid level in the blood using a radioimmunoassay. During a follow-up of twenty-eight alcoholic patients participating in inpatient detoxifying treatment, sialic acid levels were decreased after three weeks. However, elevated sialic acid content may also be encountered in patients suffering from tumor, diabetes, inflammation, and cardiovascular diseases.[22]

Acetaldehyde-Protein Adducts as Alcohol Biomarkers

Acetaldehyde is the first degradation product of alcohol formed by the metabolism of alcohol in the liver by alcohol dehydrogenase. Acetaldehyde is highly reactive and is rapidly converted into acetic acid by another liver enzyme, acetaldehyde dehydrogenase, and then acetic acid is rapidly converted into water and carbon dioxide by further degradation. Acetaldehyde, being highly reactive, also rapidly forms stable adducts with a number of compounds, including proteins such as albumin (most abundant protein in the blood) and hemoglobin (hemoglobin is also a protein). These adducts are found mostly in chronic heavy consumers of alcohol because acetaldehyde levels are more significantly elevated in these individuals than in moderate or social drinkers. Hemoglobin-acetaldehyde adduct has received more attention in the scientific community as a biomarker of alcohol abuse. In addition to blood, this marker is also found in elevated levels in urine.

Aldehyde hemoglobin adducts can be formed within thirty minutes of drinking, and the first adduct formed is called reversible hemoglobin-acetaldehyde adduct because it can break down into acetaldehyde and hemoglobin. This adduct is formed by the reaction of hemoglobin inside the red blood cell (erythrocyte) with acetaldehyde. These reversible adducts can be detected up to forty-eight hours after the last drink. Then the reversible adduct is converted into irreversible adduct, which does not break down into hemoglobin and acetaldehyde. The irreversible (stable) hemoglobin acetaldehyde adducts accumulate in the blood of chronic drinkers and remain detectable in blood for at least twenty-eight days. Hemoglobin-acetaldehyde adduct concentration is higher in men than women because men usually have higher blood levels of hemoglobin. In addition, hemoglobin-acetaldehyde adduct concentrations are significantly higher in alcohol abusers than nondrinkers.[23] The chemistry of hemoglobin-acetaldehyde adduct is complex because there is more than one type of adduct. This is because acetaldehyde, being very reactive, can form adducts by bonding with hemoglobin at different parts of the molecule.[24]

Measurement of hemoglobin-acetaldehyde adduct in human blood is difficult. Initial techniques involved high-performance liquid chromatography with isoelectric focusing gel and affinity chromatography, but very low levels of such adducts pose a technical challenge. A complex immunoassay method known as enzyme-linked immunosorbent assay (ELISA) has been developed more recently for detecting hemoglobin-acetaldehyde adducts in blood. However, the major advantage of this biomarker is that it is a direct biomarker of alcohol abuse, because acetaldehyde is derived from consuming alcohol. In addition, false positive results are rarely encountered. Niemela et al. (1991) reported that this is an excellent marker for detecting pregnant women who abuse alcohol, because the highest concentrations of hemoglobin-acetaldehyde adduct were observed in women who delivered babies with fetal alcohol syndrome.[25]

Ethyl Glucuronide and Ethyl Sulfate as Alcohol Biomarkers

Ethyl glucuronide and ethyl sulfate are minor degradation products (metabolite) of alcohol that are found in various body fluids and also in human hair. Ethyl glucuronide is formed by direct conjugation of ethanol and glucuronic acid through the action of a liver enzyme. Ethyl sulfate is also formed directly by the conjugation of ethanol with a sulfate group. These compounds are water soluble. Ethyl glucuronide can be detected after eighty hours post-alcohol consumption and is found shortly after drinking even small amounts of alcohol. Therefore, ethyl glucuronide is considered a sensitive and specific marker for alcohol consumption, as well as a direct biomarker of alcohol.

Ethyl glucuronide can be measured in urine, blood, and hair specimens. Ethyl glucuronide can be determined using a variety of methods, including gas chromatography coupled with mass spectrometry, liquid chromatography combined with mass spectrometry, and immunoassay. In one study (Schmitt et al. 1997) healthy moderate drinkers who ingested one standard drink showed a maximum ethyl glucuronide level of 3.7 mg/L in serum, and ethyl glucuronide was detected eight hours after alcohol was completely eliminated from the body and no longer detectable in the blood. In serum samples of nondrinkers, no ethyl glucuronide can be detected. In thirty-seven out of fifty drivers suspected of driving under the influence of alcohol, serum ethyl glucuronide concentration ranged from 0.1 to 20 mg/L. The authors concluded that if serum ethyl glucuronide level exceeds 5 mg/L, it can be assumed that the person is misusing alcohol.[26]

Concentration of ethyl glucuronide and ethyl sulfate in serum is higher than concentration in whole blood because both compounds are readily soluble in water and therefore found in higher amounts in serum (the water part of the blood) than in blood cells (red blood cells, white blood cells, and other blood cells). In general, ethyl glucuronide concentrations are higher than ethyl sulfate concentrations. In one study using thirteen subjects (Hoiseth et al. 2009), the ethyl glucuronide concentrations ranged from 0.63 to 9.81 mg/L in serum and 0.39 to 5.53 mg/L in whole blood. The median serum to whole blood ratio was 1.69 and the range was 1.33 to 1.90.

Similarly, for ethyl sulfate, the serum concentration in thirteen volunteers ranged from 0.11 to 2.64 mg/L and whole blood ethyl sulfate concentrations ranged from 0.10 to 1.82 mg/L. The median serum to whole blood ethyl sulfate concentration was 1.30 and the range was 1.08 to 1.47. Because both whole blood and serum ethyl glucuronide, as well as ethyl sulfate values, are determined in deceased in forensic investigations, the authors stressed the need of understanding that serum levels of both ethyl glucuronide and ethyl sulfate are substantially higher than whole blood values in interpreting such results.[27]

Because alcohol is produced by bacterial action after death, ethyl glucuronide and ethyl sulfate are postmortem markers of antemortem alcohol ingestion. A small amount of alcohol is produced by the action of bacteria in a deceased person not consuming any alcohol, but neither ethyl glucuronide nor ethyl sulfate is formed after death. In one study (Hoiseth et al. 2009) involving thirty-six death investigations where postmortem ethanol production was suspected, ethyl glucuronide and ethyl sulfate were measured in both urine and blood of the deceased. In nineteen out of thirty-nine deceased, the range of ethyl glucuronide in blood ranged from 0.1 to 23.2 mg/L, while urinary ethyl glucuronide concentrations ranged from 1.9 to 182 mg/L. For ethyl sulfate, the blood concentration ranged from 0.04 to 7.9 mg/L, while urine concentrations ranged from 0.3 to 99 mg/L. In sixteen other individuals no ethyl glucuronide or ethyl sulfate was detected. The authors concluded that in thirty-six cases, alcohol consumption before death was likely in nineteen deceased who showed positive ethyl glucuronide and ethyl sulfate concentrations in blood and urine.[28]

Ethyl glucuronide is a sensitive marker for alcohol consumption and can be detected even after small amounts of alcohol are ingested, such as 1 gm to 3 gm of alcohol where a standard drink contains 14 gm of alcohol. In a study (Thierauf et al. 2009) involving thirty-one volunteers who drank either 1 or 3 gm of alcohol, maximum amount of ethyl glucuronide in urine was 0.32 mg/L after drinking only 1 gm of alcohol. Similarly, maximum ethyl glucuronide after drinking 3 gm of alcohol was 1.53 mg/L. The corresponding ethyl sulfate levels were 0.15 mg/L (after 1 gm of alcohol) and 1.17 mg/L (after 3 gm of alcohol). These maximum achieved concentrations are considered positive by many laboratories testing urine for ethyl glucuronide and ethyl sulfate for workplace alcohol testing and noncompliance of patients undergoing alcohol rehabilitation therapy.[29] Therefore no alcohol consumption is safe to drink, at least for a day or two prior to taking preemployment alcohol tests (see more on this in chapter 9).

Determination of ethyl glucuronide in hair specimens has merit to identify heavy drinkers because ethyl glucuronide can be determined for a longer time in hair than in blood or urine. Morini et al. (2009) used liquid chromatography combined with mass spectrometry to determine hair concentrations of ethyl glucuronide in ninety-eight volunteers, including nondrinkers, social drinkers, and heavy drinkers. The authors concluded that ethyl glucuronide levels of 27 picogram/milligram of hair can be achieved in a person drinking 60 gm or higher amount of alcohol (five or more drinks) per day for at least three months. Age, gender, body mass index, smoking, hair color, and cosmetic treatment appear to have no effect on ethyl glucuronide level detected in hair specimen.[30]

In another report (Lamoureaux et al. 2009), the authors determined concentrations of ethyl glucuronide in hair using only 30 mg of hair specimen and liquid chromatography combined with mass spectrometry. The method was applied to analyze hair samples taken from four fatalities with documented excessive drinking habits, twelve heavy drinkers, and seven social drinkers. Ethyl glucuronide concentrations in hair of social drinkers were less than 10 picogram/milligram of hair, while ethyl glucuronide concentrations were above 50 picogram/milligram of hair (range 54–497) in hair specimens of heavy drinkers and deceased known to abuse alcohol.[31]

Fatty Acid Ethyl Esters as Alcohol Biomarkers

Fatty acid ethyl esters are direct markers of alcohol abuse because they are formed due to a chemical reaction between fatty acids and alcohol (ethanol). Fatty acids are an integral part of the structures of triglycerides (fats), but a small amount of fatty acids, also known as free fatty acids, are found in circulation. The chemical reaction between alcohol and fatty acid is known as esterification, which is mediated by fatty-acyl-ethyl-ester synthase (FAEE synthase), an enzyme found in abundance in the liver and pancreas. Carboxylesterase lipase, another enzyme that liberates free fatty acids from complex lipids, can also induce the reaction between alcohol and fatty acids, generating fatty acid ethyl esters. Therefore, hydrolysis of triglycerides and phospholipids generating fatty acids in the presence of alcohol may eventually be converted into fatty acid ethyl esters. Fatty acid ethyl esters are also known as nonoxidative metabolites of ethanol, while acetaldehyde and acetic acid are oxidative metabolites of ethanol, which are formed by the action of liver enzymes.

Fatty acid ethyl esters are formed primarily in the liver and pancreas and then are released into circulation. These compounds are also incorporated into hair follicle through sebum and can be used as a biomarker of alcohol abuse. There are four major fatty acid ethyl esters: ethyl myristate, ethyl palmitate, ethyl stearate, and ethyl oleate. These compounds are measured after extraction from hair or blood and analyzed using a sophisticated instrument known as gas chromatography/mass spectrometry. Then results are usually expressed as the sum of all four fatty acid ethyl ester concentrations.

It has long been known that ethanol abuse leads to severe damage of the liver and pancreas. Although acetaldehyde, the oxidative metabolite of alcohol, was long thought as the mediator of organ damage, more recent studies indicate that fatty acid ethyl esters are also responsible for damaging the liver and pancreas, because enzymes that facilitate formation of fatty acid ethyl esters are found in the highest concentrations in the pancreas and liver. In addition, the total concentration of major fatty acid ethyl esters in blood is a good marker for both acute and chronic alcohol intake. Fatty acid ethyl esters can be detected in blood for up to twenty-four hours after drinking. In contrast, blood alcohol level declines more rapidly and can be undetectable even four to twelve hours after drinking, depending on the amount consumed. A negative blood alcohol with a positive fatty acid ethyl ester test is consistent with ethanol intake four to twenty-four hours prior to blood collection. If fatty acid ethyl ester and carbohydrate-deficient transferrin tests are both positive, a patient can be suspected as a chronic consumer of alcohol.[32]

Analysis of fatty acid ethyl esters in hair is a good marker of alcohol abuse because these compounds can be detected in hair for a much longer time than in blood. In one study (Auwarter et al. 2001), the authors analyzed hair specimens from nineteen alcoholics enrolled in a treatment program, ten fatalities with verified excess alcohol consumption, thirteen moderate social drinkers who consumed up to 20 gm of alcohol per day (1.5 drinks on average), and five nondrinkers for fatty acid ethyl esters (ethyl myristate, ethyl palmitate, ethyl stearate, and ethyl oleate). The total concentration ranged from 2.5 to 13.5 ng/milligram of hair (mean 6.8) for fatalities, 0.92–11.6 ng/milligram of hair in alcoholics (mean 4.0), 0.20 to 0.85 ng/milligram of hair in social drinkers (mean 0.41), and 0.06–0.37 ng/milligram of hair in nondrinkers (mean 0.16). The authors concluded that despite large individual differences, fatty acid ethyl esters can be used as markers of excessive alcohol consumption.[33]

In another report (Pragst and Yegles 2008), the authors suggested that moderate and social drinkers should have hair fatty acid ethyl ester concentrations below 0.5 ng/milligram and ethyl glucuronide concentrations in hair below 25 pg/milligram. Above these values, alcohol abuse is possible.[34]

Fatty acid ethyl esters can be used for evaluating drinking problems with pregnant women and can aid in diagnosis of fetal alcohol spectrum disorders. Fatty acid ethyl esters detected in meconium can be related to exposure of the fetus to alcohol due to maternal consumption of alcohol. Fatty acid ethyl esters may be markers for identifying newborns who are at risk of neurodevelopmental delay due to alcohol exposure in utero.[35]

Phosphatidyl ethanol, which is formed due to a reaction between phosphatidylcholine and ethanol mediated by the enzyme phospholipase D, is an emerging biomarker of alcohol abuse. Phosphatidylcholine is an important lipid that plays an essential role in forming cell membranes.

CONCLUSION

Alcohol abuse is a serious public health concern, and it is important to screen patients who are at risk of alcohol abuse by using appropriate biomarkers so that early intervention can be achieved to treat such individuals. At present there is no unique marker for determining alcohol abuse, and various markers have their advantages and limitations. Ethyl glucuronide, ethyl sulfate, and fatty acid ethyl esters are valuable markers for assessing alcohol abuse because these markers are direct markers for alcohol consumption and are specific in nature. However, determining such markers in blood or hair is technically difficult and not feasible to perform in small hospital laboratories. In contrast, liver enzymes and MCV are routinely determined in most hospital laboratories and are cost-effective. However, such indirect markers are not specific for alcohol abuse and can be elevated in certain disease conditions.

NOTES

1. A. S. St. Leger, A. L. Cochrane, and F. Moore, "Factors Associated with Cardiac Mortality in Developed Countries with Particular Reference to the Consumption of Wine," *Lancet* 1979 (1): 1017–20.

2. Alcohol and Public Health, Center for Disease Control, Atlanta, Georgia, http://www.cdc.gov/.

3. S. E. Foster, R. D. Vaughan, W. H. Foster, and J. A. Califano, "Alcohol Consumption and Expenditures for Underage Drinking and Adult Excessive Drinking," *Journal of the American Medical Association* 289, no. 8 (February 2003): 989–95.

4. S Anai, C. S. West, M. Chang, K. Nakamura, et al., "Outcome of Men Who Present with Elevated Serum PSA (>20 ng/ml) to an Inner City Hospital," *Journal of National Medical Association* 99, no. 8 (August 2007): 895–99.

5. N. Alkan and T. Demircan, "Determination of Blood Alcohol Level in People Who Are Involved in a Judicial Event of Medical Importance (Case Report),"

Ulusal Travma Dergisis [The Turkish Journal of Trauma] 7, no. 4 (October 2001): 277–81. [Article in Turkish.]

6. P. M. Miller, S. M. Ornstein, P. J. Nietert, and R. Anton, "Self-Reporting and Biomarker Alcohol Screening by Primary Care Physicians: The Need to Translate Research Guidelines and Practice," *Alcohol and Alcoholism* 39, no. 4 (2004): 325–28.

7. P. M. Miller, C. Spies, T. Neumann, M. Javor, et al. "Alcohol Biomarker Screening in Medical and Surgical Settings," *Alcoholism Clinical and Experimental Research* 30, no. 2 (February 2006): 185–93.

8. P. Alatalo, H. Kovistro, K. Puuka, J. Hietala, et al., "Biomarkers of Liver Status in Heavy Drinkers, Moderate Drinkers and Abstainers," *Alcohol and Alcoholism* 44, no. 2 (March–April 2009): 199–203.

9. G. Targher, "Review: Elevated Gamma Glutamyltransferase Activity Is Associated with Increased Risk of Mortality, Incidence of Diabetes, Cardiovascular Events, Chronic Kidney Disease and Cancer," *Clinical Chemistry and Laboratory Medicine* 48, no. 2 (February 2010): 147–57.

10. H. Koivistro, J. Hietala, P. Anttila, S. Parkkila, et al., "Long-Term Ethanol Consumption and Macrocytosis: Diagnosis and Pathogenic Implications," *Journal of Laboratory and Clinical Medicine* 147, no. 4 (April 2006): 191–96.

11. J. R. Delanghe, A. Helander, J. P. Wielders, J. M. Pekelharing, et al., "Developmental and Multicenter Evaluation of N-latex CDT Direct Immunonephelometric Assay for Serum Carbohydrate-Deficient Transferrin," *Clinical Chemistry* 53, no. 6 (June 2007): 1115–21.

12. J. R. Delanghe and M. L. De Buyzere, "Carbohydrate-Deficient Transferrin and Forensic Medicine," *Clinica Chimica Acta* 406, nos. 1–2 (August 2009): 1–7.

13. K. Sorvajärvi, J. E. Blake, Y. Israel, and O. Niemelä, "Sensitivity and Specificity of Carbohydrate-Deficient Transferrin as a Marker of Alcohol Abuse Are Significantly Influenced by Alteration in Serum Transferrin: Comparison of Two Methods," *Alcoholism: Clinical and Experimental Research* 20, no. 3 (May 1996): 449–54.

14. S. B. Rosalki, "Carbohydrate-Deficient Transferrin: A Marker of Alcohol Use," *International Journal of Clinical Practice* 58, no. 4 (April 2004): 391–93.

15. J. B. Whitfield, V. Dy, P. A. Madden, A. C. Heath, et al., "Measuring Carbohydrate-Deficient Transferrin by Direct Immunoassay: Factors Affecting Diagnostic Sensitivity for Excessive Alcohol Intake," *Clinical Chemistry* 54, no. 7 (July 2008): 1158–65.

16. K. Golka and A. Wiese, "Carbohydrate-Deficient Transferrin (CDT): A Biomarker for Long Term Alcohol Consumption," *Journal of Toxicology Environmental Health, Part B: Critical Review* 7, no. 4 (August 2004): 319–37.

17. H. Wehr, B. Czartoryska, D. Gorska, H. Matsumoto, et al., "Serum Beta-Hexosaminidase and Alpha-Mannosidase Activities as a Marker of Alcohol Abuse," *Alcoholism: Clinical and Experimental Research* 15, no. 1 (February 1991): 13–15.

18. L. Stowell, A. Stowell, N. Garrett, and G. Robinson, "Comparison of Serum Beta-Hexosaminidase Isoenzyme B Activity with Serum Carbohydrate-Deficient Transferrin and Other Markers of Alcohol Abuse," *Alcohol and Alcoholism* 32, no. 6 (December 1997): 703–14.

19. P. Kärkkäinen, "Serum and Urine Beta-Hexosaminidase as Markers of Heavy Drinking," *Alcohol and Alcoholism* 25, no. 4 (July–August 1990): 365–69.

20. N. Waszkiewicz, S. D. Szajda, A. Jankowska, A. Kepka, et al., "The Effect of the Binge Drinking Session on the Activity of Salivary, Serum and Urinary Beta-Hexosaminidase: Preliminary Data," *Alcohol and Alcoholism* 43, no. 4 (July–August 2008): 446–50.

21. P. Karkkainen, K. Poikolainen, and M. Salaspuro, "Serum Beta-Hexosaminidase as Markers of Heavy Drinking," *Alcoholism: Clinical and Experimental Research* 14, no. 2 (April 1990): 187–90.

22. P. Sillanaukee, M. Ponnio, and K. Seppa, "Sialic Acid: A New Potential Marker of Alcohol Abuse," *Alcoholism Clinical and Experimental Research* 23, no. 6 (June 1999): 1039–43.

23. S. K. Das, L. Dhanya, and D. M. Vasudevan, "Biomarkers of Alcoholism: An Updated Review," *Scandinavian Journal of Clinical and Laboratory Investigation* 68, no. 2 (April 2008): 81–92.

24. M. D. Gross, R. Hays, S. M. Gapstur, M. Chaussee, et al., "Evidence for the Formation of Multiple Types of Acetaldehyde Hemoglobin Adducts," *Alcohol and Alcoholism* 29, no. 1 (January 1994): 31–41.

25. O. Niemela, E. Halmesmaki, and O. Yikorkala, "Hemoglobin-Acetaldehyde Adducts Are Elevated in Women Carrying Alcohol-Damaged Fetus," *Alcoholism: Clinical and Experimental Research* 15, no. 6 (December 1991): 1007–10.

26. G. Schmitt, P. Droenner, G. Skopp, and R. Aderjan, "Ethyl Glucuronide Concentration in Serum of Human Volunteers, Teetotalers, and Suspected Drinking Drivers," *Journal of Forensic Sciences* 42, no. 6 (November 1997): 1099–1102.

27. G. Hoiseth, L. Morini, A. Polettini, A. S. Christophersen, et al., "Serum/Whole Blood Concentration Ratio for Ethyl Glucuronide and Ethyl Sulfate," *Journal of Analytical Toxicology* 33, no. 4 (May 2009): 208–11.

28. G. Hoiseth, R. Karinen, A. Christophersen, and J. Morland, "Practical Use of Ethyl Glucuronide and Ethyl Sulfate in Postmortem Cases as Markers of Antemortem Alcohol Ingestion," *International Journal of Legal Medicine* 124, no. 2 (March 2010): 143–48.

29. A. Thierauf, C. C. Halter, S. Rana, V. Auwaerter, et al., "Urine Tested Positive for Ethyl Glucuronide after Trace Amounts of Ethanol," *Addiction* 104, no. 12 (December 2009): 2007–12.

30. L. Morini, L. Politi, and A. Polettini, "Ethyl Glucuronide in Hair: A Sensitive and Specific Marker of Heavy Drinking," *Addiction* 104, no. 6 (June 2009): 915–20.

31. F. Lamoureux, J. M. Gaulier, F. L. Sauvage, M. Mercerolle, et al., "Determination of Ethyl Glucuronide in Hair for Heavy Drinking Detection Using Liquid Chromatography-Tandem Mass Spectrometry Following Solid-Phase Extraction," *Annals of Bioanalytical Chemistry* 394, no. 7 (August 2009): 1895–1901.

32. M. Laposata, "Fatty Acid Ethyl Esters: Short-Term and Long-Term Serum Markers of Ethanol Intake," *Clinical Chemistry* 43, no. 8 (August 1997): 1527–34.

33. V. Auwarter, F. Sporkert, S. Harting, F. Pragst, et al., "Fatty Acid Ethyl Esters in Hair as Markers of Alcohol Consumption: Segmental Hair Analysis of Alcoholics, Social Drinkers and Teetotalers," *Clinical Chemistry* 47, no. 12 (December 2001): 2114–23.

34. F. Pragst and M. Yegles, "Determination of Fatty Acid Ethyl Esters (FAEE) and Ethyl Glucuronide (EtG) in Hair: A Promising Way for Retrospective Detec-

tion of Alcohol Abuse during Pregnancy?" *Therapeutic Drug Monitoring* 30, no. 2 (April 2008): 255–63.

35. J. Peterson, H. L. K. Kirchner, W. Xue, S. Minnes, et al., "Fatty Acid Ethyl Esters in Meconium Are Associated with Poorer Neurodevelopmental Outcomes to Two Years of Age," *Journal of Pediatrics* 152, no. 6 (June 2008): 788–92.

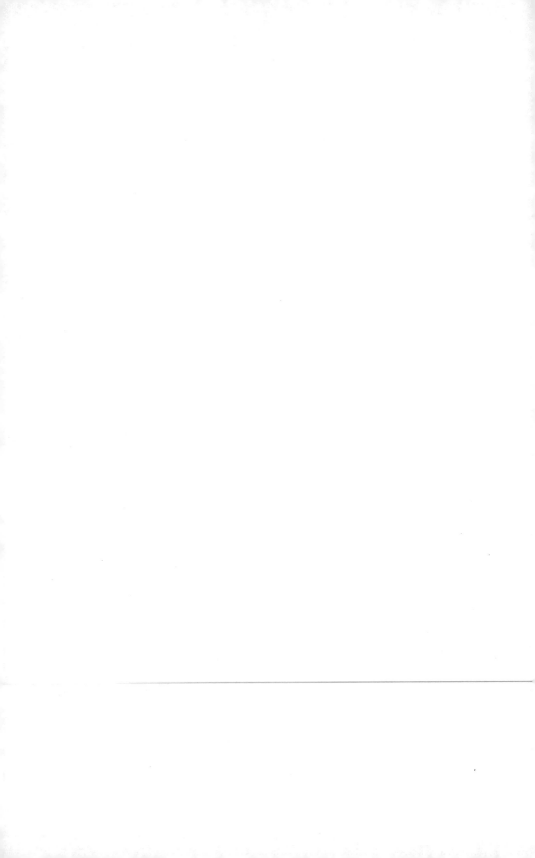

8

Pharmaceuticals, Drugs of Abuse, and Alcohol

A Potentially Deadly Mix

We are all aware of the warning labels of many over-the-counter (OTC) cold and allergy medications that state, "Avoid alcoholic beverages while taking this medication." The reason is that many allergy medications and cold medications contain antihistamine drugs that cause drowsiness, and alcohol can significantly enhance this effect. Combining alcohol and antihistamines makes driving and/or operating machinery much more difficult and not advisable. Many prescription medications have similar warning labels. There are many reported interactions between various drugs and alcohol. In general, drug-alcohol interactions cause only adverse effects and can be deadly.

HOW COMMON IS DRUG-ALCOHOL INTERACTION?

More than 2,800 prescription medications are available in the United States, and physicians write 14 billion prescriptions annually. In addition, approximately 2,000 formulations are available over the counter.[1] Approximately 70 percent of the U.S. population consumes alcohol occasionally, and about 10 percent drink daily.[2] So concurrent use of alcohol and drugs can be construed as common among Americans. According to the Substance Abuse and Mental Health Services Administration (SAMHSA), 36 percent of all patients (1.4 million) who visited emergency rooms in 2005 had overdosed with a combination of alcohol, pharmaceuticals, and/or illicit drugs.[3] The rest of the patients had overdosed with pharmaceuticals or drugs of abuse. Alcohol was most frequently combined with cocaine (estimated 86,482 visits), marijuana (33,643 visits), both cocaine and marijuana (22,377 visits), and heroin (12,797 visits). Another government report indicates that in 2004, an estimated 363,641 emergency room visits by people of all ages involved the use of alcohol combined with a drug.[4] Elderly people in particular are at higher risk from alcohol-drug interactions. Major drug-alcohol interactions are listed in table 8.1. Few drugs enhance the effect of alcohol. These drugs are listed in table 8.2.

CAN ALCOHOL-DRUG INTERACTION CAUSE DEATH?

Fatal toxicities frequently occur from alcohol and drug overdoses. In many instances, in the presence of alcohol, a lower concentration of drug may cause fatality due to drug-alcohol interactions. In a Finnish study (Koski et al. 2005), it was found that median amitriptyline (an antidepressant drug) and propoxyphene (a pain medication) concentrations were lower in alcohol-related fatal cases compared to cases where no alcohol was involved. The authors concluded that when alcohol is present, a relatively small overdose of a drug may cause fatality.[5] Although death is more frequently observed in people abusing both alcohol and illicit drugs, death due to consumption of alcohol and prescription medication has also been reported.

> In general, the toxicity of a particular drug is observed at a much lower blood concentration in the presence of alcohol. In other words, alcohol enhances the toxic effect of a drug it interacts with. Therefore, a person who died from a drug and alcohol overdose probably would have survived if alcohol was not consumed.

It has been well documented that heroin abusers who drink require less heroin to overdose. In general, postmortem blood levels of morphine are much lower than expected in tolerant individuals who died from a combined morphine and alcohol overdose.[6]

A combination of alcohol and drugs is also a leading cause of death in adolescence. In one report analyzing the causes of death among an adolescent population, the authors observed that 20.8 percent of fatalities were related to drug and alcohol combined overdose.[7]

Table 8.1. Major Drug-Alcohol Interactions

Drug Class	Trade Name	Generic Name	Drug-Alcohol Interaction
Allergies/colds/flu	Alavert	loratadine	Drowsiness, dizziness; increased risk for overdose
	Allegra, Allegra-D	fexofenadine	Avoid driving or operating heavy machinery.
	Benadryl	diphenhydramine	
	Clarinex	desloratadine	
	Claritin, Claritin-D	loratadine	
	Dimetapp Cold & Allergy	brompheniramine	
	Sudafed Sinus & Allergy	chlorpheniramine	
	Triaminic Cold & Allergy	chlorpheniramine	
	Tylenol Allergy Sinus	chlorpheniramine	
	Tylenol Cold & Flu	chlorpheniramine	
	Atarax	hydroxyzine	
Angina (chest pain), coronary heart disease	Isordil	isosorbide	Rapid heartbeat, sudden changes in blood pressure, dizziness, fainting
		nitroglycerin	
Anxiety and epilepsy	Ativan	lorazepam	Drowsiness, dizziness; increased risk for overdose; slowed or difficulty breathing; impaired motor control; unusual behavior; and memory problems
	Klonopin	clonazepam	
	Librium	chlordiazepoxide	
	Paxil	paroxetine	
	Valium	diazepam	
	Xanax	alprazolam	
	Herbal preparations (kava kava)		Liver damage, drowsiness
Arthritis	Celebrex	celecoxib	Ulcers, stomach bleeding, liver problems
	Naprosyn	naproxen	
	Voltaren	diclofenac	

(continued)

Table 8.1. (continued)

Drug Class	Trade Name	Generic Name	Drug–Alcohol Interaction
Blood clots	Coumadin	warfarin	Occasional drinking may lead to internal bleeding; heavier drinking may cause bleeding or may have the opposite effect, resulting in possible blood clots, strokes, or heart attacks
Cough	Delsym, Robitussin Cough	dextromethorphan	Drowsiness, dizziness; increased risk for overdose
	Robitussin A–C	guaifenesin + codeine	Avoid driving
Depression	Anafranil	clomipramine	Drowsiness, dizziness; increased risk for overdose; increased feelings of depression or hopelessness in adolescents (suicide)
	Celexa	citalopram	
	Desyrel	trazodone	Avoid driving
	Effexor	venlafaxine	
	Elavil	amitriptyline	
	Lexapro	escitalopram	
	Luvox	fluvoxamine	
	Norpramin	desipramine	
	Paxil	paroxetine	Serious episode of high blood pressure if beer or wine contains tyramine, which interacts with phenelzine and other drugs of this class.
	Prozac	fluoxetine	
	Serzone	nefazodone	
	Wellbutrin	bupropion	
	Zoloft	sertraline	
	Monoamine oxidase inhibitor	phenelzine	
	Nardil		
Diabetes	Glucophage	metformin	Liver toxicity and possibility of lactic acidosis with metformin.
	Micronase	glyburide	Hypoglycemia or lack of sugar control with other drugs
	Orinase	tolbutamide	

Enlarged prostate	Cardura Flomax Hytrin Minipress	doxazosin tamsulosin terazosin prazosin	Dizziness, light-headedness, fainting
Heartburn, indigestion, sour stomach	Axid Reglan Tagamet Zantac	nizatidine metoclopramide cimetidine ranitidine	Rapid heartbeat, sudden changes in blood pressure (metoclopramide); increased alcohol effect
High blood pressure	Accupril Capozide Cardura Catapres Cozaar Hytrin Lopressor HCT Lotensin Minipress Vaseretic	quinapril hydrochlorothiazide doxazosin clonidine losartan terazosin hydrochlorothiazide benazepril prazosin enalapril	Dizziness, fainting, drowsiness; heart problems such as changes in the heart's regular heartbeat (arrhythmia)
High cholesterol	Advicor Altocor Crestor Lipitor Mevacor Niaspan Pravachol Pravigard Vytorin Zocor	lovastatin + niacin lovastatin rosuvastatin atorvastatin lovastatin niacin pravastatin pravastatin + aspirin ezetimibe + simvastatin simvastatin	Liver damage (all medications); increased flushing and itching (niacin); increased stomach bleeding (pravastatin + aspirin)

(continued)

Table 8.1. (continued)

Drug Class	Trade Name	Generic Name	Drug-Alcohol Interaction
Infections	Acrodantin Flagyl Grisactin Nizoral Nydrazid Seromycin Tindamax	nitrofurantoin metronidazole griseofulvin ketoconazole isoniazid cycloserine tinidazole	Fast heartbeat, sudden changes in blood pressure; stomach pain, upset stomach, vomiting, headache, flushing, or redness of the face; liver damage (isoniazid, ketoconazole)
Muscle pain	Flexeril Soma	cyclobenzaprine carisoprodol	Drowsiness, dizziness; increased risk of seizures; increased risk for overdose; slowed or difficulty breathing; impaired motor control; unusual behavior; memory problems
Nausea, motion sickness	Antivert Atarax Dramamine Phenergan	meclizine hydroxyzine dimenhydrinate promethazine	Drowsiness, dizziness; increased risk for overdose
Pain (such as headache, muscle ache, minor arthritis pain), fever, inflammation	Advil Aleve Excedrin Motrin Tylenol	ibuprofen naproxen aspirin, acetaminophen ibuprofen acetaminophen	Stomach upset, bleeding, and ulcers; liver damage (acetaminophen); rapid heartbeat. Chronic alcohol user may experience severe overdose from small dosage of acetaminophen.

Condition	Brand name	Generic name	Effects
Seizures	Dilantin Klonopin	phenytoin clonazepam phenobarbital	Reduced effect of phenytoin; drowsiness with other drugs
Severe pain from injury, postsurgical care, oral surgery, migraines	Darvocet-N Demerol Fiorinal with codeine Percocet Vicodin	propoxyphene meperidine butalbital + codeine oxycodone hydrocodone	Drowsiness, dizziness; increased risk for overdose; slowed or difficulty breathing; impaired motor control; unusual behavior; memory problems, increased risk of death from overdose
Sleep problems	Ambien Lunesta ProSom Restoril Sominex Unisom	zolpidem esopiclone estazolam temazepam diphenhydramine doxylamine	Drowsiness, sleepiness, dizziness; slowed or difficulty breathing; impaired motor control; unusual behavior; memory problems Avoid driving
	Herbal preparations (chamomile, valerian, lavender)		Increased drowsiness Avoid driving

Source: National Institute of Alcohol Abuse and Alcoholism (NIH Publication No. 03-5329, revised 2007), http://pubs.niaaa.nih.gov/publications/Medicine/medicine.htm.

Table 8.2.   Drugs That May Increase Blood Alcohol Level and Prolong the Effect of Alcohol

Drug Class	Specific Drug
Cardiovascular drug	Verapamil increases blood alcohol concentration and prolongs its effect.
Antibiotic	Erythromycin increases alcohol absorption when low amount of alcohol is consumed.
Antiemetic	Metoclopramide enhances the effect of alcohol.
Antiulcer drug	Cimetidine increases blood alcohol level more than ranitidine.

Case Reports

Case Report 1: A twenty-eight-year-old man was found dead by his girlfriend. The postmortem analysis of the heart blood showed 90 mg/dL (0.09 percent) of alcohol, which was slightly above the legal limit for driving (0.08 percent). The heart blood also showed the presence of cyproheptadine (0.46 mg/L), a medication prescribed to his girlfriend. Cyproheptadine (trade name Periactin) is an antihistamine, anticholinergic, and antiserotonergic agent that is used in treating allergies (especially hay fever), for stimulating appetite in underweight people, and for the management of nightmares and post-traumatic stress disorder. This drug is safe but may cause drowsiness. The level of the drug found in this individual was moderate, and this drug rarely causes severe toxicity. However, in this case, the medical examiner concluded that the person died from a combined alcohol and cyproheptadine overdose.[8]

Case Report 2: Pure overdose from the antidepressant moclobemide (Aurorix) is not considered life threatening. However, one person died from a combined overdose of moclobemide and alcohol. This person died after consuming half a bottle of whiskey after ingesting this medication. The authors concluded that whiskey consumption played an important role in this case of fatal overdose.[9]

MECHANISM OF ALCOHOL-DRUG INTERACTIONS

Many different classes of drugs, including antibiotics, antidepressants, antidiabetic medications, antihistamines, antipsychotic drugs, anticonvulsants, antiulcer medications, cardiovascular drugs, narcotic analgesics, non-narcotic analgesics, and sedative hypnotic drugs, interact with alcohol. The mechanism of interaction of these drugs with alcohol can be classified under two broad categories: pharmacokinetic interaction and pharmacodynamic interaction.

- *Pharmacokinetic Interaction:* In this type of drug interaction, alcohol affects the blood level and/or distribution of an interacting drug by altering absorption, metabolism, or excretion of the drug. Alcohol interferes with hepatic metabolism of many drugs and may increase or decrease its blood concentration. The increased or decreased level of the drug in the blood alters its pharmacological effects, that is, less therapeutic benefits for reduced concentration or drug toxicity due to increased concentration. For example, chronic alcohol consumption can reduce the blood level of the antibiotic doxycycline by increasing its metabolism by the liver. Therefore, efficacy of doxycycline is reduced in people who consume alcohol regularly.
- *Pharmacodynamic Interaction:* This interaction occurs when alcohol increases or decreases the action of an interacting drug without altering its concentration. In general, alcohol and an interacting drug with similar pharmacological actions may have an additive effect or synergistic effect (the combined effect is more significant than the pharmacological actions of each drug). For example, the popular antiallergy medicine Benadryl (generic name diphenhydramine) is an antihistamine that causes drowsiness, and alcohol acts synergistically with Benadryl to enhance this effect.

Interaction of Alcohol with OTC Allergy/Cold Medications

Many cold and allergy medications are available over the counter, and some of these medications also carry a warning label stating that you should not consume alcohol if you are taking this formulation. Alcohol interacts with many first-generation antihistamines, which are found in both cold and allergy formulations. In addition, alcohol also interacts with analgesics, such as acetaminophen (active component of Tylenol) and salicylate (aspirin), which are present in many cold formulations.

> If you are taking any over-the-counter cold or allergy formulations, it is advisable to limit drinking to not more than one glass of wine or a bottle of beer per day. If you can avoid drinking altogether during this time, it will be in your best interest.

First-generation antihistamines, such as diphenhydramine and chlorpheniramine, are present in many over-the-counter allergy, cold, and sleeping aid formulations. In addition, hydroxyzine (Atarax) is a prescription medication that is widely prescribed for treating various types of allergic reactions. All these medications cross the blood-brain barrier and cause drowsiness by depressing the central nervous system (CNS). In addition, these drugs also cause some impairment of motor function. Therefore, caution must be exercised when driving or operating heavy machinery when you are taking one of these drugs. Alcohol is also a CNS depressant and enhances the drowsiness caused by these drugs. In addition, alcohol acts synergistically with these drugs in impairing motor function. Therefore, if you are taking one of these drugs, you must limit your alcohol consumption. In addition, it is advisable not to drive at all if you are taking any of these drugs and consuming any amount of alcohol.

Many cold medications contain acetaminophen or salicylate. Acetaminophen, when consumed in recommended dosage (not exceeding four 500 mg capsules a day), is a safe analgesic and antipyretic agent (reduces fever). However, overdose of acetaminophen is dangerous because it causes liver damage. When a person consumes excess acetaminophen, a toxic metabolite of acetaminophen is formed, and the liver does not have enough supply of glutathione (an endogenously found tripeptide containing three amino acids) to detoxify that toxic metabolite. This toxic metabolite then damages hepatocytes (cells found in the liver). If an acetaminophen overdose is not treated in a timely manner using a specific antidote (N-acetylcysteine; trade name Mucomyst), acetaminophen overdose could cause death.

If a person is a social drinker (one or two drinks a week), the risk of toxicity from consuming alcohol and acetaminophen is low. Some reports indicate that consuming one drink after ingesting acetaminophen may even reduce the formation of toxic metabolite of acetaminophen by the liver. On the other hand, chronic alcoholics are at an increased risk of developing liver toxicity from consuming even therapeutic dosages of acetaminophen. Chronic alcohol consumption reduces the storage of glutathione in the liver, which detoxifies the toxic metabolite of acetaminophen. In addition, chronic alcoholism may also trigger the liver to produce more toxic metabolite via induction of CYP2E1, a member of liver enzymes (cytochrome P-450 mixed-function oxidase) responsible for drug metabolism.

> If you consume more than two to three drinks a day, you should not take any medication containing acetaminophen without consulting your doctor.

In one study (Wootton and Lee 1990), the authors identified seven alcoholics who had severe liver injury soon after using acetaminophen for therapeutic purposes. All showed markedly high serum levels of liver enzymes indicative of severe liver injury, and three individuals died. The authors concluded that use of acetaminophen by an alcoholic patient is potentially lethal.[10] Furthermore, the elderly population is at higher risk from acetaminophen-alcohol interaction.

Salicylate (aspirin) is a nonsteroidal anti-inflammatory drug that is used in many over-the-counter pain medications. It is normally safe to drink alcohol while you are taking aspirin or ibuprofen if you drink in moderation (up to three drinks of alcohol a day for men, and two to three drinks for women, two to three times in one week). If you drink every day and consume more than three drinks of alcohol, then alcohol may increase the risk of stomach irritation and may even cause gastric bleeding. Regular intakes of salicylate in large dosages may cause gastric irritation, heartburn, and even an ulcer. Alcohol enhances these negative effects of salicylate. Intake of high doses of aspirin (1 gm) increases the blood alcohol level by inhibiting the gastric enzyme alcohol dehydrogenase, which metabolizes alcohol.[11] This enzyme is also present in the liver. On the other hand, low-dose aspirin (usually available in 75 or 81 mg), which is taken by many people on a regular basis to prevent heart attack and stroke, actually decreases one's blood alcohol level. Low-dose aspirin delays the gastric absorption of alcohol when consumed in moderate dosages.[12] Older people who mix alcoholic beverages with large amounts of aspirin for pain relief are at high risk of experiencing an episode of gastric bleeding.[13]

> If you drink regularly and consume more than three alcoholic drinks each day, consult with your physician before taking aspirin or ibuprofen.

Interaction of Alcohol with OTC Pain Medications

Other than acetaminophen and salicylate, ibuprofen, ketoprofen, and naproxen are also available as analgesics in many over-the-counter medications. Like salicylate, all these drugs are classified as "nonsteroidal anti-inflammatory drugs" because they control pain by inhibiting cyclooxygenase enzyme. All these drugs can cause gastric irritation. People who drink in moderation can consume these medications safely, but heavy drinkers should not use these medications without consulting with their physicians because of increased risk of developing gastric bleeding and ulcers. With relatively stronger medications like naproxen and ketoprofen, it is advisable not to drink at all when taking such medications.

Interaction of Alcohol with Prescription Pain Medications

Prescription pain medications can be classified under two broad categories: (1) nonsteroidal anti-inflammatory medications, such as indomethacin, diclofenac, mefenamic acid, and so on; and (2) narcotic analgesics, which are natural opiates such as morphine and codeine, as well as synthetic opiates, such as hydromorphone, oxycodone, hydrocodone, oxymorphone, meperidine, methadone, and propoxyphene.

In general, prescription nonsteroidal anti-inflammatory drugs are much stronger than their OTC counterparts. These drugs also cause gastric irritation, bleeding, and ulcers, and consumption of alcohol increases this risk greatly. Consuming one or two drinks occasionally is not going to cause any harm if you take these medications, but even if you consume two to three drinks on a regular basis, you must discuss this with your physician when such medications are prescribed for you.

Interactions between narcotic analgesics and alcohol cause more serious adverse effects than interactions between alcohol and nonsteroidal anti-inflammatory drugs. These drugs are prescribed in patients to control moderate to severe pain. The combination of alcohol and these narcotic analgesic drugs enhances the sedative and respiratory depression effects of both substances, and may cause severe overdose, prompting a situation that could require hospital admission. Death may occur at a much lower blood morphine level if an individual consumes alcohol.[14] Alcohol interacts with the extended-release mechanism of many opiate narcotic analgesics, causing excessive release of the drug (dose-dumping effect). As a result, coma or even death may occur from an excessive blood level of the opiate medication. Recently, hydromorphone extended-release capsules (Palladone) were withdrawn from the market because of the dose-dumping effect. Alcohol enhances the CNS depression effect of oxymorphone, and such interaction may cause slow respiration, lower blood pressure, and, in some cases, coma. Alcohol increases blood concentration of propoxyphene by reducing its first-pass metabolism. In addition, alcohol also reduces the psychomotor skill of a person by acting in synergy with the opiate pain medication.

If you are taking any narcotic analgesic for pain management, please do not consume alcohol.

Interaction of Alcohol with Sleeping Aids

Insomnia is the most frequently reported sleep symptom, severely affecting up to 15 percent of the U.S. population.[15] Many sleeping aids are available for treating insomnia. Over-the-counter sleeping aids sometimes contain antihistamines, such as diphenhydramine, and interaction of this drug with alcohol has been discussed earlier in the section dealing with the interaction of alcohol with allergy/cold medication. The most important class of drug in treating insomnia is the benzodiazepine class of drugs. There are more than fifty benzodiazepines, although only about fifteen of them are available in the United States. The most commonly prescribed benzodiazepines in the United States are diazepam, temazepam, alprazolam, lorazepam, and clonazepam.

Dosages of benzodiazepines that are sedatives may increase drowsiness if alcohol is consumed. Nobody taking any prescription tranquilizer should be drinking at all. It increases the risk of household and automobile accidents.

> Even a glass of wine may produce enough drowsiness, dizziness, and lack of motor coordination due to interaction with a benzodiazepine drug to make driving a hazard.

A low dose of flurazepam (Dalmane) interacts with a low dose of alcohol to impair driving ability even when alcohol is consumed long after taking the medication.[16] The hazard of interaction between benzodiazepines and alcohol is magnified in elderly people who demonstrate an increased response to benzodiazepines. In the presence of enough alcohol, severe CNS depression may occur in a patient taking any benzodiazepine medication. Acute ingestion of alcohol combined with benzodiazepines is responsible for several toxicological interactions that may have serious clinical consequences. Fatal poisoning involving alcohol and benzodiazepines, especially triazolam, continues to be a serious problem.[17]

Even non-benzodiazepine sleeping aids such as zolpidem (Ambien), zaleplon (Sonata), and eszopiclone (Lunesta) should not be combined with alcohol, because interaction between alcohol and any of these drugs increases the risk of driving when not fully awake (sleep-driving).

Although with the introduction of benzodiazepines old barbiturates are rarely prescribed, alcohol and barbiturates do not mix well at all. A combination of barbiturate and alcohol causes excessive CNS depression and impaired psychomotor performance. There are even reports of death due to concomitant use of alcohol and barbiturates due to severe respiratory depression.[18]

Interaction of Alcohol with Antidepressants

Antidepressant drugs include old monoamine oxidase inhibitors, tricyclic antidepressants, tetracyclic antidepressants, and newer antidepressants, such as selective serotonin reuptake inhibitors (SSRI) and serotonin-norepinephrine reuptake inhibitors (SNRI). Older tricyclic antidepressants such as amitriptyline, nortriptyline, doxepin, and so on are prescribed less frequently than newer SSRI medications. Alcohol increases the sedative effect of tricyclic antidepressants, for example, amitriptyline (Elavil), and also inhibits psychomotor skills, thus making driving hazardous. A chemical called tyramine, found in some beer and wine, interacts with antidepressants (which are monoamine oxidase inhibitors) and can cause a dangerous rise in blood pressure even after a single drink. Tailor et al. (1994) reported a case of hypertensive crisis resulting from drinking tap beer in a patient taking monoamine inhibitor antidepressant phenelzine.[19]

Alcohol heightens the negative side effects of SSRI drugs. The combination of alcohol and any of these drugs may produce increased drowsiness, clouded judgment, slower reflexes, and even suicidal thoughts. Alcohol may also interfere with the clinical efficacy of these drugs.

> Just one alcoholic drink may lead to DWI (driving with impairment) if you are taking an SSRI. Your level may be below the legal limit for driving, but if both alcohol and any SSRI drugs are found in your blood, you may be charged with a DWI because your driving is impaired.

Serotonin is a neurotransmitter that plays a role in one's mood. SSRI medications inhibit serotonin reuptake by presynaptic nerve cells, and higher serotonin levels available outside the nerve cells can bind with specific serotonin receptors to elevate our mood. However, in the presence of excess extracellular serotonin, a life-threatening medical condition known as "serotonin syndrome" may arise. The symptoms include very high heart rate, high blood pressure, severe twitching, and convulsion. If untreated, this syndrome can be fatal. It is unusual to observe serotonin syndrome in a patient receiving a single SSRI medication, but if a patient consumes alcohol in large amounts, especially hard liquor, serotonin syndrome may occur even if one medication is prescribed to the patient. In one report (Velez et al. 2004), the authors described life-threatening serotonin syndrome in a fifty-seven-year-old man who was taking paroxetine (Paxil) and who consumed a pint of hard liquor.[20]

Interaction of Alcohol with Antidiabetic Medications

Antidiabetic medications, also known as oral hypoglycemic agents, are prescribed to patients with type 2 diabetes (non-insulin-dependent diabetes) in order to lower serum concentration of sugar (glucose). Metformin (Glucophage) is a popular first-line oral hypoglycemic agent, and one potential side effect of this medication is to increase the concentration of lactic acid in the blood, causing a syndrome called lactic acidosis. If the concentration of lactic acid is very high in the blood, it may even cause a medical emergency. A person taking metformin should only drink in moderation, because excess alcohol intake may cause lactic acidosis due to the interaction of excess alcohol with metformin.

Alcohol may also interact with various sulfonylureas, another popular class of oral hypoglycemic agent. The effects are sometimes opposite. For example, a patient taking glipizide (Glucotrol) may find his or her blood sugar concentration stays low longer (hypoglycemia), while a person taking tolbutamide (Orinase) may find a lack of glucose control because alcohol reduces the effectiveness of this drug. Even two to three drinks may trigger this effect.

Alcohol also enhances the glucose-lowering effect of insulin. Therefore, a person with diabetes taking either insulin or oral hypoglycemic agents should only drink occasionally and limit themselves to no more than two standard drinks. Drinking hard liquor may be dangerous for these patients, because alcohol content may be higher than the standard drink. Caution should also be exercised if you drink mixed drinks, because one drink may be equivalent to two to three standard drinks in terms of alcohol content. Please tell your physician if you drink on a regular basis, so that your doctor can properly select your medication and guide you in how much drinking is safe when you are taking an oral hypoglycemic agent.

Interaction of Alcohol with Antibiotics

There are many classes of antibiotics, including aminoglycosides, cephalosporins, macrolide antibiotics, penicillins, quinolones, sulfonamides, and tetracycline. Each of these classes of drugs contains many members, and there are also other classes of antibiotics with few members. Fortunately, only a few antibiotics approved for use in the United States show clinically significant drug interaction with alcohol, and drinking must be avoided when taking any of these medications. These antibiotics carry a warning label stating that if you are taking the medication, you should avoid alcohol consumption altogether as long as you are taking that medication. Even one drink may potentiate an adverse effect if you are taking one of these specific antibiotics. Cephalosporins, such as cefamandole, cefotetan, and cefoperazone, interact with alcohol even after one drink. Symptoms include flushing, wheezing, breathing difficulty, rapid heartbeat, and profound sweating, as well as nausea and vomiting, and such symptoms may develop within fifteen to thirty minutes after drink-ing.[21] It is advisable not to drink for an additional two to three days after you complete the course of one of these cephalosporins. Alcohol reduces blood concentration, thus the effectiveness of doxycycline may also in-terfere with the absorption of erythromycin. Alcohol must be avoided if you take metronidazole (Flagyl), tinidazole (Tindamax), ketoconazole (Nizoral), furazolidone (Furoxone), griseofulvin (Grisactin), and the anti-malarial drug quinacrine (Atabrine).

Interaction between metronidazole and alcohol (consuming high amounts of alcohol) may even cause fatality. In one case report, a thirty-one-year-old woman died from taking metronidazole and drinking heav-ily. Her blood alcohol was elevated to 162 mg/dL (more than double the legal limit of drinking, 80 mg/dL).[22]

Interaction of Alcohol with Antiulcer Medications

The commonly prescribed antiulcer medications (also used in treating acid reflux), such as cimetidine (Tagamet) and ranitidine (Zantac), may prolong the effect of alcohol. DiPadova et al. (1992) studied the interac-tions between alcohol and cimetidine, ranitidine, and famotidine using human subjects. Cimetidine showed a greater effect on blood alcohol levels compared to ranitidine, but famotidine showed no significant ef-fect. The authors concluded that patients taking cimetidine or ranitidine should be warned of possible impairments after consumption of alcohol in quantities usually considered safe when not taking these medications.[23]

Interaction of Alcohol with Anticoagulants

Warfarin (Coumadin) is prescribed to reduce blood clotting. However, excessive action of warfarin is dangerous, because a patient may bleed to death (life-threatening hemorrhages). Acute alcohol consumption increases the effectiveness of warfarin, while chronic alcohol consump-tion reduces the effectiveness of warfarin therapy. This opposing effect of acute versus chronic alcohol consumption on warfarin therapy is a medical challenge.[24] Warfarin therapy must be monitored very carefully in patients who drink on a regular basis.

Interaction of Alcohol with Cardiovascular Medications

This class of drugs includes a wide variety of medications prescribed to treat ailments of the heart and the circulatory system. Acute alcohol con-sumption interacts with some of these drugs, causing dizziness or faint-ing upon standing. These drugs include nitroglycerin, methyldopa (Al-domet), hydralazine (Apresoline), and guanethidine (Ismelin). Chronic alcohol consumption also reduces the efficacy of propranolol. Verapamil increases blood alcohol level and prolongs its effect.

Interaction of Alcohol with Miscellaneous Drugs

Phenytoin (Dilantin) is used to treat patients with seizure disorders. People who drink regularly may experience a decreased effect of this medication and may require a higher dosage. Regular drinkers may also require a higher dosage of propofol (Diprivan). Metoclopramide (Reglan) increases absorption of alcohol and prolongs its effect. A patient taking this medication and consuming alcohol may experience additional sedation and may be unable to drive. Methotrexate is an anticancer drug. A low dose of methotrexate is also used in treating patients with rheumatoid arthritis. Alcohol consumption increases the risk for methotrexate-induced liver toxicity. The manufacturer of this drug advises against prescribing this drug to patients who drink alcohol excessively.

ABUSING ALCOHOL AND DRUGS
SIMULTANEOUSLY: A RECIPE FOR DEATH

A 2006 survey indicated that about 20.4 million Americans (8.3 percent) ages twelve and older were currently illicit drug abusers, meaning they abused drugs during the month prior to the survey. The survey also revealed that marijuana was the most common illicit drug abused, followed by cocaine, ecstasy, and methamphetamine.[25] Other drugs abused include various benzodiazepines, barbiturates, opiates (heroin, morphine, codeine, oxycodone, and methadone), and phencyclidine. In addition, various young people also abuse rave party drugs, mainly ecstasy (3,4-methylenedioxymethamphetamine), ketamine, gamma-hydroxybutyric acid (GHB), and flunitrazepam (Rohypnol). In order to enhance the experience of abused drugs, people also consume large amounts of alcohol.

Abusing alcohol and drugs at the same time is a recipe for death. All of these drugs can cause death due to drug overdose. Alcohol significantly enhances the adverse effects of these abused drugs, accelerating death from overdose. There are numerous reports in the medical literature documenting significantly lesser amounts of various abused drugs present in the postmortem blood of the victim when alcohol was also present in the blood.

Think twice before you abuse any drug, and think at least ten times before you abuse alcohol and drugs at the same time. It could be your last night on this planet if you do not think about the possible consequences.

Cocaethylene: A Messenger of Death

Although a combination of any abused drug and alcohol is potentially lethal, the combination of cocaine and alcohol is probably the most dangerous recipe for death. The body detoxifies cocaine into a harmless compound called benzoylecgonine. Unfortunately, when cocaine and alcohol are consumed at the same time, this metabolic detoxification of cocaine is altered, and a dangerous active metabolite of cocaine is formed due to an interaction with alcohol. This dangerous metabolite is called cocaethylene. Alcohol also increases other toxic metabolites of cocaine, for example norcocaine. Alcohol also increases the blood level of cocaine, thus prolonging its toxicity. In general, if a person who overdoses on cocaine is admitted to the hospital in a timely fashion, the victim has a good chance of survival. In contrast, later rebound toxicity causing fatality may occur in a victim abusing both cocaine and alcohol.[26]

CONCLUSION

Out of almost 5,000 drugs (combining prescription and OTC drugs), only a small fraction of drugs demonstrate a clinically significant interaction with alcohol. However, when such an interaction is present, extreme care must be exercised when you drink. If you are taking an over-the-counter cold or allergy medication, the best place to start is to study the medication label and talk to the pharmacist on staff in the store. Your pharmacist is very familiar with all drug-drug and drug-alcohol interactions. If the advice is not to drink at all, please follow the advice—it can save you from all sorts of trouble. If you are a heavy drinker, you may get liver damage from simply consuming Tylenol. Consult with your pharmacist to see if ibuprofen is more appropriate for pain relief. If you are taking a prescription drug, consult with your physician about whether you can drink alcohol occasionally or not when taking this medication. If you are a heavy drinker, tell your doctor, because you may need a different drug or a higher dosage of a drug. Again, studying the label on your medication is a good idea. If you do your homework and study all warning labels on medications and abide by the warnings, you can avoid almost all troubles with drug-alcohol interactions.

Do not abuse drugs. Abusing drugs does not solve any problems or help you get through any difficulty. It only makes matters worse. Talk to your parents, relatives, teachers, and friends or loved ones for help. Do not abuse drugs and alcohol at the same time—unless you have a death wish.

NOTES

1. B. F. Sands, C. M. Knapp, and D. A. Ciraulo, "Medical Consequence of Alcohol-Drug Interaction," *Alcohol Health & Research World* 17, no. 4 (December 1993): 316–20.

2. L. T. Midanik and R. Room, "The Epidemiology of Alcohol Consumption," *Alcohol Health & Research World* 16, no. 3 (September 1993): 183–90.

3. See http://www.samhsa.gov/newsroom/advisories/0703135521.aspx.

4. See http://www.samhsa.gov/news/newsrelease/060510_dawn2htm (accessed June 26, 2009).

5. A. Koski, E. Vuori, and I. Ojanpera, "Relation of Postmortem Blood Alcohol and Drug Concentrations in Fetal Poisonings Involving Amitriptyline, Propoxyphene and Promazine," *Human and Experimental Toxicology* 24, no. 8 (August 2005): 389–96.

6. M. Hickman, A. Longford-Hughes, C. Bailey, J. Macleod, et al., "Does Alcohol Increase the Risk of Overdose Death? The Need for a Translational Approach," *Addiction* 103, no. 7 (July 2008): 1060–62.

7. V. Valle, H. Gosney, and J. Sinclair, "Qualitative Analysis of Coroners' Data into the Unusual Deaths in Children and Adolescents," *Child Care and Health Development* 34, no. 6 (November 2008): 721–31.

8. B. Levine, D. Green-Johnson, S. Hogan, and J. E. Smialek, "A Cyproheptadine Fatality," *Journal of Analytical Toxicology* 22, no. 1 (January–February 1998): 72–74.

9. G. S. Bleumink, A. C. van Vliet, A. van der Tholen, and B. H. Stricker, "Fatal Combination of Moclobemide Overdose and Whiskey," *Netherlands Journal of Medicine* 61, no. 3 (March 2003): 88–90.

10. F. T. Wootton and W. M. Lee, "Acetaminophen Hepatotoxicity in the Alcoholic," *Southern Medical Journal* 83, no. 9 (September1990): 1047–49.

11. R. T. Gentry, E. Baraona, I. Amir, R. Roine, et al., "Mechanism of the Aspirin-Induced Rise in Blood Alcohol Levels," *Life Sciences* 65, no. 23 (October 1999): 2505–12.

12. S. Kechagias, K. A. Jonsson, B. Norlander, B. Carisson, et al., "Low-Dose Aspirin Decreases Blood Alcohol Concentrations by Delaying Gastric Emptying," *European Journal of Clinical Pharmacology* 53, nos. 3–4 (December 1997): 241–46.

13. M. C. Dufour, L. Archer, and E. Gordis, "Alcohol and the Elderly," *Clinical and Geriatric Medicine* 8, no. 1 (February 1992): 127–41.

14. F. Johnson, G. Wagner, S. Sun, and J. Stauffer, "Effect of Concomitant Ingestion of Alcohol on the In Vivo Pharmacokinetics of KADIAN (Morphine Sulfate Extended Release) Capsules," *Journal of Pain: Official Journal of American Pain Society* 9, no. 4 (April 2008): 330–36.

15. G. S. Richardson, T. Roth, and J. A. Kramer, "Management of Insomnia: The Role of Zaleplon," *Medscape General Medicine* 4, no. 1 (March 2002): 9.

16. M. Linnolia, M. J. Mattila, and B. S. Kitchell, "Drug Interactions with Alcohol," *Drugs* 18, no. 4 (October 1979): 299–311.

17. E. Tanaka, "Toxicological Interactions between Alcohol and Benzodiazepines," *Journal of Toxicology: Clinical Toxicology* 40, no. 1 (January 2002): 69–75.

18. H. Kinoshita, M. Nishiguchi, S. Kasuda, H. Quchi, et al., "An Autopsy Case of Poisoning with Ethanol and Psychotropic Drugs," *Soudni Lekkarstivi* 53, no. 2 (April 2008): 16–17.

19. S. A. Tailor, K. I. Shulman, S. E. Walker, J. Moss, et al., "Hypertensive Crisis Associated with Phenelzine and Tap Beer: A Reanalysis of the Role of Pressor Amines in Beer," *Journal of Clinical Psychopharmacology* 14, no. 1 (February 1994): 5014.

20. L. I. Velez, G. Shepherd, B. S. Roth, and F. L. Benitez, "Serotonin Syndrome with Elevated Paroxetine Concentrations," *Annals of Pharmacotherapy* 38, no. 2 (February 2004): 269–72.

21. H. Portier, J. M. Chalopin, M. Freysz, and Y. Tanter, "Interaction between Cephalosporins and Alcohol," *Lancet* 2, no. 8188 (August 1980): 263.

22. S. J. Cina, R. A. Russell, and S. E. Conradi, "Sudden Death Due to Metronidazole/Ethanol Interaction," *American Journal of Forensic Medicine and Pathology* 17, no. 4 (December 1996): 343–46.

23. C. DiPadova, R. Roine, M. Frezza, R. T. Gentry, et al., "Effects of Ranitidine on Blood Alcohol Levels after Ethanol Ingestion: Comparison with H-2 Receptor Antagonists," *Journal of the American Medical Association* 267, no. 1 (January 1992): 83–86.

24. D. E. Havrda, T. Mai, and J. Chonlahan, "Enhanced Antithrombotic Effect of Warfarin Associated with Low-Dose Alcohol Consumption," *Pharmacotherapy* 25, no. 2 (February 2005): 303–7.

25. National Survey on Drug Use and Health, U.S. Department of Health and Human Services, Washington, D.C., Government Printing Office, 2006, http:// oas.samhsa.gov.

26. M. B. Patel, M. Opreanu, A. J. Shah, K. Pandya, et al., "Cocaine and Alcohol: A Potential Lethal Duo," *American Journal of Medicine* 122, no. 1 (January 2009): e5–6.

9

Workplace Alcohol and Drug Testing

When Not to Drink at All

By far the most common legal substance that can affect job performance is alcohol (ethyl alcohol). Many studies have clearly documented that heavy drinking and misuse of alcohol over time is associated with absenteeism, industrial accidents, poor job performance, job turnover, lack of self direction, poor interpersonal relations with coworkers, and lower level of job satisfaction, as well as theft, vandalism, and negative work behavior.[1] Historically, employers have relied on supervisors to identify such problem employees. Later, workplace drug and alcohol testing programs evolved to address these issues using a more rigorous, direct approach. The anticipated effect of workplace alcohol and drug testing is to deter employees from abusing alcohol and drugs and to prevent workplace accidents, as well as to improve productivity and morale.

Workplace drug testing has evolved from virtually nonexistent in the 1980s to a point where there is widespread acceptance of drug testing programs by employers, both in the public and private sector. The federal drug testing programs applied to 1.8 million employees in 2005. The types of testing conducted have included job applicants, postaccident/ unsafe practice, reasonable suspicion, follow-up to treatment, random, and voluntary testing.[2]

Private employers also embrace the practice of preemployment and workplace drug testing in order to achieve a drug-free workplace. Workplace drug testing deters employees from abusing drugs, as reflected in the Drug Testing Index published by Quest Diagnostics, a reputable national reference laboratory performing workplace drug testing. According to the Drug Testing Index published on March 12, 2008, among the combined U.S. workforces, only 3.8 percent of the drug tests had positive results in 2007 compared to 13.6 percent test results that were positive in 1988. In addition, amphetamine, methamphetamine, and cocaine abuse by American workers is also in decline.[3]

Nevertheless, according to a 2007 federal government report, drug and alcohol abuse continues to be a serious problem in the United States, with an estimated 9.4 million workers between the ages of eighteen and sixty-four reporting illicit drug use in the past month of the survey, while an estimated 10.6 million workers were dependent on or abused alcohol. The prevalence of drug abuse was highest among workers who were between eighteen and twenty-five. In addition, food service workers and construction workers showed a higher prevalence of drug abuse than other occupational groups. The prevalence of alcohol use was also highest in workers between the ages of eighteen and twenty-five. Construction workers had the highest prevalence of past-month heavy alcohol use, followed by workers in installation, maintenance, and repair businesses.[4] However, it is undisputed that workplace drug testing deters employees from drug abuse.[5]

Preemployment drug testing is more common than alcohol testing. However, both alcohol and drug tests are mandated by the federal government for personnel in safety-sensitive positions. These personnel include: aviation personnel, commercial drivers and personnel working in commercial transportation, pipeline workers and personnel involved in transporting hazardous materials, maritime personnel, and military personnel.

Many employers in the private sector also implement both alcohol and drug testing for employees in security-sensitive positions or jobs related to public safety or health, such as hospital nurses and related health care providers. Although the focus of this book is on alcohol, because workplace alcohol and drug testing are interrelated, in this chapter, I discuss both topics so that readers can get familiar with the current practice of workplace alcohol and drug testing. Detailed discussions on workplace alcohol and drug testing, including applicable laws, technical aspects of such testing, the role of medical review officers, and the consequences of positive alcohol and drug testing results in the workplace, is beyond the scope of this book. This chapter provides only an overview.

HOW WORKPLACE DRUG AND ALCOHOL TESTING EVOLVED

On September 15, 1986, President Reagan issued Executive Order No. 12564, which directed all federal employees involved in law enforcement, national security, protection of life and property, and public health and safety, as well as other functions requiring a high degree of public trust, to be subjected to mandatory drug testing. Following this executive order, the U.S. Department of Health and Human Services developed guidelines and protocols on testing for drugs of abuse. The overall testing process under mandatory drug testing guidelines consists of proper collection of specimens, initiation of a chain of custody (record of personnel who have possession of the specimen from the time of collection to the time of analysis), and analysis of the specimen by a Substance Abuse and Mental Health Services Administration (SAMHSA) certified laboratory.

Commercial motor vehicles make up about 4 percent of police-reported crashes and 12 percent of traffic fatalities. The role of alcohol in commercial motor vehicle accidents was first recognized in 1970, and then subsequent studies showed that a blood alcohol level of 0.1 percent (100 mg/100ml of blood: 100 mg/dL) was consistently associated with fatally injured drivers. Prompted by some highly publicized alcohol-related commercial transportation accidents, including the 1989 Exxon Valdez oil spill in Alaska, the 1990 conviction of three Northwest Airlines pilots for having significant blood alcohol while on duty, and a 1991 New York subway derailment, the U.S. Congress passed the Omnibus Transportation Employee Testing Act in 1991, which requires drug and alcohol testing of safety-sensitive employees working in aviation, trucking, railroads, mass transit, pipeline, and other transportation industries.[6] The U.S. Department of Transportation (DOT) publishes rules on who must conduct drug testing, what procedures to use, and when such testing should be done. These regulations are applicable to roughly 12.1 million people and are encompassed in 49 Code of Federal Regulations Part 40 (49CFR40). The Office of Drug and Alcohol Policy and Compliance (ODAPC) publishes, implements, and provides authoritative interpretations of these results.

The Department of Defense also developed its own regulations for contractors working in the national security arena (Section 48 CFR 252, 223-7004). Under these regulations defense contractors must maintain a drug-free workplace that includes a comprehensive employee assistance program, provision for self-referral and supervisory referrals for drug testing, supervisory training on detecting and responding to illegal drug use, and a carefully controlled and monitored employee drug testing policy. The U.S. Department of Energy, the National Aeronautics and Space Administration (NASA), and the Nuclear Regulatory Commission (NRC) all have drug testing requirements for safety-sensitive contractors.

In addition to federal laws and regulations, many states have their own drug laws. In general, three types of state legislation may affect workplace drug testing policy:

1. State and local laws regulating drug testing
2. State worker's compensation laws
3. State unemployment insurance laws

In the interest of promoting a safer work environment, some states offer employer discounts on their workers' compensation insurance premium, and many states deny workers' compensation where injuries are determined to be related to substance abuse. In addition, some states have policies to deny unemployment benefits to people who are fired due to positive drug testing results or drug abuse.

CURRENT PRACTICES OF WORKPLACE
DRUG AND ALCOHOL TESTING

Preemployment drug testing is the most common type of workplace drug testing; alcohol testing along with drug testing is less common, unless the position is security sensitive. In general, a person undergoing preemployment drug testing has few legal rights, and in most cases, employment is denied if the drug test is failed. An employer may also conduct drug testing and alcohol testing under the following circumstances, especially for employees who are working in safety-sensitive positions:

- Annual physical test
- Pre-promotion test
- Postaccident drug testing
- Treatment follow-up test
- Return to duty drug testing
- Random, unannounced drug testing

Usually five drug classes are tested, including amphetamine and methamphetamine, cocaine, marijuana, opiates, and phencyclidine, in federally mandated workplace drug testing programs. Private employers may also test for additional drugs, such as benzodiazepines, barbiturates, methadone, methaqualone, and propoxyphene.

The Federal Motor Carrier Safety Administration (FMCSA) issues guidelines regarding alcohol and drug testing rules for people required to obtain a commercial driver's license. The Department of Transportation (DOT) rules include procedures for urine drug testing and breath alcohol testing. Initially, the agency issued urine drug testing rules in December 1989, and then in 1994 the rules were amended to add breath alcohol testing procedures because alcohol is widely consumed by the general population in the United States.

In December 2000, modification of the initial guidelines was published in order to incorporate input from the public sector concerning the final rules. In August 2001, the FMCSA revised modal-specific drug and alcohol testing regulations (published in 49 Code of Federal Regulations Part 382) to reflect the revisions made in 2000. Finally, in 2008 the DOT amended certain provisions of its drug and alcohol testing procedures to change instructions to collectors, laboratories, medical review officers, and employers regarding adulterated, substituted, diluted, and invalid urine specimen results. These changes were intended to create consistency with specimen validity requirements established by the U.S. Department of Health and Human Services. The final rule was published in the *Federal Register* on June 25, 2008.[7] Although meant for drug and alcohol testing for appropriate federal employees, many private corporations also use these guidelines to develop their own workplace drug and/or alcohol testing policies.

Who Is Tested?

In general, any person seeking employment in the public or private sector may be subjected to preemployment drug testing. However, only certain personnel hired for security-sensitive positions are subjected to both alcohol and drug testing. The FMCSA rules apply to safety-sensitive employees. Those who operate commercial motor vehicles that require a commercial driver's license may be subjected to both alcohol and drug testing. These personnel are listed in table 9.1.

Use of alcohol is prohibited while working in such security-sensitive jobs. In addition, alcohol should not be consumed for at least four hours before reporting for such jobs. Abuse of any illicit drug is not permitted under any circumstances.

Table 9.1. Personnel Subjected to Workplace Alcohol and Drug Testing

Commercial Motor Vehicle–Related Personnel
Anyone who owns or leases commercial motor vehicles
Anyone who assigns drivers to operate commercial motor vehicles
Federal, state, and local governments
For-hire motor carriers
Private motor carriers
Civic organizations (disabled veteran transport, Boy/Girl Scouts, etc.)
Church bus drivers

Aviation Personnel
Flight crew, including pilots
Flight attendants
Flight instructors
Aircraft dispatch personnel
Aircraft maintenance and preventive maintenance personnel
Ground security coordinators
Aviation screening personnel
Air traffic controllers

The Federal Aviation Administration (FAA) determines drug and alcohol testing guidelines applicable to airline personnel and air traffic controllers. The guidelines were published in the DOT's workplace drug and alcohol testing programs (Title 49, CFR Part 40).

HOW WORKPLACE ALCOHOL AND
DRUG TESTING ARE CONDUCTED

The current guidelines allow for screening tests to be conducted using saliva devices or appropriate breath analyzers approved by the National Highway Traffic Safety Administration in order to determine the blood alcohol level of the person being tested. Direct determination of blood alcohol by drawing blood from the arm of a person is not done. Two tests are required to determine if a person has a prohibited alcohol concentration. A screening test is conducted first. Any result less than 0.02 percent (20 mg/dL) alcohol concentration is considered a "negative" test. If the alcohol concentration is 0.02 percent or greater, a second confirmation test must be conducted after a waiting period of at least fifteen minutes, but the confirmation must be performed within thirty minutes of the initial screening test. A new mouthpiece and an evidential breath testing device must be used to assure proper registering of the results. The person undergoing drug testing and the individual conducting the confirmation breath test (called a breath alcohol technician or BAT) must complete the alcohol testing form to ensure that the results are properly recorded. It is also important to print out the results, including date and time, a sequential test number, and the name and serial number of the instrument to ensure the reliability of the results. The confirmation test results determine if any actions must be taken.

In the United States, Intoximeter, Alcosensor, Alcotest, Intoxilyzer, and DataMaster are commonly used breath analyzers. A person being tested blows into a breath analyzer, and the results are reported as blood alcohol concentration. Breath analyzers do not directly measure the blood alcohol level, but rather estimate blood alcohol levels indirectly by measuring the amount of alcohol in one's breath (see chapter 6 for a more in-depth discussion on breath analyzers).

Drug testing is conducted by analyzing urine specimens. The analysis is performed at laboratories certified and monitored by the SAMHSA, an agency under the Department of Health and Human Services (DHHS). The specimen collection procedures and chain of custody ensure that the specimen's security, proper identification, and integrity are not compromised. The Omnibus Transportation Employee Testing Act of 1991 requires that drug testing procedures for commercial motor vehicle drivers include split specimen procedures. Each urine specimen is subdivided into two bottles labeled as a "primary" and a "split" specimen. Both bottles are sent to a laboratory. Only the primary specimen is opened and used for the urinalysis. The split specimen bottle remains sealed and is stored at the laboratory. If the analysis of the primary specimen confirms the presence of illegal, controlled substances, the driver has seventy-two hours to request the split specimen be sent to another DHHS-certified laboratory for analysis. This split specimen procedure essentially provides the driver with an opportunity for a "second opinion." All urine specimens are analyzed for marijuana, cocaine (as benzoylecgonine, a cocaine metabolite), amphetamines, opiates, and phencyclidine. The testing is a two-stage process. First, a screening test is performed. If it is positive for one or more of the drugs, then a confirmation test is performed for each identified drug using state-of-the-art gas chromatography/mass spectrometry (GC/MS) analysis. GC/MS confirmation ensures that over-the-counter medications or preparations are not reported as positive results. After conducting the drug test, the laboratory reports the result to the appropriate agency personnel. All drug test results are reviewed and interpreted by a physician (medical review officer [MRO]) before they are reported to the employer. If the laboratory reports a positive result to the MRO, the MRO contacts the person and conducts an interview to determine if there is an alternative medical explanation for the drugs found in the driver's urine specimen.

All alcohol and drug testing results are confidential. Employees failing workplace alcohol and/or drug testing may be given an opportunity to undergo drug or alcohol rehabilitation. After successful drug rehabilitation, a person is eligible to work again depending on the position under the Americans with Disabilities Act.

LEGAL GUIDELINES FOR WORKPLACE
ALCOHOL AND DRUG TESTING

The legal limit for driving in all states in the United States is 0.08 percent blood alcohol (80 mg/dL) or less. However, personnel involved in safety-sensitive positions are subjected to more stringent requirements. As implemented on January 1, 1995, the mandatory alcohol testing program for commercial motor vehicle drivers includes preemployment testing, random testing, reasonable suspicion testing, and postaccident testing. Random testing requires that randomly sampled employees report to the job site immediately before, during, or after their driving shift to be tested for the presence of drugs and/or alcohol. Commercial drivers with a blood alcohol level of 0.04 percent (40 mg/dL) or higher should be suspended immediately. Those who register a blood alcohol between 0.02 to 0.03 percent should be removed from their duties for twenty-four hours. In the case of an accident, all involved drivers are required to submit to alcohol testing within two hours. Reasonable suspicion testing allows an employer to test an employee if appearance, behavior, speech, or breath/body odor shows signs of alcohol use.[8] The employee's refusal to be tested for blood alcohol or not cooperating with the testing proposal is considered a violation of the rule, and under such circumstances the breath analyzer test should be considered positive and appropriate action taken against the person refusing to take the test.

According to a news report published recently in the *St. Petersburg Times*, a school superintendent recommended that the school board fire a bus driver who failed an alcohol breath test. On the evening of September 17, 2009, the driver sat down for dinner with her husband and consumed a couple of 16-ounce beers. After the meal she had three or four cocktails, the last one at 11 PM. Bus drivers are forbidden from consuming alcohol within twelve hours of getting behind the wheel. The driver started her pre-trip preparation at 5:55 AM and admitted that she violated the twelve-hour rule. She was selected for a random alcohol test, and when she returned to the bus depot, her first test showed a blood alcohol concentration of 0.057 percent (57mg/dL). A second test a few minutes later showed a blood alcohol level of 0.053 percent, and, finally, another test at 10:17 AM showed a level of 0.043 percent. Two more tests on a second breath testing machine tested within the next forty-five minutes demonstrated blood alcohol levels of 0.029 percent and 0.028 percent, respectively. The driver was suspended and the school superintendent recommended that the school board terminate her employment.[9]

The Federal Aviation Administration also has strict guidelines for alcohol consumption for security- and safety-sensitive personnel involved in the aviation industry. Airline pilots must abide by the current regulations governing alcohol use, and the FAA can even take emergency revocation action against a pilot's airman certificate when a pilot is in violation of the agency's alcohol and drug policy. The FAA has a long-standing policy of eight hours of prohibition against pre-duty alcohol consumption. Different airlines may have policies where pilots must refrain from consuming alcohol longer than eight hours. Because of extremely low acceptable limits for blood alcohol in pilots, it is possible that a pilot may not be able to fly the airplane despite not consuming alcohol for eight hours. The current regulation prohibits pilots from performing safety-sensitive duties with a blood alcohol level of 0.02 percent or higher. A reported alcohol level between 0.02 and 0.039 percent, while not a rule violation, may result in the pilot being grounded for an additional eight hours, or until the alcohol level is reduced below the 0.02 percent limit. Reporting for duty or being on duty with a blood alcohol level of 0.04 percent or higher as measured by a breath analyzer or other method is a serious violation of FAA regulations, and the pilot may be subject to stiff penalties.

A United Airlines pilot was pulled from his transatlantic flight from London to Chicago after a coworker suspected him of being drunk. He failed the breath test, and a subsequent blood alcohol test showed a level of 0.05 percent (50 mg/dL), well above the acceptable limit of 0.02 percent (20 mg/dL), at or below which a pilot is eligible to fly the aircraft. The United flight carrying 124 passengers was canceled, and passengers were put on different carriers. The pilot was remorseful and pleaded guilty to the charges against him. Washington lawyer Chris Humphreys commented that an American Airlines pilot who recorded a blood alcohol level of 0.039 percent (39 mg/dL) was given a fine in July 2009. Another pilot with a blood alcohol level of 0.06 percent (60 mg/dL) was given a suspended sentence.[10]

Legal limits for blood alcohol levels in pilots, commercial drivers, and other personnel involved in safety-sensitive positions, such as miners, mariners, and so on, are extremely low, and consuming just one drink prior to reporting for duty is enough to get a blood alcohol level above the acceptable limit. Even consuming moderate to high amounts of alcohol the night before (eight to twelve hours prior to reporting to duty) may be problematic. Caution must be exercised by these personnel regarding alcohol consumption prior to reporting for duty. Any presence of illicit drugs in the urine of a person undergoing workplace alcohol or drug testing is a violation. However, some prescription drugs, such as narcotic analgesics, may cause a positive workplace drug testing result. The person must establish during his or her interview with the medical review officer (MRO) that such prescription drugs are being taken under the supervision of a licensed medical practitioner. In addition, the MRO may verify that information independently with the individual's physician in order for that individual to pass the drug test.

The U.S. Department of Homeland Security also enforces a strict policy to ensure military personnel are not affected by alcohol and drug abuse. Individuals applying for active duty in the U.S. Army, U.S. Army Reserves, Army National Guard, U.S. Navy, U.S. Marines, or the U.S. Air Force are given a drug and alcohol test as a part of their initial physical exam at the Military Entrance Processing Station. If any individual tests positive for alcohol or marijuana, he or she cannot join the military and, at the discretion of the commander, may receive a waiver for being tested after waiting for forty-five days. If still testing positive, a final waiver may be granted again at the discretion of the commander. After waiting for one year, if the individual fails the test, the person is permanently disqualified from joining the military. If a person tests positive for cocaine, a waiver may be granted and the person must wait for a year before being retested. If the second test is positive, that person is permanently disqualified from joining any active duty. However, during the first test, if a person tests positive for any drug other than alcohol, marijuana, or cocaine, that person is permanently disqualified. The Department of Defense mandates that several drugs must be tested for, including marijuana, cocaine, amphetamine, and opiates, while tests for barbiturates, phencyclidine, and LSD (lysergic acid diethylamide) are done on a random rational basis. Steroids can also be tested for if indicated.

Active duty members are not allowed to consume any alcohol if below the age of twenty-one. In addition, alcohol cannot be consumed twelve hours prior to joining active duty, while in uniform, within twelve hours of operating a motor vehicle, and any other time as restricted by the commander. Possession or sales of illegal drugs, as well as abuse of prescription medications, are not tolerated in the military, and active duty personnel are subjected to regular alcohol and drug testing, at least once a year. Failure to pass an alcohol or drug test may lead to disciplinary action. Military personnel are usually younger than the general U.S. population, and there are more men than women. However, due to strict drug and alcohol testing policies in place since December 1981, drug abuse among military personnel is much lower than the general U.S. population. According to the latest report available, in 2005, 4.6 percent of military personnel admitted drug abuse based on an anonymous survey by the Department of Defense, while in the general American population, 8.3 percent admitted drug abuse based on an anonymous survey conducted by the federal government. Drug abuse is also higher among the younger population (ages eighteen to twenty-five). In that group, 6.8 percent of military personnel admitted abuse of a drug compared to 18.8 percent of people in the general population.[11]

Alcohol Testing in Urine

Federal workplace alcohol and drug testing programs use breath tests for alcohol and urine tests for drugs of abuse. However, an extensive number of commercial international maritime workplace alcohol and drug testing programs utilize urine samples for both alcohol and drugs (amphetamines, barbiturates, benzodiazepines, buprenorphine, marijuana, cocaine, methadone, opiates, and propoxyphene).[12] In addition, administrators of many hospitals use urine specimens for both alcohol and drug testing. Alcohol may appear in the urine within two hours of consumption and may be detected in the urine longer than in the blood, up to twelve to twenty-four hours after consumption of alcohol. Just after drinking, in the early absorption phase, the urine alcohol concentration (UAC) to blood alcohol concentration (BAC) ratio is less than in the late absorption phase when the UAC to BAC is between 1.0 and 1.2. After absorption is complete, UAC to BAC ratio is around 1.3 to 1.4.[13] Urine concentrations of ethanol, as reported by some laboratories, can be convertible to blood levels by the following formula: divide the urine concentration by 1.3, provided alcohol is not in the early absorptive stage. For instance, the urine concentration of 0.08 percent is equivalent to a blood concentration of 0.06 percent. There is, however, some individual variation in this ratio, and urine alcohol measurement can only provide an approximate level of blood alcohol. Ethanol is screened in urine using an automated alcohol dehydrogenase–based enzymatic assay and confirmed by quantitative gas chromatography. This method also allows the separation and quantitation (amount present) by many volatile substances such as methanol, isopropyl alcohol, and ethylene glycol, if present in the urine.

However, false positive results in urine alcohol tests may be encountered in patients suffering from diabetes, because sugar present in the urine specimen can be converted into alcohol by bacteria or yeast. Jones et al. (2000) reported high urinary alcohol concentrations of 82 mg/dL and 102 mg/dL in two victims of date rape who denied any alcohol consumption. Both girls (ages fifteen and eighteen) suffered from diabetes mellitus. The presence of glucose in urine and the high risk of yeast (fungus) infection in female diabetics suggests that ethanol was produced by fermentation after the collection of the urine specimens, and positive ethanol results in their urine specimens was an artifact. Therefore, it is important to add a preservative like sodium fluoride to the collection cup in order to avoid such false positive urine alcohol results.[14]

In another report (Helander et al. 2009), one subject demonstrated a urine ethanol concentration of 10.8 gm/L (1080 mg/dL), a concentration not physiologically possible. Low levels of ethyl glucuronide and ethyl sulfate, minor metabolites of ethanol, were also detected, raising suspicion regarding unexpectedly high urine alcohol level. The urine tested positive for *Candida albicans*, fermenting yeast causing yeast infection in humans, thus further raising the suspicion that the alcohol level detected in the urine was due to postcollection formation of ethanol by the yeast found in the specimen. In order to investigate this false positive case of urinary ethanol determination, the authors analyzed another twenty-four specimens collected from other individuals and observed the presence of ten of fifteen ethanol positive specimens and four of nine ethanol negative specimens where yeast and/or bacteria were present. In four ethanol positive specimens, no ethanol metabolite was found (ethyl glucuronide or ethyl sulfate), indicating that these urine specimens had false positive results for ethanol. When yeast negative but bacteria positive specimens were supplemented with glucose and stored for a week, ethanol was formed in some of these specimens, indicating that even bacteria such as *E. coli* and *P. aeruginosa* can produce ethanol from sugar. The authors concluded that false positive ethanol urine tests may result if urine specimens are collected without using proper preservatives.[15]

Drug Testing Using Urine

The majority of workplace drug testing is carried out using urine. As mentioned earlier, federally mandated drug testing requires testing for five drugs, including amphetamines, cocaine, marijuana, opiates, and phen-cyclidine, which are commonly referred to as the five SAMHSA drugs. In addition to these five drugs, private employers at their discretion may test for additional drugs, such as barbiturates, benzodiazepines, metha-done, oxycodone, propoxyphene, and methaqualone. These drugs are generally referred to as non-SAMHSA drugs. Among the five SAMHSA drugs, the amphetamine class of drugs includes both amphetamine and methamphetamine, while opiates include morphine, codeine, and heroin. Similarly, among non-SAMHSA drugs, the barbiturate class includes various drugs, including secobarbital, pentobarbital, phenobarbital, and butalbital. There are more than fourteen approved benzodiazepines in the United States, but the most commonly abused benzodiazepines are alpra-zolam, diazepam, clonazepam, halazepam, lorazepam, and oxazepam.

Most drugs stay in the urine for two to three days, while some drugs, such as marijuana metabolite, may stay for up to thirty days in chronic abusers. The window of detection of various illicit drugs is given in table 9.2. Some drugs, such as amphetamines, are detected unchanged in urine drug tests. However, some drugs are detected in urine as their metabolite;

Table 9.2.   Window of Detection of SAMHSA and Commonly Monitored Non-SAMHSA Drugs

Drug	Detection Window in Urine
SAMHSA drugs	
Amphetamine	2 days
Methamphetamine	2 days
Cocaine (as benzoylecgonine)	2 days after single use; 4 days after repeated use
Morphine	2–3 days
Codeine	2 days
Heroin (as morphine)	2 days
Phencyclidine	14 days
Marijuana	2–3 days after single use
(as marijuana metabolite 11-nor-Δ^9-tetrahydrocannabinol- 9-carboxylic acid; THC-COOH)	30 days in chronic abuser
Non-SAMHSA drugs	
Barbiturates	
Short-acting (pentobarbital, secobarbital etc.)	1 day
Long-acting (phenobarbital)	21 days
Benzodiazepines	
Short-acting (alprazolam, lorazepam, etc.)	3 days
Long-acting (diazepam, lorazepam, etc.)	30 days
Methadone	3 days
Methaqualone	3 days
Oxycodone	2–4 days
Propoxyphene	6 hours–2 days

Table 9.3. Cutoff Concentrations of Various SAMHSA and non-SAMHSA drugs

Drug or Drug Class	Immunoassay (ng/mL)	GC-MS Confirmation (ng/mL)	
SAMHSA Drugs			
Amphetamines	1000	Amphetamine	500
		Methamphetamine	500
Cannabinoids	50	THC-COOH	15
Cocaine metabolites	300	Benzoylecgonine	150
Opiates	2000	Morphine	2000
		Codeine	2000
		6-Acetylmorphine	10*
Phencyclidine	25	Phencyclidine	25
Non-SAMHSA Drugs			
Barbiturates	200	Barbiturates	150^
Benzodiazepines	200	Benzodiazepines	150^
Methadone	300	Methadone	200
Methaqualone	300	Methaqualone	200
Propoxyphene	300	Propoxyphene	300
Oxycodone	100 or 300 ng/mL	Oxycodone	100

*6-monoacetyl morphine is a specific metabolite indicating heroin abuse.
^Individual drug in this class of drug can be confirmed at 150 ng/mL cutoff concentration.

for example, cocaine is determined as benzoylecgonine, a major cocaine metabolite. Similarly, marijuana is determined as 11-nor-Δ9-tetrahydro-cannabinol- 9-carboxylic acid or THC-COOH, the major metabolite of marijuana.

Like alcohol testing where most tests cannot accurately determine blood alcohol level below 0.02 percent (20 mg/dL), assays employed for detection of various drugs in urine specimens also have detection limits. Usually screening assays are done using immunoassays and automated analyzers, and if a screening assay is positive, the presence of a particular drug in the urine specimen must be confirmed by a second analytical method. The gold standard for confirmation of drugs in urine specimens is gas chromatography/mass spectrometry (GC/MS). This is a very sophisticated analytical instrument costing between $75,000 and $100,000. In general, GC/MS is capable of confirming drug concentrations in much lower levels than immunoassays. Screening and confirmation cutoff concentrations of various drugs are given in table 9.3. If the screening test is positive but the confirmation test is negative, the drug testing result should be considered negative.[16]

LIMITATIONS OF ALCOHOL AND DRUG TESTING

Breath analyzers are widely used for determination of alcohol use among employees working in security- and safety-sensitive positions.

Breath analyzers, although based on robust analytical principles, are occasionally subject to certain limitations, including false positive and false negative test results. Derogis et al. (1995) reported that out of 204 patients studied using the breath analyzer, three patients showed false positive ethanol levels and another three patients showed false negative results.[17] Blood alcohol determination using gas chromatography is very accurate and is the method of choice in laboratories performing legal alcohol determinations (please see chapter 6 for more in-depth discussion on breath analyzers and various methods for determining blood alcohol concentrations).

Workplace drug testing also has certain limitations. For example, immunoassays are used for screening tests and such assays are subject to interferences, meaning that another drug may trigger a positive result. Amphetamine immunoassays are subject to interferences from many over-the-counter cold medications, such as brompheniramine, ephedrine, phentermine, phenylpropanolamine, pseudoephedrine, and phenylephrine.[18] Fortunately, such false positive test results can be eliminated in the GC/MS confirmation step.

Consuming food containing poppy seeds is legal, but poppy seeds contain both morphine and codeine, and urine opiate drug testing can be positive after consuming such foods (depending on the amount consumed and the time elapsed after eating). Because the GC/MS confirmation step also targets morphine (heroin abusers also show morphine in their urine because heroin is finally metabolized to morphine) and codeine, eating poppy seeds may result in a positive drug test. A morphine concentration of 5,880 ng/mL after ingestion of poppy seed cake in one subject was reported by Thevis et al. (2003). Other subjects in this study also showed significant amounts of morphine, which was confirmed in the urine by the GC/MS method.[19] Although in November 1998, SAMHSA increased the cutoff concentration for screening (as well as the GC/MS confirmation cutoff) for opiates to 2000 ng/mL, it is still possible to get positive test results from consuming poppy seed products, especially if the opiate concentrations (morphine and codeine) are relatively high in the seeds. Australian, Turkish, and Dutch poppy seeds are available in the market, and Australian poppy seeds usually have high amounts of opiates (90 to 200 microgram of morphine per gram of poppy seeds), while Turkish and Dutch poppy seeds contain only 4 to 5 microgram of morphine per gram of seeds.[20] Some private employers still use the old 300 ng/mL cutoff for both screening and confirmation of opiates in workplace drug testing. Such levels of morphine and codeine can be easily achieved by eating one poppy seed muffin prior to a pre-employment drug test. After eating food containing poppy seeds, urine may test positive at 300 ng/mL cutoff level for a day or two. Therefore, it is important not to consume such food several days prior to taking a preemployment drug test.

Although less common than positive workplace drug testing results due to eating food containing poppy seeds, certain herbal teas originating from South America, especially mate de coca tea and health Inca tea, may be contaminated with cocaine. Usually one tea bag contains 1 gm of dried plant material and may contain between 1.4 and 5 mg of cocaine. Drinking such tea prior to workplace drug testing may result in a positive cocaine test because sufficient amounts of cocaine are usually present in the tea for urinary concentrations of benzoylecgonine (cocaine metabolite) to exceed the cutoff concentration of 300 ng/mL. Although U.S. customs regulations require that no cocaine should be present in any herbal tea, literature references indicate that some health Inca tea sold in the United States contains cocaine. Jackson et al. (1991) reported urinary concentration of benzoylecgonine after ingestion of one cup of health Inca tea by volunteers. Benzoylecgonine was detected up to twenty-six hours postingestion. Maximum urinary benzoylecgonine concentration ranged from 1400 ng/mL to 2800 ng/mL after ingestion of health Inca tea. The total excretion of benzoylecgonine in thirty-six hours ranged from 1.05 to 1.45 mg, which correlated with 59–90 percent of the ingested cocaine dose from drinking such tea prepared using one tea bag.[21]

In addition, taking certain prescription medications, such as a narcotic analgesic, may cause positive workplace drug testing. Common prescription medications that result in positive workplace drug testing are listed in table 9.4. It is important to disclose use of any such medication prior to submitting urine specimen for workplace drug testing.

Table 9.4. Prescription Drugs that May Cause a Positive Result in Workplace Drug Testing

Positive Workplace Test	Generic Name of the Drug
Amphetamines	amphetamine, amphetaminil, clobenzorex, ethylamphetamine, fenoproporex, mefenorex, prenylamine, methamphetamine, benzphetamine, famprofazone, furfenorex, selegiline
Opiates	codeine, morphine, hydromorphone
Benzodiazepine	estazolam, flurazepam, temazepam, triazolam, midazolam, alprazolam, chlordiazepoxide, clorazepate, clonazepam, diazepam, halazepam, lorazepam, nitrazepam, prazepam, oxazepam quazepam

Author's Note: Oxycodone does not interfere with workplace opiate testing.

TIPS TO PASS WORKPLACE ALCOHOL AND DRUG TESTS

For passing alcohol tests, do not drink at all for at least twelve hours and do not consume more than two standard drinks between twelve hours and twenty-four hours before testing. Most workplace alcohol tests have very strict requirement and even a single drink a few hours prior to alcohol testing can push blood alcohol over the acceptable limit of 0.02 percent (20 mg/dL) or less.

To pass preemployment drug tests do not drink too much water before testing due to being nervous. Because people try to beat drug tests by diluting urine so that drug concentrations can be pushed below the detection threshold, all drug testing facilities follow strict criteria to determine which specimens are not acceptable for analysis. Creatinine below 20 mg/dL and specific gravity below 1.003 may be considered an indication of intentionally diluted urine. Drinking too much water (more than 3 liters in twenty-four hours) may cause such dilution of urine. Therefore, drink normal amounts of fluid before workplace drug testing and do not consume too much caffeine. In addition, do not eat any poppy seed–containing food at least three to four days prior to drug testing and do not drink any herbal tea, especially any herbal tea coming from South America, because it may be contaminated with cocaine.

CONCLUSION

Workplace alcohol and drug testing are common practice in today's work environment in order to achieve a drug- and alcohol-free workplace. Workplace drug testing is more prevalent than combined alcohol and drug testing. Usually personnel employed in security- and safety-sensitive positions are subjected to both alcohol and drug testing. As a result of implementing such programs, alcohol- and drug-related workplace injuries are declining in the United States.

There are very strict criteria for blood alcohol limits in personnel working in security-sensitive positions, and it is advisable not to drink at all before reporting for such work. For workplace drug testing, any positive test may cause adverse action against the person, and abusing drugs is a bad idea. Although there are many products advertised on the Internet as effective to beat drug tests, in reality none of them work because drug testing facilities routinely screen for such adulterants, and if detected, the drug testing may be considered positive.

NOTES

1. T. C. Blum, P. M. Roman, and J. K. Martin, "Alcohol Consumption and Work Performance," *Journal of Studies on Alcohol* 44 (1993): 61–70.

2. D. Bush, "The U.S. Mandatory Guidelines for Federal Workplace Drug Testing Programs: Current Status and Future Considerations," *Forensic Science International* 174 (2008): 111–19.

3. Drug Testing Index, Quest Diagnostics, March 12, 2008.

4. Substance Abuse and Mental Health Services Administration, *News* 15, no. 5 (September/October 2007).

5. C. S. Carpenter, "Workplace Drug Testing and Worker Drug Use," *Health Services Research* 42, no. 2 (April 2007): 795–810.

6. J. E. Brady, S. P. Baker, C. Dimaggio, M. L. McCarthy, et al., "Effectiveness of Mandatory Alcohol Testing Programs in Reducing Alcohol Involvement in Fatal Motor Carrier Crashes," *American Journal of Epidemiology* 170, no. 6 (September 2009): 775–82.

7. "Procedures for Transportation Workplace Drug and Alcohol Testing Programs: Final Rule," *Federal Register* 73, no. 123 (June 25, 2008): 35961–75.

8. J. E. Brady, S. P. Baker, C. Dimaggio, M. L. McCarthy, et al., "Effectiveness of Mandatory Alcohol Testing Programs in Reducing Alcohol Involvement in Fatal Motor Carrier Crashes," *American Journal of Epidemiology* 170, no. 6 (September 2009): 775–82.

9. T. Marrero, "Hernando Superintendent Recommends School Board Fire Bus Driver Who Failed Alcohol Breath Test," *St. Petersburg* (Florida) *Times*, October 16, 2009.

10. Associated Press, "United Pilot Charged with Being over Alcohol Limit," *New York Times*, January 5, 2010.

11. J. F. Jemionek, C. L. Copley, M. L. Smith, and M. R. Past, "Concentration Distribution of the Marijuana Metabolite Delta 9-Tetrahydrocannabinol-9-Carboxylic Acid and Cocaine Metabolite Benzoylecgonine in the Department of Defense Urine Drug Testing Program," *Journal of Analytical Toxicology* 32, no. 6 (July–August 2008): 408–16.

12. A. Helander, C. A. Hagelberg, O. Beck, and B. Petrini, "Unreliable Alcohol Testing in a Shipping Safety Program," *Forensic Science International* 189, nos. 1–3 (August 2009): e45–47.

13. A. W. Jones, "Urine as a Biological Specimen for Forensic Analysis of Alcohol and Variability in the Urine to Blood Relationship," *Toxicological Review* 25, no. 1 (January 2006): 15–35.

14. A. W. Jones, A. Eklund, and A. Helander, "Misleading Results of Ethanol Analysis in Urine Specimens from Rape Victims Suffering from Diabetes," *Journal of Clinical and Forensic Medicine* 7, no. 3 (September 2000): 144–46.

15. A. Helander, C. A. Hagelberg, O. Beck, and B. Petrini, "Unreliable Alcohol Testing in a Shipping Safety Programme," *Forensic Science International* 189, no. 10 (August 2009): e45–47.

16. A. Dasgupta, *A Health Educator's Guide to Understanding Drugs of Abuse Testing* (Sudbury, MA: Jones and Bartlett, 2009), 55–91.

17. V. Derogis, P. Bourrier, O. Douay, A. Turcant, et al., "Ethyl Alcohol Levels in Expiratory Air vs. Blood Alcohol Levels in 204 Cases in an Emergency Unit," *Presse Medicale* 24, no. 23 (June 1995): 1067–70.

18. A. Dasgupta, S. Saldana, G. Kinnaman, M. Smith, et al., "Analytical Performance Evaluation of EMIT II Monoclonal Amphetamine/Methamphetamine Assay: More Specificity than EMIT D.A.U. Monoclonal Amphetamine/Methamphetamine Assay," *Clinical Chemistry* 39, no. 1 (January 1993): 104–8.

19. M. Thevis, G. Opfermann, and W. Schanzer, "Urinary Concentrations of Morphine and Codeine after Consumption of Poppy Seeds," *Journal of Analytical Toxicology* 27, no. 1 (January 2003): 53–56.

20. M. G. Pelders and J. J. W. Ross, "Poppy Seeds: Difference in Morphine and Codeine Content and Variation in Inter- and Intra-individual Excretion," *Journal of Forensic Sciences* 41 (1996): 209–12.

21. G. F. Jackson, J. J. Saady, and A. Poklis, "Urinary Excretion of Benzoylecgonine Following Ingestion of Health Inca Tea," *Forensic Sciences International* 49 (1991): 57–64.

10

Why Not to Drink at All
When You're Pregnant

Pregnancy and drinking do not mix at all. Alcohol use among women of childbearing age is a leading preventable cause of birth defects and developmental disabilities. Ethyl alcohol, which is commonly referred to as alcohol, is a well-documented teratogen. A teratogen is an agent that can cause birth defects if the mother is exposed to that agent during pregnancy. After conception (when the egg is fertilized), it takes about six to nine days for the embryo to anchor to the uterus, and then a common blood supply line is developed (placenta) between the mother and the embryo so that nutrients can flow to the embryo for its development into a fetus. This supply line lasts until delivery of the baby when the placenta is cut from the newborn after birth. A teratogen can cross over from the mother to the developing embryo (or fetus) and cause birth defects. Alcohol is a small molecule, so it can easily pass through the placenta to the embryo and cause birth defects. These defects are collectively called "fetal alcohol spectrum disorders." If more severe signs of these birth defects are present in a newborn, the condition may be called "fetal alcohol syndrome." Drinking alcohol during pregnancy may cause stillbirth, and a newborn may even die from fetal alcohol syndrome shortly after birth. Poor outcomes associated with drinking alcohol during pregnancy include but are not limited to

- Stillbirth/death of the baby shortly after birth
- Preterm baby
- Smaller birth weight/growth retardation of the baby
- Neurological abnormality/intellectual impairment
- Facial abnormalities

DRINKING DURING PREGNANCY
AND STILLBIRTH/INFANT MORTALITY

Drinking during pregnancy, especially heavy drinking (for women seven drinks per week or three or more drinks per occasion) or binge drinking (drinking alcohol in order to get intoxicated—four drinks in two hours for a female; see also chapter 2), is associated with very poor outcomes of pregnancy, including stillbirth and high infant mortality. A study by Marbury et al. (1983) involving 12,440 pregnant women clearly established that drinking fourteen or more drinks per week was associated with stillbirth, low birth weight, and preterm babies (gestational age under thirty-seven weeks).[1] A recent epidemiological study involving 79,216 mothers concluded that intake of four drinks of alcohol per week or binge drinking on more than three occasions during pregnancy is associated with an increased risk of infant mortality among full-term infants, especially soon after birth.[2]

Despite the risk associated with binge or heavy drinking with poor pregnancy outcomes, a double-digit percentage of women in the United States are involved in binge drinking during their childbearing years. In a study based on women between the ages of eighteen and forty-four who participated in the CDC Behavioral Risk Factors Surveillance System (58,431 women in 2001, 64,181 in 2002, and 65,678 in 2003), the authors reported that the percentage involved in binge drinking was 11.9 percent, 12.4 percent, and 13.0 percent in 2001, 2002, and 2003. The authors concluded that health care providers must identify and intervene with these binge drinkers who engage in alcohol use in pregnancy, in order to reduce the risk of alcohol-exposed pregnancy.[3] Although the percentage of pregnant women involved in binge drinking is substantially lower than the percentage of women in childbearing age involved in binge drinking, the average annual percentage of alcohol use among pregnant women was 12.2 percent in one report (Denny et al. 2007), and 1.9 percent of pregnant women were involved in binge drinking according to the same report. Surprisingly, the highest percentages of pregnant women reporting alcohol use during the survey period of 2001–2005 were women ages thirty-five to forty-four (17.7 percent), college graduates (14.4 percent), employed (13.7 percent), and unmarried (13.4 percent), and average alcohol use among these groups was higher than the overall average of 12.2 percent of pregnant women who used any alcohol during pregnancy.[4]

Although binge drinking and heavy drinking are dangerous practices during pregnancy, some studies have discovered that even moderate or infrequent drinking during pregnancy may cause adverse outcomes, including death of the baby. In one study (Kesmodel et al. 2002), the authors investigated 24,768 pregnant women and found that the risk of stillbirth among women who consumed five or more drinks per week was three times higher than women who consumed less than one drink per week. The rate of stillbirth was 1.37 per 1,000 births among women who consumed less than one drink per week to 8.83 per 1,000 births among women who consumed five or more drinks per week.[5]

A recent study (Aliyu et al. 2008) reported that mothers who consumed any alcohol during pregnancy were 40 percent more likely to have stillbirths compared to nondrinking mothers. In addition, mothers who consumed five or more drinks per week during pregnancy experienced a 70 percent elevated risk of stillbirth compared to pregnant women who did not consume any alcohol during pregnancy. These findings reinforce current counseling strategies toward pregnant women—and women who intend to get pregnant—of the detrimental effect of drinking during pregnancy.[6] In addition, women giving birth to children with fetal alcohol syndrome also have a higher risk of early mortality.[7]

FETAL ALCOHOL SYNDROME, FETAL ALCOHOL SPECTRUM DISORDERS, AND EPIDEMIOLOGY

Fetal alcohol syndrome due to prenatal alcohol exposure was first reported by Jones and Smith in 1973.[8] Since then many publications have documented the teratogenic effect of alcohol in both human and animal studies. This syndrome is the most common noninherited (nongenetic) cause of mental retardation in the United States. "Fetal alcohol spectrum disorders" was a term described in 2004 to convey that exposure of the fetus to alcohol produces a continuum of effects, and that many babies who do not fulfill all criteria for a diagnosis of fetal alcohol syndrome may nevertheless be profoundly impacted negatively throughout their lives due to exposure to alcohol. Therefore, fetal alcohol spectrum disorders include a wide range of permanent birth defects due to maternal consumption of alcohol during pregnancy, which also includes all serious complications found in babies born with fetal alcohol syndrome.

Other medical terminology related to birth defects in babies caused by maternal alcohol consumption during pregnancy include partial fetal alcohol syndrome, fetal alcohol effect, alcohol-related neurodevelopmental disorders, and alcohol-related birth defects. Approximately 1 to 4.8 of every 1,000 children born in the United States has fetal alcohol syndrome, while as many as 9.1 babies out of 1,000 babies born have fetal alcohol spectrum disorder. This is an alarming statistic because nearly 1 in every 100 babies born in the United States is born with fetal alcohol spectrum disorders. Therefore, fetal alcohol spectrum disorders are a major public health issue, affecting up to 1 percent of the U.S. population.[9] Recent school studies indicate that the prevalence of fetal alcohol syndrome in the United States is at least 2 to 7 per 1,000 babies, and current prevalence of fetal alcohol spectrum disorders may be as high as 2 to 5 percent in the United States among school population. Such prevalence of alcohol-related complications in newborns is higher among school populations than in the general population.[10]

IS ANY AMOUNT OF ALCOHOL SAFE DURING PREGNANCY?

Drinking is a risk factor for poor outcome of pregnancy, including the possibility of a child born with fetal alcohol syndrome or a related disorder. A risk factor means that chances of adverse outcome is high if such a factor is present in a person. For example, if an individual has an elevated cholesterol level (over 200 mg/100 milliliter of blood; 200 mg/dL), that person has an increased risk of myocardial infarction (heart attack). That does not mean that every person with a cholesterol value over 200 mg/dL has a higher chance of a heart attack than a person with a desirable cholesterol level (less than 200 mg/dL). Because heart attacks are not desirable, physicians always advise their patients to keep cholesterol levels below 200 mg/dL by changing their diet and lifestyle and, if necessary, taking medication. Similarly, not every woman who drinks alcohol during pregnancy will have a poor outcome. However, it is impossible to predict which women will be affected by drinking and which women will not be affected by drinking based on any laboratory tests or any other means. In addition, it is also impossible to predict if even one episode of drinking during pregnancy is going to hurt the fetus. Although fetal alcohol syndrome and less severe fetal alcohol spectrum disorders are strongly associated with higher levels of alcohol consumption during pregnancy, animal studies have suggested that even a single episode of alcohol consumption equivalent to two standard drinks during pregnancy may lead to loss of fetal brain cells. Maternal factors that increase the risk of a baby being born with fetal alcohol spectrum disorders include maternal age (thirty and older), history of binge drinking, and low socioeconomic status.[11]

Adverse pregnancy outcomes due to use of alcohol have been noted very early in history, and Aristotle's warning of adverse effects of alcohol associated with pregnancy was probably one of the earliest observations regarding alcohol and pregnancy. However, the majority of documented adverse outcomes of pregnancy associated with alcohol use began with the eighteenth-century London Gin Epidemic (ca. 1720–1750), when newer distillation techniques entered into England from the Netherlands with the ascent of William and Mary to the throne of England. At that time a ban was placed on imported French wine, and plenty of distilled liquor in the form of gin was available in England at low cost because taxes were lowered on the sale of such liquors. Crime rates were high in England, probably due to increased drinking of gin, and physicians in London also blamed alcohol for a higher death rate compared to birth rate. By 1725 the damage caused by alcohol was so significant that the London College of Physicians presented their concerns to the House of Commons and commented that the frequent use of several sorts of distilled liquors resulted in the birth of weak, feeble, distempered children who became burdens to society rather than assets. Fearing the loss of their workforce, combined with poor pregnancy outcomes due to alcohol use and related factors, the elites of London became vocal on the abuse of distilled alcohol and caused the eventual repeal of the law that helped increase the production of cheap alcohol.[12]

Modern research on understanding fetal alcohol syndrome started in the 1970s. Although earlier publications indicated that fetal alcohol syndrome was associated with heavy drinking, and modest drinking during pregnancy may be relatively safe, more recent in-depth studies indicate that at this point we do not know for sure how much alcohol is safe for a pregnant woman to consume to avoid adverse effects on the developing fetus or newborn. A 2002 study found that fourteen-year-old children whose mothers drank as little as one drink a week were significantly shorter and leaner and had a smaller head circumference than children of women who were nondrinkers.[13] This research is in contrast to the earlier studies that reported that up to two drinks per day were safe during pregnancy.

Based on the body of literature on poor pregnancy outcomes associated with alcohol use, the American Academy of Pediatrics (AAP) and the American College of Obstetricians and Gynecologists (ACOG) have for many years recommended alcohol abstinence for both pregnant women and women trying to become pregnant, because no safe threshold for drinking during pregnancy can be established. In 1994, the AAP and the ACOG released a joint statement advising physicians to question all pregnant women at their first visits regarding their current and past consumption of alcohol. Because drinking during pregnancy is associated with a negative social stigma, denial is not uncommon, especially among minority women. Fortunately, screening tools have been developed to help clinicians accurately identify pregnant women who consume alcohol during pregnancy. One such tool is a four-item questionnaire called T-ACE, which is validated for use with pregnant women, including minority women. The T-ACE is the tool that is recommended by the ACOG and the National Institute on Alcohol Abuse and Alcoholism for screening pregnant women for potential alcohol consumption. The questions asked in this test are given in table 10.1. A total score of two or more is considered positive for risk of drinking.[14]

Table 10.1.   T-ACE Scoring Tool for Assessing Risk of Drinking in a Pregnant Woman

Question	Scoring
How many drinks does it take to make you feel high?	Score 2 if more than 2 drinks, or 1 for 1 drink
Have people annoyed you by criticizing your drinking?	Yes answer score 1
Have you felt you need to cut down on your drinks?	Yes answer score 1
Have you ever had a drink first thing in the morning to steady your nerves?	Yes answer score 1

A total score of 2 or more is indicative of drinking risk in pregnancy.

The 2005 U.S. surgeon general, Dr. Richard H. Carmona, issued an advisory warning to pregnant women and women who may become pregnant to abstain from alcohol consumption in order to eliminate the chance of giving birth to a baby with any harmful effects of fetal alcohol spectrum disorders. This updates a 1981 surgeon general's advisory that suggested that pregnant women should limit alcohol consumption. Dr. Carmona said,

> We must prevent all injury and illness that is preventable in society, and alcohol-related birth defects are completely preventable. We do not know what, if any, amount of alcohol is safe. But we do know that the risk of a baby being born with any of the fetal alcohol spectrum disorders increases with the amount of alcohol a pregnant woman drinks, as does the likely severity of the condition. And when a pregnant woman drinks alcohol, so does her baby. Therefore, it's in the child's best interest for a pregnant woman to simply not drink alcohol.

In addition, studies indicate that a baby can be affected by alcohol consumption within the earliest weeks after conception, even before a woman knows she is pregnant. The surgeon general also recommended that women who plan to become pregnant should abstain from consuming alcohol.[15] The Healthy People 2010 objectives include increasing the percentage of pregnant women who report abstinence from alcohol use to 95 percent and increasing the percentage who report abstinence from binge drinking to 100 percent, because binge drinking is particularly harmful to the fetal brain.

FETAL ALCOHOL SYNDROME AND FETAL ALCOHOL SPECTRUM DISORDERS: CLINICAL FEATURES

Fetal alcohol syndrome usually presents with three major features: growth retardation; some degree of brain damage, such as small head size at birth; and characteristic facial features.

Diagnosis of fetal alcohol syndrome and related disorders are based on the following criteria:[16]

- **Category 1:** Confirmed maternal consumption of alcohol
- **Category 2:** Fetal alcohol syndrome may be confirmed without established maternal alcohol consumption if major features of fetal alcohol syndrome, including growth retardation, facial abnormalities, and neurodevelopmental abnormalities are observed.
- **Category 3:** Partial fetal alcohol syndrome with confirmed maternal exposure to alcohol
- **Category 4:** Alcohol-related birth defect if maternal alcohol consumption is confirmed and one or more congenital defects characteristic of fetal alcohol syndrome is present in the newborn
- **Category 5:** Alcohol-related neurodevelopmental disorders if maternal consumption of alcohol is confirmed and neurodevelopmental abnormalities or cognitive disorders are present. Any obvious physical characteristics of fetal alcohol syndrome may be absent.

The most common deformity seen in fetal alcohol syndrome is moderate to severe growth retardation during pregnancy and also after the birth of the newborn. This is manifested by the crown-rump length of the infant (measurement of the infant from the top of the head to the bottom of the buttocks), head circumference, and body weight due to irreversible change in body structure from fetal exposure to alcohol. Other facial abnormalities observed in these babies include microcephaly (small head, a neurodevelopmental disorder where the circumference of the head is significantly smaller than the head of the average person in the same age-group and gender), long and narrow forehead, frontal bossing (unusually prominent forehead), and a variety of other deformities (table 10.2). Facial abnormalities common in fetal alcohol

Table 10.2. Abnormalities Present in Babies with Fetal Alcohol Syndrome

Abnormality	Comments
Growth retardation	Low birth weight, lack of weight gain over time, low weight-to-height ratio
Facial abnormalities	Small head circumference, small eye opening, small midface, flat midface, flat upper lip, low nasal bridge, short nose
Neurodevelopmental problems	Abnormalities of central nervous system, small head size at birth, impaired motor skills, poor eye-hand coordination, hearing loss
Behavioral and cognitive problems	Mental retardation, learning disability, poor memory, language deficiency, poor judgment, problem with reasoning and math
Cardiac malfunctions	Atrial septal defect, ventricular septal defect, and other malfunctions
Other organ problems	Renal insufficiency, endocrine disorders, various problems with eyes

syndrome are shown in figure 10.1. Mental retardation is the major complication of fetal alcohol syndrome due to impaired neurodevelopment of the fetus associated with the maternal use of alcohol during pregnancy. The brain of the fetus is the organ that is most vulnerable to prenatal alcohol across a wide range of regions. However, other complications found in babies born with fetal alcohol syndrome include cardiac malformations, bone and joint problems, endocrine disorders, and eye and hearing problems. Some of these complications may also be found in babies born with fetal alcohol spectrum disorders.

Alcohol can easily cross the placenta and enter fetal circulation and can also easily cross the fetal blood-brain barrier. Alcohol has a direct toxic effect on the developing brain of the fetus, including developing neurons. The hippocampus is one of the major targets for alcohol to exert its toxic effect on the developing brain. The hippocampus is a major part of the limbic system of the brain ("limbic" can be loosely translated to "belt," and the limbic system has a beltlike structure) and plays an important role in forming long-term memory and orientation. The limbic system is a major part of the brain structure that controls emotion, behavior, long-term memory, and olfaction (sense of smell). Ethanol can release L-glutamate, an amino acid that also acts as a neurotransmitter, in the hippocampus of the fetal brain, and toxicity of ethanol may be mediated through the release of L-glutamate. In addition, acetaldehyde, a metabolite of alcohol, may play a role in the teratogenic effect of alcohol on the fetus.[17] Ethanol also triggers widespread suicide by developing neurons (neurodegenera-

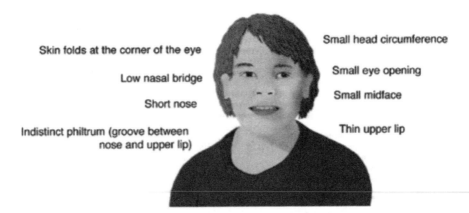

Skin folds at the corner of the eye

Low nasal bridge

Short nose

Indistinct philtrum (groove between nose and upper lip)

Small head circumference

Small eye opening

Small midface

Thin upper lip

Figure 10.1. Facial features associated with fetal alcohol syndrome

Source: Alcohol Research and Health Journal, reference 20. The National Institute of Alcohol Abuse and Alcoholism (NIAAA) website. Information in the public domain.

tion due to neural apoptosis), thus causing degeneration of the developing fetal brain. Based on rat experiments, it has been postulated that neural apoptosis is due to the blockage of N-methyl-D-aspartate glutamate receptors and excessive activation of GABA (gamma-aminobutyric acid) receptors.[18]

In addition, alcohol impairs placental blood flow to the fetus by constricting blood vessels, causing fetal hypoxia (lack of oxygen) and malnutrition. Oxidative stress normally experienced by the fetus may also be increased due to the maternal use of alcohol. Major problems associated with fetal alcohol syndrome and fetal alcohol spectrum disorders are discussed below.

Mental Health Issues and Fetal Exposure to Alcohol

Mental retardation is the major complication associated with fetal alcohol syndrome, as well as fetal alcohol spectrum disorders. In addition, a variety of behavioral problems may be associated in children where the fetus was affected to a lesser degree by the maternal use of alcohol during pregnancy. Fetal alcohol syndrome is a devastating developmental disorder, and it is now a leading cause of mental retardation. In addition to structural abnormalities and growth deficit, fetal alcohol syndrome is associated with a broad spectrum of neurobehavioral abnormalities, including lower IQ, hyperactivity, attention deficit disorder, learning disabilities, memory and language problems, and reduced visuospatial ability (mental capacity to visualize objects and their spatial arrangement) in children born with this syndrome.[19]

In addition, children with fetal alcohol spectrum disorders also have significant impairments in memory that negatively affect their academic performance and daily functioning. Verbal memory is one of the main areas of memory affected by gestational alcohol exposure, especially in forming memory, as well as recall. Spatial memory is also impaired, and such impairment is found among children, adolescents, and adults who were exposed to alcohol in utero. Animal research has documented that key areas of the brain involved in memory functioning are affected by alcohol if the fetus is exposed to alcohol due to maternal drinking.[20] In addition, the odds of appearance of many psychiatric illnesses, including substance abuse, depression, anxiety, paranoid behavior, antisocial behavior, obsessive-compulsive disorders, and psychotic disorders are higher in adults whose mothers were involved in one or more episode of binge drinking while pregnant.[21] Mental health issues associated with fetal alcohol syndrome are listed in table 10.3.

Table 10.3.   Mental Health Issues Associated with Fetal Alcohol Syndrome

Mental retardation
Attention deficit disorder/hyperactivity disorder
Memory impairment
Learning disability
Behavior/learning problems causing dropping out of school
Depression/anxiety
Paranoid behavior
Obsessive-compulsive disorders
Alcohol/substance abuse problems
Inappropriate sexual behavior
Antisocial trends/trouble with the law

Cardiac Malformations and Fetal Exposure to Alcohol

The common cardiac malfunctions associated with fetal alcohol syndrome are ventricular septal defects (VSD) and atrial septal defects (ASD). Both defects are due to the presence of a hole or holes in the heart. The human heart has four chambers, two upper chambers known as the left and right atria and two lower chambers known as the left and right ventricles. Ventricular septal defect means that one or more holes are present in the wall that separates the right and left ventricles of the heart. Ventricular septal defect is one of the most common congenital (present from birth) heart defects. In the fetus, the right and left ventricles of the heart are not separate, but as it grows to a full-term baby, a wall is formed to separate these two ventricles. If the wall formation is incomplete, VSD occurs, while in ASD the wall between the left and right atrium is incomplete. If the hole is small (both VSD and ASD), it may close as the baby grows, but if the hole is large, both defects may cause the heart to work harder, causing heart failure. Major symptoms of VSD are shortness of breath, fast breathing, hard breathing, and pounding heart. Similar symptoms may also be observed in patients with ASD. Although VSD and ASD are the major congenital heart defects associated with fetal alcohol syndrome, other cardiac malfunctions may also be observed with fetal alcohol syndrome.[22]

Other Problems Associated with Fetal Alcohol Syndrome

Alcohol is capable of causing deformation of all cells and organs. Significant skeletal deformity, such as cervical spine fusion (developmental deformity of vertebrate), microcephaly (small head size), and abnormal thoracic cage development are frequently associated with fetal alcohol syndrome.[23] A delayed bone age (delayed bone development) has been observed in children with fetal alcohol syndrome. The effect is more significant in the long bones, which explains the shorter height of children born with fetal alcohol syndrome compared to normal children of the same age-group. The eyes may also be affected by fetal alcohol syndrome. The cornea may be smaller and cloudy at birth. Other eye problems include nystagmus (involuntary eye movement), microphthalmos (abnormal smallness in the dimensions of one or both eyes), coloboma (a hole in the structure of the eye, such as in the eyelid, iris, retina, or other structure), and epicanthus (skin fold of the upper eyelid).

Renal abnormality or renal impairment may also be present in a child with a history of maternal drinking during pregnancy. Some hearing impairment may also be present in these children.[24] Prenatal alcohol exposure also causes abnormalities in endocrine functions. Alcohol abuse is known to result in abnormalities of endocrine function. Alcohol is not only able to cross the placenta and directly affect fetal cells; it can also cause disruption in the mother's endocrine function, thus disrupting maternal-fetal hormonal interactions, which may affect the ability of the mother to maintain a successful pregnancy.

Alcohol-induced endocrine imbalance may play a major role in the mechanism by which alcohol harms the fetus. The hypothalamic-pituitary-adrenal (HPA) axis is programmed during fetal development, and alcohol can reprogram this axis, causing hyperactivity of this axis in the baby born with fetal alcohol syndrome; such effects may last for the lifetime of the child. Fetal reprogramming of the HPA axis due to fetal alcohol exposure may be responsible for many problems, including behavior, endocrine, cognitive, and immune deficiencies.[25]

The hypothalamic-pituitary-adrenal (HPA) axis is a complex set of direct influence and feedback mechanisms between the hypothalamus (a funnel-shaped part of the brain), the pituitary gland (a small gland located below hypothalamus in the brain), and the adrenal glands (small conical-shaped glands on top of kidneys), which control many essential body functions, including the immune system, digestion, sexuality, mood, and stress level. This system also controls the level of various hormones and cortisol in the body. Reprogramming of this axis during fetal growth may cause many problems throughout the life of an affected individual.

HOW DOES PRENATAL EXPOSURE TO ALCOHOL AFFECT THE CHILD THROUGH ADULTHOOD?

Exposure of the fetus to alcohol affects the newborn throughout its entire life. A newborn baby may be born with a small head and be fussy and may also suffer from feeding problems (poor sucking). In addition, such a baby may bond poorly with the mother and have an abnormal sleep cycle, frequently waking up during the night. The baby may also have poor muscle tone and may appear floppy. As a toddler, language delays, poor coordination and balance, poor memory, head banging, and hyperactivity may be observed. As the baby grows older (ages four to twelve) learning disabilities, short attention span, frequent temper tantrums, and aggressiveness are commonly observed features. At this stage, a baby born with fetal alcohol syndrome may also experience difficulty in getting along with others. As an adolescent, poor judgment, memory impairment, poor problem-solving ability, and poor social skills are common among children born with this syndrome. Dropping out of school, trouble with the law, developing drug and alcohol dependence, and a variety of other problems may develop when these children reach adulthood.

Exposure of the fetus to alcohol results in lifelong consequences that affect physical development, intellectual development, behavior, social development, occupation, independent living, and sexual behavior. Babies born with fetal alcohol syndrome or fetal alcohol spectrum disorders may even need lifelong assistance and are often prone to suicide.[26] The devastating effects of exposure of the fetus to alcohol last a lifetime, and abstinence from alcohol consumption during pregnancy is the best way to prevent such detrimental effects. There is no good therapy that is able to reverse the ill effects of fetal alcohol syndrome or fetal alcohol spectrum disorders.

SMOKING, DRINKING, AND DRUG ABUSE DURING PREGNANCY AND POOR OUTCOME

Smoking is hazardous to health, and maternal smoking during pregnancy is associated with several adverse developmental outcomes in the offspring. These include preterm delivery, spontaneous abortion, growth restriction, and increased risk of sudden infant death syndrome, as well as long-term behavioral and psychiatric disorders in the offspring.[27] An increase in congenital abnormalities (birth defects) associated with cigarette smoking and the use of alcohol during pregnancy has been reported in many scientific studies. Smoking and drinking during pregnancy also increases the risk of many complications in pregnancy, including placental abruption, unexplained stillbirth, preterm labor, and intrauterine growth restrictions. In one report (Odendaal et al. 2009), the authors concluded that preterm labor leading to delivery of premature babies occurs more frequently in women who smoke and drink during pregnancy, and the risk was more than the sum of the effects of either smoking or drinking. Therefore, smoking and drinking have synergistic effects that greatly increase the risk of preterm labor. Smoking and drinking also have synergistic effects for delivering babies with low birth weight and growth restriction.[28]

Substance abuse during pregnancy has devastating effects on pregnancy outcome, including stillbirth, preterm labor, and various birth defects. Babies born to cocaine-addicted mothers often have congenital abnormalities and low birth weight. One of the most devastating effects of fetal cocaine exposure is damage to the developing heart. In addition, substance abuse during pregnancy is associated with significant maternal and fetal morbidity.[29] In some states exposure of a fetus to illicit drugs due to maternal abuse is considered a form of child neglect and abuse and can lead to losing custody of the child and the potential for prosecution. Concurrent abuse of illicit drugs and alcohol has synergistic effects associated with poor outcomes in pregnancy. Detailed discussion of the effect of substance abuse on poor pregnancy outcome is beyond the scope of this book, but many studies are available on this subject.

IS IT SAFE TO DRINK DURING BREAST-FEEDING?

Ample evidence indicates that drinking alcohol during pregnancy is associated with severe risks of poor pregnancy outcome, which is preventable by abstinence, but the risks of consumption of alcohol during breast-feeding are not as well defined. Alcohol is a small molecule and can easily pass from the mother's blood into her milk. A nursing infant is exposed to only a fraction of the alcohol that the mother drinks, but the infant detoxifies alcohol at a much slower rate than the mother. Adverse effects of alcohol on suckling infants include changes in sleep pattern with much-reduced sleep and waking up more frequently, decrease in milk intake, and risk of developing low blood sugar (hypoglycemia). When alcohol appears in breast milk, it alters the natural flavor of the milk and may explain why an infant might consume less milk. Currently, there is no known benefit of exposing the infant to alcohol. In contrast, most likely no level of alcohol in breast milk is safe for the infant. Drinking water and pumping and dumping breast milk will not accelerate elimination of alcohol from the breast milk, because alcohol is not trapped in the breast milk but is constantly removed as it moves back into the bloodstream. Therefore, the only way to ensure that there is no alcohol in breast milk is to wait long enough after consumption of alcohol before the next breast-feeding.

Elimination of alcohol from the body depends on body weight and number of drinks consumed. For example, if a 90-pound woman drinks two drinks in an hour, it will take approximately five hours and forty minutes for the body to clear all of the alcohol. However, if the woman's weight is 150 pounds, it will take four hours and thirty minutes for alcohol elimination after consuming two standard drinks in an hour. Nursing mothers who choose to consume alcohol should carefully plan a breast-feeding schedule by storing milk before alcohol consumption and then waiting for complete elimination of alcohol from the breast milk before resuming breast-feeding.[30] Contrary to popular belief, which encourages women to drink alcohol as an aid to lactation, alcohol consumption in reality disrupts breast milk production.[31]

CONCLUSION

Due to devastating and lifelong effects of maternal consumption of alcohol on the offspring, pregnant women must abstain from drinking alcohol. In addition, smoking and substance abuse are also associated with stillbirth, spontaneous abortion, and other poor outcomes in pregnancy. Contrary to earlier guidelines where moderate alcohol consumption during pregnancy was considered relatively safe, in 2005 the U.S. surgeon general issued an advisory strongly recommending pregnant women to refrain from consuming alcohol because no safe limit of alcohol during pregnancy has been established. Fetal alcohol syndrome and less severe fetal alcohol spectrum disorders are completely preventable if pregnant women practice total abstinence.

NOTES

1. M. C. Marbury, S. Linn, R. Monson, S. Schoenbaum, et al., "The Association of Alcohol Consumption with Outcome of Pregnancy," *American Journal of Public Health* 73, no. 10 (October 1983): 1165–68.

2. K. Strandberg-Larsen, A. Gronboek, A. M. Anderson, P. K. Andersen, et al., "Alcohol Drinking Pattern during Pregnancy and Risk of Infant Mortality," *Epidemiology* 20, no. 6 (November 2009): 884–91.

3. J. Tsai, R. L. Floyd, and J. Bertrand, "Tracking Binge Drinking among U.S. Childbearing Age Women," *Preventive Medicine* 44, no. 4 (April 2007): 298–302.

4. C. H. Denny, J. Tsai, R. L. Floyd, P. P. Green, et al., "Morbidity and Mortality Weekly Report," 58, no. 19 (May 2009): 529–32.

5. U. Kesmodel, K. Wisborg, S. F. Olsen, T. B. Henriksen, et al., "Moderate Alcohol Intake during Pregnancy and the Risk of Stillbirth and Death in the First Year of Life," *American Journal of Epidemiology* 155, no. 4 (February 2002): 305–12.

6. M. H. Aliyu, R. E. Wilson, R. Zoorob, S. Chakrabarty, et al., "Alcohol Consumption during Pregnancy and the Risk of Early Stillbirth among Singletons," *Alcohol* 42, no. 5 (August 2008): 369–74.

7. J. P. Berg, M. E. Lynch, and C. D. Coles, "Increased Mortality among Women Who Drank Alcohol during Pregnancy," *Alcohol* 42, no. 7 (November 2008): 603–10.

8. K. L. Jones and D. W. Smith, "Recognition of the Fetal Alcohol Syndrome in Early Infancy," *Lancet* 302, no. 7836 (November 1973): 999–1001.

9. P. D. Sampson, A. P. Streissguth, and F. L. Bookstein, "Incidence of Fetal Alcohol Syndrome and Prevalence of Alcohol-Related Neurodevelopmental Disorder," *Teratology* 56, no. 5 (November 1997): 317–26.

10. P. A. May, J. P. Gossage, W. O. Kalberg, L. K. Robinson, et al., "Prevalence and Epidemiological Characteristics of FASD from Various Research Methods with an Emphasis on Recent in School Studies," *Developmental Disability Research Review* 15, no. 3 (2009): 176–92.

11. D. J. Wattendorf and M. Muenke, "Fetal Alcohol Spectrum Disorders," *American Family Physicians* 72, no. 2 (July 2005): 279–82.

12. K. R. Warren and B. G. Hewitt, "Fetal Alcohol Spectrum Disorders: When Science, Medicine, Public Policy, and Laws Collide," *Developmental Disabilities and Research Reviews* 15, no. 3 (September 2009): 170–75.

13. N. L. Day, S. L. Leech, G. A. Richardson, M. D. Cornelius, et al., "Prenatal Alcohol Exposure Predicts Continued Deficits in Offspring Size at 14 Years of Age," *Alcohol Clinical and Experimental Research* 26, no. 10 (October 2002): 1584–91.

14. B. A. Bailey and R. J. Sokol, "Pregnancy and Alcohol Use: Evidence and Recommendations for Prenatal Care," *Clinical Obstetrics and Gynecology* 51, no. 2 (June 2008): 436–44.

15. "U.S. Surgeon General Releases Advisory on Alcohol Use in Pregnancy," U.S. Department of Health and Human Services, Washington D.C., 2005, http://www.surgeongeneral.gov/pressreleases/sg02222005.html.

16. D. J. Wattendorf and M. Muenke, "Fetal Alcohol Spectrum Disorders," *American Family Physicians* 72, no. 2 (July 2005): 279–82.

17. J. D. Reynolds and J. F. Brien, "Ethanol Neurobehavioral Teratogenies and the Role of L-glutamate in the Fetal Hippocampus," *Canadian Journal of Physiology and Pharmacology* 73, no. 9 (September 1995): 1209–23.

18. C. Ikonomidou, P. Bittigau, M. J. Ishimaru, D. F. Wozniak, et al., "Ethanol-Induced Apoptotic Neurodegeneration and Fetal Alcohol Syndrome," *Science* 287, no. 5455 (February 2000): 1050–60.

19. S. N. Mattson and E. P. Riley, "A Review of the Neurobehavioral Deficits in Children with Fetal Alcohol Syndrome or Prenatal Exposure to Alcohol," *Alcohol Clinical and Experimental Research* 22, no. 2 (April 1998): 279–94.

20. S. Manji, J. Pei, C. Loomes, and C. Rasmussen, "A Review of the Verbal and Visual Memory Impairments in Children with Foetal Alcohol Spectrum Disorder," *Developmental Neurorehabilitation* 12, no. 4 (October 2009): 239–47.

21. H. M. Barr, F. L. Bookstein, K. D. O'Malley, P. D. Connor, et al., "Binge Drinking during Pregnancy as a Predictor of Psychiatric Disorders on the Structured Clinical Interview for DSM-IV in Young Adult Offspring," *American Journal of Psychiatry* 163, no. 6 (June 2006): 1061–65.

22. L. Burd, E. Deal, R. Rios, E. Adickes, et al., "Congenital Heart Defects and Fetal Alcohol Spectrum Disorders," *Congenital Heart Disease* 2, no. 4 (July 2007): 250–55.

23. D. F. Smith, G. G. Sandor, P. M. MacLeod, S. Tredwell, et al., "Intrinsic Defects in the Fetal Alcohol Syndrome: Studies on 76 Cases from British Columbia and the Yukon Territory," *Neurobehavioral Toxicology and Teratology* 3, no. 2 (Summer 1981): 145–52.

24. J. D. Chaudhuri, "Alcohol and the Developing Fetus: A Review," *Medical Science Monitor* 6, no. 5 (2000): 1031–41.

25. X. Zhang, J. H. Sliwowska, and J. Weinberg, "Prenatal Alcohol Exposure and Fetal Programming: Effects on Neuroendocrine and Immune Function," *Experimental Biology and Medicine* (Maywood) 230, no. 6 (June 2005): 376–88.

26. J. Merrick, E. Merrick, M. Morad, and I. Kandel, "Fetal Alcohol Syndrome and Its Long-Term Effects," *Minerva Pediatrica* 58, no. 3 (June 2006): 211–18.

27. A. K. Shea and M. Steiner, "Cigarette Smoking during Pregnancy," *Nicotine and Tobacco Research* 10, no. 2 (February 2008): 2657–78.

28. H. J. Odendaal, D. W. Steyn, A. Elliott, and L. Burd, "Combined Effects of Cigarette Smoking and Alcohol Consumption on Perinatal Outcome," *Gynecologic and Obstetric Investigation* 67, no. 1 (January 2009): 1–8.

29. K. M. Kuczkowski, "The Effects of Drugs Abuse on Pregnancy," *Current Opinion in Obstetrics and Gynecology* 19, no. 6 (December 2007): 578–85.

30. G. Koren, "Drinking Alcohol While Breastfeeding: Will It Harm My Baby?" *Canadian Family Physician* 48, no. 1 (January 2002): 39–41.

31. J. A. Mannella and M. Y. Pepino, "Biphasic Effects of Moderate Drinking on Prolactin during Lactation," *Alcohol Clinical and Experimental Research* 32, no. 11 (November 2008): 1899–1908.

11

Dangers of Moonshine Whiskey and Related Illegally Produced Liquors

"Moonshine" is an old term for smuggled liquor because such liquors were transported at night under moonlight to avoid detection by any law enforcement agents. In a broad sense, moonshine whiskey or moonshine liquors are defined as alcoholic drinks that are produced illegally without proper license and sold to consumers without paying any taxes. The people involved in producing such liquors are called "moonshiners." In the United States, moonshine whiskeys have been prepared since the late eighteenth century, mostly in the Appalachian Mountains region and the South. At that time, fermentation of mostly corn, but also apples and peaches, followed by distillation to produce whiskey and other alcoholic beverages became a cottage industry among farmers who profited from selling such liquors when corn prices were relatively low and it was unprofitable to sell corn.

The federal government first implemented taxes on liquors in 1790. Farmers producing moonshine whiskey protested and resentment finally exploded in 1794, with angry farmers seizing the city of Pittsburgh, Pennsylvania. At that time, President Washington sent troops to control the volatile situation and arrested leaders of the uprising. During the Civil War (1861–1865), the federal government imposed taxes on liquor production to collect extra revenue in order to help pay for the war. However, after the Civil War was over, the federal government continued to collect revenue on alcohol and tobacco, and many small farmers producing moonshine whiskey and related liquors refused to pay such taxes. Thus, the production of moonshine whiskey was performed at night under moonlight using equipment known as a still, and wood fire was used for distillation. In order to avoid detection of the smoke, such production was carried out in remote areas.

Production of such illegal liquors increased during the 1920s when alcohol consumption was illegal in the United States. Although producers of moonshine whiskey and related liquors were called "moonshiners," people who smuggled such products were called "bootleggers," because they often concealed the liquor in their long boots. In the 1920s and later, bootleggers used cars for transportation of illegally produced alcohols and drove at night at high speed to escape detection by law enforcement agencies. This created a culture of car racing, which eventually evolved into the popular National Association for Stock Car Auto Racing (NASCAR). Although a ban on alcohol consumption was no longer present in 1933, the moonshine whiskey culture continued, and even today, moonshine liquors are produced in the United States and the rest of the world. Although moonshine whiskey is the most popular term, it is also called mountain dew, hooch, white lightning, rotgut, happy Sally, stump, and white mule.

Current U.S. laws permit home production of beer and wine by fermentation for personal use. An individual may produce up to 100 gallons of beer or wine per year for personal use, and a family of two can produce up to 200 gallons of such alcoholic beverages per year. No permit or record is needed, and no tax is payable to either state or federal authorities. However, selling such alcoholic beverages is not permitted, and federal law does not permit production of distilled liquor such as whiskey without a valid permit, because distillation of alcohol requires skill, and if not done properly, it can cause harm to consumers. Despite legal sanctions, illegal whiskey production and subsequent consumption, mostly by people with low incomes, continues to occur even today.

Not all moonshine whiskeys are illegal. Certain brands produced by local distillers with proper licensing may be legally available in certain states, such as Virginia. Today, moonshine liquors are defined as any illegally produced alcohol worldwide. In addition, the broader term "surrogate alcohol" is used to define moonshine liquors, as well as any alcoholic product not designated for human consumption. Consumption of such products may cause severe toxicity and even death.

MOONSHINE WHISKEY: CURRENT STATUS

When the prohibition of alcohol was repealed in 1933, illegally produced moonshine whiskey was on the decline. Nevertheless, in the 1960s and 1970s, moonshine continued to be a problem to federal authorities. Production and consumption of moonshine whiskey has been on decline in the United States since 1990, but such illegally produced liquors are still encountered in the United States. Currently, consumption of moonshine whiskey is mostly found in rural populations in Alabama, Georgia, South Carolina, and Mississippi. However, consumption of moonshine whiskey has also been reported in the urban populations of the District of Columbia, Michigan, Pennsylvania, and Virginia.[1] The main reason for the decline in production of illegally produced alcohol is that large commercial breweries can buy raw material in bulk at such a cheap price that even after paying taxes, the cost of such liquors is not that much higher than illegally produced moonshine liquors. However, moonshine whiskey is still cheaper than legal alcohol, and many consumers of moonshine whiskey simply do it to get a kick.

According to a March 23, 2000, report by the *New York Times*, 130 proof alcohol was produced for three dollars a gallon, bottled in six-pack plastic jugs, and sold for ten to twelve dollars a gallon in the back rooms of bars known as "nip joints" or "shot houses" in big mid-Atlantic cities such as Richmond, Virginia, Washington, D.C., Baltimore, Maryland, and Philadelphia, Pennsylvania. Such illegally produced alcohol was sold for one dollar per shot, which was much lower in price than legal whiskey. The major manufacturing places for such illegal liquors were Rocky Mount, Virginia, and the surrounding areas. Since the federal excise tax on a gallon of whiskey at that time was $13.50, the U.S. Bureau of Alcohol, Tobacco, Firearms and Explosives (ATF) estimated a loss of $19.6 million in tax revenue between 1992 and 1999 that was related to the sale of moonshine liquors. The task force of state and federal agents applying federal law rather than weaker anti-moonshiner state laws made its first arrest in March 2000.[2] Federal agents also closed illegal moonshine whiskey production facilities in Virginia and North Carolina. Since moonshining carries a sentence of five years in prison, federal agents often use other charges, such as tax evasion and money laundering, which carry stiffer (longer) sentences.

WHY ARE MOONSHINE WHISKEY AND RELATED ALCOHOLS DANGEROUS?

Like any whiskey production, moonshine whiskey is produced by the fermentation of sugar using yeast followed by distillation using a still. Moonshine whiskey is mainly made from corn. After the corn is ground into meal, sugar is sometimes added, and then it is soaked in hot water. Malt may also be added in order to convert cornstarch into sugar. Then yeast is added to start the fermentation process; this mixture is called "mash." The mash is heated in a still for a set amount of time (usually two days) where the fermentation process is nearly complete. The still is heated (in the past by using wood fire, but today moonshiners may use propane gas) a final time to distill the alcohol, which is collected as clear liquid. Commercial liquors often have a golden or amber color, which is due to the aging and storage process in oak barrels. Moonshine whiskey is always clear like water, because it is not aged prior to sale. Moonshine and related alcohols are dangerous for the following reasons:

- Poor production conditions and lack of quality control
- High alcohol content
- Presence of various harmful contaminants, including lead
- Harmful substances added to these products to increase "kick"

Because moonshine whiskeys and related liquors are produced illegally, there is no federal inspector who can ensure that proper sanitary conditions are met to produce such products. Often impure water is used for production, and insects may even get into the product. Moreover, the distillation process requires skill, and it usually takes two to three passes through the still to remove impurities from distillated liquors. Moonshiners may not be careful in the manufacturing process, so contaminants may be present in such products. Some moonshiners add harmful substances such as manure, embalming fluid, bleach, rubbing alcohol (isopropyl alcohol), and even paint thinner to increase the kick from consumption of such liquors (see table 11.1).

Serious toxicity and even death may occur from consuming moonshine whiskey and related illegally produced liquors. The major dangers of

Table 11.1. Potential Contaminants Found in Moonshine Liquors

Heavy Metals
Mostly lead,* but arsenic, zinc, and copper may also be found in high amounts.

Other Contaminants
  Methanol^
  Formaldehyde
  Acetaldehyde
  Ethylene glycol
  Embalming fluid
  Insecticide
  Herbicide, such as paraquat
  Paint thinner
  Manure

*Most commonly encountered contaminant.
^ Not commonly encountered in the United States but major contaminant added to illegally produced liquors in many countries.

moonshine whiskey and related products are high alcohol (ethanol) content—sometimes as high as 75 percent (150 proof)—and lead contamination. Methanol, a harmful alcohol, is sometimes added (a more common practice in third world countries because it is cheap) as a contaminant in moonshine liquors to reduce the cost as well as to increase the kick. Methanol is dangerous and may cause death or total blindness (see chapter 12).

The alcohol content of moonshine whiskey is usually quite high, but it may vary widely. In one report (Holstege et al. 2004), the authors found that ethanol content of various moonshine whiskey specimens (forty-eight samples analyzed) varied from 10.5 percent to 66 percent, with a mean alcohol content of 41.2 percent. In addition, lead was found as a contaminant in forty-three out of forty-eight samples analyzed. Toxic methanol was found in one specimen.[3] In another report (Morgan et al. 2004), the alcohol content of 115 moonshine samples seized by the authorities from nine states showed alcohol content between 3.85 percent and 65.80 percent, with a median alcohol content of 44.75 percent (middle value). The lead content in these moonshine liquor specimens varied from 5302 micrograms/100 milliliter (dL), and in thirty-three samples (28.7 percent of all samples), lead concentrations exceeded 300 micrograms/dL, the limit designated potentially hazardous by the Food and Drug Administration. Drinking one liter of such liquor per day may cause lead toxicity.[4]

> Lead toxicity is the major complication of consuming moonshine whiskey and related illegally distilled liquors.

The elevated lead content in moonshine whiskey and other illegally produced liquors is related to the stills being made from automobile radiators. Multiple copper tubes are attached to the unit and sealed with lead soldering. An automobile radiator often contains lead, and the lead leaches out into the moonshine during the production process, especially when the radiator is taken from an older used car.[5] Although lead is the main contaminant found in moonshine whiskey and related illegally produced liquors, other contaminants may also be present in such products (see table 11.1).

Moonshine Liquors and Lead Poisoning

Lead is a heavy metal that has been used by humans for a long time. The early victims of lead poisoning were workers involved in lead mining or lead-related work, as well as wine drinkers. Lead's sweet taste made it useful in winemaking in ancient days to counteract the astringent flavor of tannic acid found in grapes. Lead-sweetened wine containing high amounts of lead was an important staple of upper-class Romans and may have caused decreased fertility and an increase in psychosis among Roman aristocrats.[6]

In modern times, major environmental exposures to lead were due to tetraethyl lead, a volatile and flammable organic lead derivative used in gasoline to improve octane numbers and in lead-based paints. In the United States, lead-based paint was banned in 1978. However, deteriorated lead-based paint in older housing remains the most common source of lead exposure in American children today. In 1986, leaded gasoline was phased out. Despite such efforts, Americans are still exposed to environmental lead through old house paint, contaminated soil, lead-contaminated water due to the use of lead pipes and solder, and food (lead-lined containers and pottery glazes made with lead).[7]

Lead enters the body either through inhalation or ingestion. Lead is distributed in the body in three main compartments: blood, soft tissue, and bone. Lead stored in bones may be resident for twenty-five to thirty years or more. Lead toxicity is serious and may be life threatening. Lead affects hematological (blood), renal, and neurological systems, with the hematological system being one of the most important targets of lead toxicity. Lead inhibits the production of hemoglobin, the major component of red blood cells that carry oxygen. Many of lead's toxic properties are due to its ability to mimic or compete with calcium, thus affecting the neurological system. Lead can also cause acute or chronic renal failure, as well as hypertension (high blood pressure). The acceptable level of lead in blood is less than 10 micrograms/dL of blood, and a blood lead level higher than 50 micrograms/dL is considered clinically significant and requires medical intervention. Blood lead concentration higher than 100 micrograms/dL may even cause death if not promptly treated.

There are many reports of lead toxicity due to consumption of moonshine whiskey and other home-brewed liquors. Morgan et al. (2003) reported four adult cases of potentially lethal lead toxicity in moonshine drinkers who were admitted in February and March 2000 to the Grady Memorial Hospital at Atlanta. The blood lead levels of these patients were 81 micrograms/dL, 190 micrograms/dL, 312 micrograms/dL, and 230 micrograms/dL. These patients were treated and eventually survived. In addition, the authors interviewed 581 patients who visited their hospital and found that 8.6 percent of these patients consumed moonshine in the past five years. Moonshine drinkers were predominantly men between the ages of forty and fifty-nine. The authors then analyzed blood specimens from the moonshine drinkers and observed that the median blood lead level among moonshine drinkers was 11.0 micrograms/dL, which was substantially greater than the median blood level of lead of 2.5 micrograms/dL among nondrinkers. The authors concluded that moonshine consumption was more prevalent than expected in their patient population. Furthermore, moonshine consumers were more likely to report heavy alcohol consumption, and such consumption was strongly associated with elevated blood levels of lead.[8]

Fatal lead poisoning due to the consumption of moonshine whiskey has also been reported in medical literature. Pegues et al. (1993) reported that blood lead concentration ranged from 16 to 259 micrograms/dL in nine patients with lead poisoning due to consumption of moonshine liquor. One patient died from lead poisoning.[9] In another report (Kaufmann et al. 1991), the authors noted that death related to lead poisoning in the United States has been rare since removing all lead-based paints and lead products from gasoline. Between 1979 and 1998, an estimated two hundred lead poisoning–related deaths occurred in the United States, but alcohol-related lead poisoning occurred in 28 percent of the adults who died from lead poisoning. Among these adults, twenty were reported to have consumed illegally produced moonshine alcohol.[10]

Although illegally produced moonshine whiskey consumption is usually associated with lead toxicity, such toxicity may also be encountered from drinking homemade wine. A potentially lethal blood lead level of 98 micrograms/dL was reported in a sixty-six-year-old man who consumed homemade red wine. A detailed investigation revealed that the wine specimen contained 14 milligrams of lead per liter of wine, a very high amount. The source of the lead was the highly corroded surface of a bathtub that was used for grape crushing, and the juice was stored there for up to one week before bottling. The homemade wine was very acidic (pH of 3.8), which would have greatly contributed to the solubilization of lead from the corroded bathtub.[11]

A moderate level of lead in blood may cause chronic lead toxicity, which in turn may lead to the development of hypertension and gout. People who consume moonshine whiskey are at higher risk of a body burden of lead, and even if they do not experience acute, life-threatening lead toxicity, they may experience many complications of lead poisoning. Symptoms of lead poisoning are listed in table 11.2.

Table 11.2. Symptoms of Lead Poisoning

Confusion
Fatigue
Impairment of verbal skills
Impaired memory
Impaired motor skills
Peripheral neuropathy
Hematological problem
Endocrine (hormone) problem
Psychiatric problem

Moonshine Liquors and Poisoning with Other Heavy Metals

Gerhardt et al. (1980) reported twelve sequential cases of arsenic poisoning, where a significant number of such cases were due to consumption of contaminated moonshine whiskey. Some specimens of confiscated whiskey demonstrated high amounts of arsenic as a contaminant.[12] In another report by Gerhardt et al. (1980), in addition to lead, the authors found copper, zinc, and arsenic in potentially toxic ranges in some samples of moonshine whiskey (a total of twelve samples analyzed). One whiskey specimen had a potentially toxic concentration of arsenic (41.5 micrograms/dL), and copper was found in a high amount (1.4 mg/dL) in another specimen. As expected, seven specimens contained lead, with amounts varying from 3.5 to 530 micrograms/dL.[13] Although copper toxicity from consuming moonshine whiskey has not been well documented in the medical literature, consuming moonshine whiskey may put an individual at a much higher risk of getting copper toxicity.

Miscellaneous Toxicity Due to Consumption of Moonshine Whiskey

Conradi et al. (1980) reported a case where a person died from paraquat poisoning, presumably from paraquat being mixed into illicit moonshine alcohol. During an autopsy investigation, this herbicide was found in major organs of the victim.[14] Methanol contamination of moonshine liquors is not commonly encountered in the United States, but cheap methanol is added to illegally produced liquors in many countries of the world. Consumption of such liquors may cause epidemics, including blindness and death. Similarly, ethylene glycol, rubbing alcohol (isopropyl alcohol), and other alcohols with higher molecular weight may also be present in moonshine liquors (the toxicity of such substances is described in detail in chapter 12). In a report by Lachenmeier et al. (2009), additives like sulfites, sorbic acid, saccharin, and artificial colors were detected in cheap fruit wine products collected from local markets in Poland. In addition, the authors also detected ethyl carbamate, a human carcinogen, in some cheap unrecorded alcohol products and concluded that the harmful effect of unrecorded alcohol products on the health of people with poor socioeconomic status should be investigated in detail.[15]

MOONSHINE LIQUORS IN OTHER NATIONS

Although research on moonshine liquors focused on lead poisoning in the United States, in Eastern Europe and other countries research on moonshine focused on volatile components other than ethanol (alcohol) in such products. Cheap, illegally produced alcohols are often adulterated with methanol, an inexpensive product, and death may occur from consuming such products. There are many reports of mass poisoning from consuming such products.

Methanol poisoning due to consumption of moonshine liquors is a major public health concern in many third world countries.

Although methanol poisoning is the major public health safety issue related to consumption of moonshine liquors in other countries, lead poisoning from drinking such products has also been reported.

Mass Methanol Poisoning from Consuming Moonshine Liquors: World Reports

A report in the *New York Times* on May 21, 2008, indicated that consumption of contaminated moonshine claimed 110 lives among poor people in Bangalore, India, nearby rural areas, and across the state border of Tamil Nadu. A vast majority of the dead lived in slums and got sick after consuming contaminated cheap moonshine. The police chief, Srikumar, stated that the liquor was spiked with camphor and tobacco and was suspected to have toxic amounts of methanol. In addition, the liquor also contained a high amount of alcohol (40 percent) according to Venugopal, the state's top liquor enforcement official.[16] In Kenya, Kabir Ahmad reported that on November 22, 2000, Kenyan courts charged 6 people with manslaughter for illegally brewing alcoholic liquor that claimed 140 lives in Nairobi and the neighboring Kiambu district around November 15. Another 20 people became irreversibly blind, and more than 400 people were admitted to the hospital. This was one of the worst poisoning incidents in Kenya from consumption of illicitly produced alcohol. Police reported that the brew had been laced with methanol to increase its potency. In 1998, a similar brew killed 100 people and in 1999, another 23 died and 5 became blind after consuming contaminated alcohol.[17]

The number of deaths due to methanol poisoning between October 1992 and May 2001 in Turkey was 271; 241 of these victims were men. In this report (Yayci et al. 2003), the authors determined that twenty-nine victims died from methanol poisoning due to the consumption of cologne, and three men died from drinking an alcoholic beverage named "Raki." The authors concluded that in order to decrease mortality due to methanol poisoning, some precautions should be developed that would help prevent the production and consumption of illegally produced alcoholic beverages.[18] Cheap eau de cologne was the major source of methanol poisoning and death in Turkey, and the authors commented that public education about colognes and legislative control of cologne production are important in preventing methanol poisoning.[19] In the Adana region of Turkey, methanol contamination occurs during home production of Raki from grapes, figs, and plums. Villagers often use wooden materials and reed pipes during the distillation process, and methanol (wood alcohol produced during wood burning) is produced automatically by the equipment during the production of alcohol. Thus, villagers unknowingly sell contaminated Raki to consumers, and severe methanol toxicity may occur after consuming such products. Gulmen et al. (2006) reported that seventeen deaths occurred in Adana, Turkey, due to consumption of such alcoholic drinks.[20]

Higher Alcohols Found in Moonshine Liquors in Other Countries

Although methanol adulteration is the major cause of mass poisoning from consumption of moonshine liquors in countries other than the United States, contamination of such products with higher alcohols (alcohols with molecular weight greater than ethyl alcohol) is another public safety concern, because some of these higher alcohols are toxic. In one study, Szucas et al. (2005) determined that in addition to methanol, isobutanol, propanol, butanol, and isoamyl, alcohol concentrations found in illegally produced spirits in Hungary were significantly higher compared to levels found in spirits produced legally. The authors concluded that their results suggest that the consumption of such homemade spirits is an additional risk factor for developing alcohol-induced cirrhosis of the liver and may have contributed to higher levels of mortality from liver cirrhosis in Central and Eastern Europe. Therefore, restriction of the supply and sale of alcohol from illicit sources is urgently needed to significantly reduce mortality from chronic liver disease.[21] Although higher alcohols are found in legally produced alcoholic beverages, much higher amounts of higher alcohols may be encountered in illegally produced alcoholic drinks, because the process of production is crude and not standardized. Narawane et al. (1998) investigated 328 patients from a public hospital in Mumbai, India, and concluded that although illicit liquors in general contain less alcohol than legally produced alcoholic drinks, alcoholic liver disease occurs more commonly with consumers of illicit liquors, and such liver diseases appear earlier than in people drinking legally produced liquors.[22]

Surrogate Alcohol

"Surrogate alcohol" is a broad term that includes illegally produced moonshine and all nonbeverage alcohols, that is, alcohols not intended for human consumption. Denatured alcohol (methylated spirit in which methanol is added to alcohol to make it nondrinkable) is a major surrogate alcohol that is sometimes consumed by alcoholics (see chapter 12 for methanol toxicity). Aftershave lotion, mouthwash, windshield wiper fluid, antifreeze, and fire lighting liquids can all be considered surrogate alcohol. In Russia, there are two types of surrogate alcohol: (1) true surrogate alcohol, that is, solutions and liquids manufactured from ethanol or containing large amounts of ethanol, and (2) false surrogate alcohol, such as methanol, propanol, and ethylene glycol.[23]

McKee et al. (2005) determined the composition of surrogate alcohols consumed in Russia, where an estimated 7.3 percent of the population drink such product. The authors identified three broad ranges of products, including *samogon* (home-produced spirits), medicinal compounds, and other alcohols not produced for human consumption (mostly aftershave). Although samogon contains less alcohol than commercially produced vodka, certain toxic higher alcohols were present in such illegally produced liquors in Russia. Medicinal compounds, however, contained more alcohol than vodka, and other nonbeverage alcohol products also contained high amounts of alcohol (ethanol). The authors concluded that a significant number of Russian men are drinking products that have either very high concentrations of ethanol or contaminants known to be toxic to humans. These products are untaxed and thus much less expensive than vodka, but consumption of such products by a significant number of people is a serious public health and safety concern.[24]

In Estonia, a wide range of nonbeverage alcoholic products are consumed by individuals. These products include aftershave lotions, fire lighting fluid, medicinal compounds, and illegally produced spirits. Lank et al. (2006) determined that the medicinal compounds contained an average 67 percent alcohol, while aftershaves contained slightly less. The illegally produced liquors contained an average of 43 percent alcohol (range 32–53 percent), but also contained detectable quantities of toxic higher alcohols. However, these products were sold at roughly half the price of commercially available vodka, and fire lighting fluids were very inexpensive. The presence of higher amounts of alcohol in these products, as well as the presence of toxic higher alcohols, can cause serious toxicity or illness and is thus a major public health concern.[25]

Surrogate alcohol use is a potential threat to public health. In general, there are two pathways by which such products exert their toxicity. First, the presence of components other than alcohol, most commonly methanol and lead, in significant amounts in such products have caused significant outbreaks of toxicity and even death after mass consumption. Methanol, the major culprit, has caused massive outbreaks of alcohol-related death and toxicity in various parts of the world after consumption of such contaminated products. Second, high alcohol content in these surrogate products, especially medicinal alcohol, is responsible for organ damage, especially liver cirrhosis and other diseases from chronic consumption of such products. Leon et al. (2007) reported that in Russia there is a strong link between consumption of surrogate alcohol and all-cause mortality among men. In addition, almost half of all deaths in working-age men in a typical Russian city may be accounted for by hazardous drinking (non-beverage alcohol consumption, problem drinking, or both).[26]

CONCLUSION

Moonshine whiskey and related illegally produced alcohol is a public safety concern even today, although production of such illegally produced liquors is on the decline at the present. The major problem of consuming such alcohol is lead toxicity. In addition, other harmful substances, such as methanol, higher alcohols, herbicides, pesticides, and various heavy metals, may also be present in such products. In other countries, adulteration of illegally produced alcohol with methanol is a major public health hazard. There are many reports of massive alcohol poisoning and death after consuming such illegally produced alcoholic products, mostly among poor people, in various parts of the world. Strict regulation and public education is urgently needed to overcome these important public safety issues.

NOTES

1. R. Montgomery and R. Finkenbine, "A Brief Review of Moonshine Use," *Psychiatric Service* 50, no. 8 (August 1999): 1088.

2. P. Kilborn, "U. S. Cracks Down on Rise in Appalachia Moonshine," *New York Times*, March 23, 2000.

3. C. P. Holstege, J. D. Ferguson, C. E. Wolf, A. B. Baer, et al., "Analysis of Moonshine Whiskey," *Journal of Toxicology: Clinical Toxicology* 42, no. 5 (August 2004): 597–601.

4. B. W. Morgan, C. S. Parramore, and M. Ethridge, "Lead Contaminated Moonshine: A Report of Bureau of Alcohol, Tobacco and Firearms Analyzed Samples," *Veterinary and Human Toxicology* 46, no. 2 (April 2004): 89–90.

5. B. W. Morgan, K. H. Todd, and B. Moore, "Elevated Blood Lead Levels in Urban Moonshine Drinkers," *Annals of Emergency Medicine* 37, no. 1 (January 2001): 51–54.

6. S. C. Gilfillan, "Lead Poisoning and the Fall of Rome," *Journal of Occupational Medicine* 7, (February 1965): 53–60.

7. M. Czachur, M. Standbury, M. Gochfield, G. G. Rhoads, and D. Wartenberg, "A Pilot Study of Take-Home Lead Exposure in New Jersey," *American Journal of Industrial Medicine* 28 (1995): 289–93.

8. B. W. Morgan, L. Barnes, C. S. Parramore, and R. B. Kaufmann, "Elevated Blood Lead Levels Associated with the Consumption of Moonshine among Emergency Department Patients in Atlanta," *Annals of Emergency Medicine* 42, no. 3 (September 2003): 351–58.

9. D. A. Pegues, B. J. Hughes, and C. H. Woernle, "Elevated Blood Lead Levels Associated with Illegally Distilled Alcohol," *Archives of Internal Medicine* 153, no. 12 (June 1993): 1501–4.

10. R. B. Kaufmann, C. J. Staes, and T. D. Matte, "Deaths Related to Lead Poisoning in the United States, 1979–1998," *Environmental Research* 91, no. 2 (February 1991): 78–84.

11. S. Mangas, R. Visvanathan, and M. van Alphen, "Lead Poisoning from Homemade Wine: A Case Study," *Environmental Health Perspective* 109, no. 4 (April 2001): 433–35.

12. R. E. Gerhardt, E. A. Crecelius, and J. B. Hudson, "Moonshine-Related Arsenic Poisoning," *Archives of Internal Medicine* 140, no. 2 (February 1980): 211–13.

13. R. E. Gerhardt, E. A. Crecelius, and J. B. Hudson, "Trace Element Content of Moonshine," *Archives of Environmental Health* 35, no. 6 (November–December 1980): 332–34.

14. S. E. Conradi, L. S. Olanoff, and W. T. Dawson, "Fatality Due to Paraquat Intoxication: Confirmation by Postmortem Tissue Analysis," *American Journal of Clinical Pathology* 80, no. 5 (November 1980): 771–76.

15. D. W. Lachenmeier, S. Granss, B. Rychak, J. Rehm, et al., "Association between Quality of Cheap and Unrecorded Alcohol Products and Public Health Consequences in Poland," *Alcohol Clinical and Experimental Research* 33, no. 10 (October 2009): 1757–69.

16. S. Sengupta, "Poison Moonshine Kills 110 of India's Poor," *New York Times*, May 21, 2008.

17. K. Ahmad, "Methanol-Laced Moonshine Kills 140 in Kenya," *Lancet* 356, no. 9245 (December 2000): 1911.

18. N. Yayci, H. Agritmis, A. Turla, and S. Koc, "Fatalities Due to Methyl Alcohol Intoxication in Turkey: An 8-Year Study," *Forensic Science International* 131, no. 1 (January 2003): 36–41.

19. S. Kalkan, A. A. Cevik, C. Cavdar, O. Aygoren, et al., "Acute Methanol Poisoning Reported to the Drug and Poison Information Center in Izmir," *Veterinary and Human Toxicology* 45, no. 6 (December 2003): 334–37.

20. M. K. Gulmen, D. Meral, A. Hilal, R. Akcan, et al., "Methanol Intoxication in Adana, Turkey," *Toxicology Mechanism and Methods* 16, no. 7 (September 2006): 508–14.

21. S. Szucas, A. Sarvary, A. McKee, and R. Adany, "Could the Higher Level of Cirrhosis in Central and Eastern Europe Be Due Partly to the Quality of Alcohol Consumed? An Exploratory Investigation," *Addiction* 100, no. 4 (April 2005): 536–42.

22. N. M. Narawane, S. Bhatia, P. Abraham, S. Sanghani, et al., "Consumption of Country Liquor and Its Relation to Alcoholic Liver Disease in Mumbai," *Journal of the Association of Physicians in India* 46, no. 6 (June 1998): 510–13.

23. D. W. Lachenmeier, J. Rehm, and G. Gmel, "Surrogate Alcohol: What Do We Know and Where Do We Go?" *Alcoholism: Clinical and Experimental Research* 31, no. 10 (October 2007): 1613–24.

24. M. McKee, S. Suzcs, A. Sarvary, R. Adany, et al., "The Composition of Surrogate Alcohols Consumed in Russia," *Alcohol: Clinical and Experimental Research* 29, no. 10 (October 2005): 1884–88.

25. K. Lank, M. Vali, S. Szucs, R. Adany, et al., "The Composition of Surrogate and Illegal Alcohol Products in Estonia," *Alcohol and Alcoholism* 41, no. 4 (July–August 2006): 446–50.

26. D. A. Leon, L. Saburova, S. Tomkins, E. Andreev, et al., "Hazardous Alcohol Drinking and Premature Mortality in Russia: A Population-Based Case-Controlled Study," *Lancet* 369, no. 9578 (June 2007): 1001–2009.

12

More Dangerous than Alcohol
Methanol and Ethylene Glycol

Methanol and ethylene glycol are sweeter tasting than ethyl alcohol but not suitable for human consumption. Both methanol and ethylene glycol are more dangerous than alcohol because the body converts both of them into very toxic compounds (metabolites), and if ingested or even inhaled for a prolonged period of time (especially methanol) serious poisoning and even death may result. According to a 2002 report by Davis et al., the average methanol exposure reported to the American Association of Poison Control Centers between 1993 and 1998 was 2,254 cases annually, and one death occurred in every 183 exposures. In this report, the authors concluded that 90.3 percent of cases of methanol toxicity were due to unintentional exposure, while 8.3 percent of cases were due to intentional exposure.[1]

In the most recent report of the American Association of Poison Control Centers (2007), substances involved in a majority of the exposures were analgesics. For children younger than six, most exposure was from cosmetics and personal care products. In 2007, 2,252 cases of methanol and 5,395 cases of ethylene glycol poisonings were reported to the U.S. Poison Control Centers. Of those intoxicated with methanol, twenty-six patients were classified as experiencing "major" disability, and eleven patients died. For those patients who were intoxicated with ethylene glycol, 135 patients were classified as having "major" disability, and sixteen patients died. Interestingly, there were more reports of exposure to isopropyl alcohol (7,447 cases) than methanol or ethylene glycol poisoning in the same year, but only thirty-six patients experienced major complications and only one patient died, because isopropyl alcohol causes less toxicity in general than either methanol or ethylene glycol. It is important to recognize that these numbers probably underestimate the true incidence of exposure, however, due to not recognizing the ingestion or failing to report the suspected or known ingestion to a poison control center.[2]

In chemical terminology alcohol is any organic compound that contains a hydroxyl group (-OH). A hydroxyl group is composed of one oxygen atom and one hydrogen atom and this group (also known as a functional group) is responsible for many properties of this class of organic compounds. There are many organic compounds that contain the hydroxyl group, and all are classified under the general term "alcohol." The simplest compound in this series is methyl alcohol or methanol, which is also referred as "wood spirit" or "wood alcohol." Methanol contains only one carbon, one oxygen, and four hydrogen atoms. The next alcohol in this series is ethyl alcohol or ethanol, which is widely referred to as "alcohol" and is the active ingredient of alcoholic beverages as well as hard liquor. Next in the series is propyl alcohol, a more complex structure that is found in two distinct forms: propyl alcohol and isopropyl alcohol. Both compounds have the same number of carbon, hydrogen, and oxygen but differ slightly in structure. Propyl alcohol and isopropyl alcohol have antiseptic properties. Propyl alcohol is used in many household products, such as shampoo, hair spray, aftershave, mouthwash, and so on. Isopropyl alcohol is also referred to as rubbing alcohol, and a 70 percent solution of isopropyl alcohol is widely used as a disinfecting agent. Isopropyl alcohol evaporates very quickly and is also used in many cleaning solutions, such as paint thinner and antifreeze. Chemical structures of common alcohols are given below.

CH_3-OH   Methanol (one carbon, four hydrogens, and one oxygen)

CH_3-CH_2-OH   Ethyl Alcohol (two carbons, six hydrogens, and one oxygen)

CH_3-CH_2-CH_2-OH   Propyl Alcohol (three carbons, eight hydrogens, and one oxygen)

CH_3
|
CH-OH   Isopropyl Alcohol (three carbons, eight hydrogens,
|
CH3   and one oxygen)

Ethylene glycol is also an alcohol and contains two hydroxyl groups. This compound is widely used as automobile antifreeze and for manufacturing plastic and polymers. Alcoholics tend to drink methanol or ethylene glycol, especially in winter, as a substitute for ethanol. The chemical structure of ethylene glycol is given below.

CH$_2$-OH   Ethylene Glycol (two carbons, six
| hydrogens, and two oxygens)
CH$_2$-OH

METHANOL: PRODUCTION

Methanol is produced when wood is burned, a process chemically termed "dry distillation of wood" or "pyrolysis." Pure methanol was first prepared in 1661 by Robert Boyle from boxwood, and later, in 1834, the chemical structure of methanol was described by Dumas and Peligot. Because methanol can be prepared from burning wood, it is also called wood alcohol or wood spirit. Today, methanol is no longer prepared from wood but is manufactured primarily from methane, which is found in natural gas or during the burning of coal. However, natural gas is preferred over burning coal to get methane because of environmental concerns, and it is the major source of raw material (methane) for industrial production of methanol. In this process, methane is converted into synthetic gas (which primarily contains carbon monoxide and hydrogen and may also contain some carbon dioxide) using steam, pressure, and high temperature with the aid of a nickel catalyst in methanol manufacturing plants. Then synthetic gas is converted into methanol using high pressure and temperature with the aid of another catalyst, such as zinc oxide or chromium oxide. A catalyst is an agent that accelerates a chemical reaction but is not consumed in the process, and it can be used over and over again.

Methane is a greenhouse gas, second only to carbon dioxide for the greenhouse effect. Methane is found in landfills, and landfills are one of the major sources of atmospheric methane.[3] Methane is the most abundant hydrocarbon in the atmosphere and has contributed to an estimated 20 percent of postindustrial global warming.

Only three types of bacteria regulate the fluxes of methane on Earth: methanotrophic bacteria, methanogenic archaea, and methanotrophic archaea.[4] Methanogenic archaea found in wetlands converts carbon dioxide and hydrogen into methane, while methanotrophic bacteria converts methane to methanol in the first step of their metabolic pathway using a specific enzyme called methane monooxygenase. One form of this enzyme is soluble, while another form is bound to cell membranes.[5] Methanol can be prepared from biogas using specific bacteria and using tools of genetic engineering. Such bacteria can be fine-tuned for the development of economically competitive bioprocesses based on methanol.[6] "Biogas" is defined as gas produced by the biological breakdown of organic matter, such as manure, municipal waste, cow dung (gobor gas in India), green waste, and farm waste, which are all rich in methane. Landfill gas is also a type of biogas.

On November 5, 2008, Professor Tsang and his group at Oxford University announced that they had successfully developed a novel method by which glycerol, the main by-product of biodiesel and oleochemical (chemicals produced from plant and animal fat) production, could be turned into methanol. For every 9 kg of vegetable oil processed, 1 kg of glycerol is produced as an unwanted by-product, and in the United States approximately 350,000 tons of glycerol are incinerated each year.[7] In this method, using a novel catalyst, conversion of glycerol to methanol can be achieved under relatively mild conditions (100°C and 20 bar of pressure). ISIS Innovation, a subsidiary of the University of Oxford, has patented this technology.

METHANOL: COMMERCIAL USE AND
USE IN HOUSEHOLD PRODUCTS

Methanol is biodegradable and is widely used in the manufacturing of a variety of chemicals including formaldehyde, which then can be used for manufacturing plastics, paints, synthetic textiles, adhesive, and foam cushions (table 12.1). Methanol is also used for producing the gasoline additive methyl-tertiary-butyl ether (MTBE, which is no longer used in the United States but is common in other parts of the world). Methanol can be used as a fuel, and during the Second World War was used in rocket fuel. Methanol is the most versatile fuel available, and its use may substitute for petroleum. If 5–15 percent methanol is added to gasoline in internal combustion engines (such as automobiles), there is an immediate reduction in atmospheric pollution, as well as improvement in the performance of the engine. Methanol can also be used in electrical power plants and for heating and other fuel applications.[8]

Pure methanol has been used as a fuel for racing cars for a long time, because methanol fire can be extinguished using water but petroleum-induced fire cannot be controlled as easily. In 1964, following a devastating crash and explosion at an Indianapolis car race, fuel for Indy cars was switched to methanol. In 2006, the fuel used in these racing cars was a blend of 90 percent methanol and 10 percent ethanol (ethyl alcohol),

Table 12.1. Methanol and Ethylene Glycol: Commercial Applications and Domestic Products

Compound	Common Sources
Methanol	
Domestic use	Windshield washer fluid, carburetor cleaner, windshield deicer, paint and varnish remover, gas line antifreeze, paint thinners, cleaning products, and Canned Heat; also used in making denatured alcohol (methylated spirit)
Commercial use	Fuel additive, fuel, preparation of formaldehyde (formalin, a tissue preservative that is 40 percent solution of formaldehyde), acetic acid, methyl methacrylate, methyl chloride, synesthetic resins, synthetic textiles, polymers, plastics, paints, adhesives, and foam cushions; also used as a solvent in chemical laboratories and industry
Ethylene glycol	
Domestic use	Automobile antifreeze (major use), hydraulic brake fluid coolant
Commercial use	Deicing fluid for aircrafts; preparation of polyester fibers, resins, polymers, dye and plastic bottles containing polyethylene tetraphthalate

while in 2007 the fuel was completely switched to 100 percent ethanol.[9] One disadvantage of methanol in its use as a fuel is its corrosive nature toward some metals, including aluminum.

Another application in producing energy is the methanol fuel cell, where methanol can be used to generate electricity. The methanol fuel cell is ideal where a small amount of electricity is required for powering a device for a long time, such as cell phones, laptops, and digital cameras. Several companies, including the Japanese company Toshiba, are actively involved in developing such fuel cells. On October 22, 2009, Toshiba Corporation announced the launch of its first direct methanol fuel cell product: Dynario, which is an external power source for mobile digital consumer products. This device, a small palm-sized product, when fueled with an injection of methanol from its dedicated cartridge can generate enough electricity to charge two mobile phones.[10]

Methanol is also found in many household products, including windshield washer fluid, carburetor cleaner, paints, varnishes, paint thinners, and various cleaning products (see table 12.1). Methanol is used in preparing denatured alcohol, because the addition of methanol to ethanol makes it toxic and undrinkable. In addition, denatured alcohol is cheap because it is exempted from the excise duty, which is applicable to ethanol. Denatured alcohol is used as a fuel for spirit burners, camping stoves, and Canned Heat, which is designed to be burned directly from its can. A popular brand is Sterno (Candle Corporation of America, a subsidy of Blyth, Greenwich, Connecticut). Denatured alcohol, which usually contains 5–10

percent methanol, is also referred to as "methylated spirit" in many countries in the world. Although not a household chemical, embalming fluid
contains methanol, along with formaldehyde, ethanol, and other chemicals.

HUMAN EXPOSURE TO METHANOL

As you can see, methanol is used in a variety of commercial and consumer products. As a result, human exposure to methanol may occur
through different routes, including inhalation, cutaneous exposure
(which is through the skin), and ingestion. Methanol is well absorbed
through all three routes and may cause toxicity regardless of the route of
exposure. In one report (Givens et al. 2008), the authors studied all cases
of methanol exposure from January 2003 to May 2005 using the Texas
Poison Center Network database. The authors reported that eighty-seven
cases of methanol exposure were through inhalation, while eighty-one
cases were through ingestion. Carburetor cleaner was responsible for
the majority of inhalation cases (seventy-nine out of eighty-seven), while
ingestion involved mostly windshield washer fluid (thirty-nine out of
eighty-one) and carburetor cleaner (twenty out of eighty-one). While
most of the inhalation exposure to methanol (78 percent) was intentional,
most ingestion of methanol cases were either accidental (65 percent) or in
suicide attempts (24 percent). A majority of these patients (56 percent of
patients in the inhalation group and 46 percent of patients in the ingestion group) were admitted to the hospital, and some patients experienced
vision loss in both groups.[11] This recent report indicates that exposure to
methanol through inhalation may cause serious toxicity, although some
of the previous reports indicated that individuals who abuse methanol-
containing products by inhalation are at low risk of developing methanol
toxicity.[12] In a report by Frenia and Schauben (1993), out of seven cases
of methanol toxicity due to inhalation abuse of carburetor cleaner, one
person died from methanol inhalation, while another person experienced
vision loss.[13] However, such serious methanol toxicity only results from
abuse of methanol-containing products. Routine occupational exposure
to methanol-containing products is relatively safe. Methanol is also absorbed through the skin and may cause methanol toxicity as reported in
the following case.

A Case Study

In the 1980s methanol production was introduced at a new petrochemical
complex in the port of Jubail, Saudi Arabia. A consultant who was super-
vising tank cleaning prior to methanol loading wore a positive-pressure

breathing apparatus but no protective clothing. After working for two to three hours in the tank, he came out and worked on deck, but unfortunately he wore his methanol-soaked clothing, which had eventually dried out because methanol is very volatile, with a boiling point of only 65°C. He developed visual disturbances, a typical symptom of methanol toxicity, eight hours after exposure, but recovered fully in the hospital.[14]

METHANOL EXPOSURE AND PREGNANCY

Exposure to both ethanol and methanol is dangerous during pregnancy because these low molecular weight substances can cross the placenta and affect the fetus. Hantson et al. (1997) reported a case where a twenty-six-year-old in her thirty-eighth week of pregnancy drank 250 to 500 mL methanol voluntarily. She was admitted to the hospital five hours after examination but gynecological examination and fetal monitoring failed to detect any fetal distress. The mother was treated for methanol poisoning and after six days delivered her baby. At that point no methanol was detected in the blood of the mother and no further complications were noted in the mother and her newborn.[15] However, in another report where a twenty-eight-year-old pregnant woman was poisoned with methanol (route of exposure not reported) and was treated aggressively, including using hemodialysis, methanol was also detected in the blood of the newborn baby. Despite aggressive therapy, both the mother and her newborn died from methanol poisoning.[16]

METHANOL CONTENT OF
ALCOHOLIC BEVERAGES AND FRUIT JUICES

A small amount of methanol is found in alcoholic beverages as a part of the natural fermentation process, and this small amount does not cause any harm because the ethanol present in the drink protects the human body from methanol toxicity. However, illicit drinks prepared from methylated spirit cause severe and even fatal illness. Illegally prepared moonshine whiskey may contain much higher amounts of methanol and cause severe toxicity (see chapter 11). In the European Union, 0.04 percent methanol at 40 percent alcohol (10 gm of methanol in one liter of ethanol) is considered the upper limit of safety.[17]

Pectin is a natural product found in plants and in many fruits. Apples, bananas, oranges, and strawberries contain significant amounts of pectin. Pectin is a polysaccharide (carbohydrate) that is often found in methylated form. When plant enzymes break down pectin, a process that occurs during the ripening of fruit, methanol is released. During the processing of fruits, especially when preparing freshly squeezed juices, pectin may be hydrolyzed, thus producing methanol. Often manufacturers treat cloudy apple juice with pectin esterase in order to get rid of the cloudiness (which is due to soluble and colloidal pectin), and slightly higher amounts of methanol can be found in processed apple juice compared to other juices. Humans cannot metabolize pectin, but bacteria in the gut can break down pectin, producing a small amount of methanol. However, the amount of methanol consumed by humans when drinking fruit juices or eating fruits is so small that it does not cause any toxicity. In a recently published article, Hang and Woodams (2010) reported that the methanol content of apple eau-de-vie (a traditional alcoholic beverage produced in France by fermented apple juice, also known as hard cider) made from apples grown in the Finger Lakes region of New York had a minimum methanol content of below 200 mg and maximum methanol content of 400 mg in 100 mL of 40 percent ethanol. The United States' legal limit of methanol for fruit brandy is 0.35 percent by volume of alcohol or 280 mg per 100 mL of 40 percent methanol. Although the methanol content of apple eau-de-vie may exceed the upper limit set by the U.S. government, the methanol content of hard cider varied from 0.037 percent to 0.091 percent, which was significantly below the upper limit of methanol content set by the U.S. government. Pasteurization of apple juice prior to preparing apple cider and the alcoholic beverage significantly reduced the methanol content of the drink.[18] In general, methanol content of processed fruit juice is lower than freshly squeezed juice.

Aspartame Controversy

Aspartame is a synthetic artificial sweetener (NutraSweet, Equal, and other brands) that is a methyl ester of a dipeptide (contains two amino acids: phenylalanine and aspartic acid). This compound has no nutritional value but is used in many diet drinks, including Diet Coca Cola. It has been estimated that aspartame is used in more than ninety countries in the world and in more than 6,000 food products. Aspartame is not absorbed and is completely broken down in the intestine into phenylalanine, aspartic acid, and methanol. Current use of aspartame, even by high user groups, remains well below the aspartame level of 50 mg/kg of body weight/day (U.S. Food and Drug Administration) and 40 mg/kg of body weight/per day (European Food Safety Authority). A critical review of all studies did not find any credible information that regular use of aspartame at recommended levels causes cancer, learning disabilities, or neurological diseases. The epidemiology and toxicological studies published so far indicate that aspartame is safe at current levels of consumption as a nonnutritive sweetener.[19]

Another controversy based on various Internet blogs regarding aspartame use is the generation of methanol, which is a toxic compound. It is true that aspartame contains 11 percent by volume of methanol, and complete breakdown of aspartame leads to methanol production in the body. Drinking a standard can of diet soda (330 mL) sweetened with aspartame will yield 20 mg of methanol; a similar amount of fruit juice will produce 40 mg of methanol; and an alcoholic beverage consumed in the same amount will produce 60–100 mg of methanol.

In addition to methanol, aspartame also produces phenylalanine, and many products containing aspartame have a warning level that the products contain phenylalanine so that an individual with phenylketonuria can be careful in consuming such products. Nevertheless, the yield of phenylalanine after drinking a can of diet soda is 100 mg compared to 500 mg of phenylalanine from consuming a glass of milk or 300 mg of phenylalanine from an egg.

Therefore, an amount of methanol and phenylalanine generated from consumption of aspartame-containing food is safe. Clinical studies have shown no evidence of toxic effect and no increase in blood methanol or phenylalanine with daily consumption of 50 mg/kg of body weight/per day (equivalent to seventeen cans of diet soft drink daily for a 70 kg adult) as documented in a report by Zehetner and McLean (1999) that was published in the prestigious medical journal the *Lancet*.[20]

ENDOGENOUS PRODUCTION OF METHANOL

A very small amount of methanol is produced in our body along with ethanol. Human blood typically contains 0.2 to 0.8 mg of methanol per liter of blood. A typical human body produces 0.3 to 0.6 gm of methanol per day and up to 30 gm of ethanol per day. Methanol is produced in trace amounts during mammalian metabolism, and ethanol may be produced in the gut by bacterial activity, but the complete mechanism by which the body produces methanol and ethanol is not fully elucidated. Methanol has also been detected in human breath in 0.2 to 0.6 parts per million (ppm). After consuming certain fruits, methanol levels in breath may increase. After eating 1 kg of apple, a total of approximately 0.5 gm of alcohol is released in the body. Therefore, daily consumption of a few apples or oranges may increase daily endogenous methanol production from 0.3 gm to 0.6 mg/per day, but such increases have no demonstrated harmful effects to the body such as nonalcoholic liver disease.[21]

A more recent study (Turner et al. 2007) demonstrated that methanol is present in the exhaled breath of all people, and its concentration is further increased after consumption of ripe fruits and fruit juices, as well as after consumption of alcoholic drinks. Methanol may remain in the body long after ethanol following heavy alcohol consumption. However, authors of this study reported that increases in methanol content of breath after consumption of fruit or fruit juice was small and less than expected based on earlier studies.[22]

How the Body Handles Methanol

Methanol is readily absorbed after ingestion or inhalation and enters into the bloodstream. A small amount of methanol is excreted unchanged in urine and also through exhaled breath, but the majority of methanol is metabolized by the same enzyme in the liver that metabolizes ethanol, namely, alcohol dehydrogenase. In this process formaldehyde is generated and further metabolized by another liver enzyme, acetaldehyde dehydrogenase, to formic acid (fig. 12.1).

Although methanol is relatively nontoxic, both methanol metabolites (formaldehyde and formic acid) are toxic and responsible for the toxicity

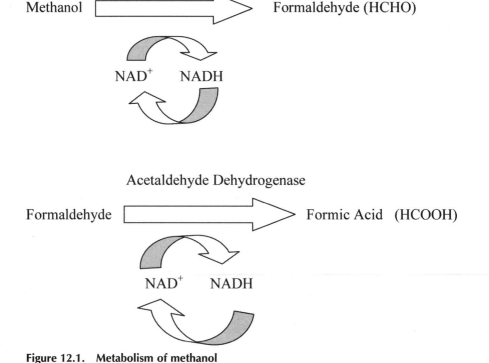

Figure 12.1. Metabolism of methanol

of methanol. Although both rodents and primates metabolize methanol into formic acid, rodents can rapidly metabolize formic acid into carbon dioxide so this end toxic metabolite of methanol metabolism does not accumulate in them and spares them from many toxic manifestations of methanol, as observed in primates. The metabolism of formaldehyde into carbon dioxide is a folate-dependent enzymatic reaction. Primates also metabolize formaldehyde into formic acid through a folate-dependent pathway; the rate of metabolism of methanol by primates is much slower than the rate observed in rodents.[23] Therefore, methanol toxicity is observed in monkeys and humans but not in rodents. Johlin et al. (1987) demonstrated that total folate was 60 percent lower in human liver than in rat liver, and tetrahydrofolate (a form of folate that is crucial for conversion of formaldehyde into carbon dioxide) is also 50 percent in human liver compared to rat liver. Additionally, the activity of 10-formyltetrahydrofolate dehydrogenase, a key liver enzyme that catalyzes the final step of conversion (oxidation) of formaldehyde into carbon dioxide, was markedly reduced in both human and monkey livers, thus explaining low-formate conversion into carbon dioxide in humans and monkeys, who are susceptible to methanol toxicity.[24]

METHANOL TOXICITY

Methanol itself is relatively nontoxic, and methanol toxicity is a classic example of "lethal synthesis," where metabolites of methanol in the body are the major cause of methanol toxicity. Formaldehyde, the end product of methanol metabolism, is the key factor in causing toxicity from methanol, including blindness and death. Because of this, methanol toxicity is not initially characterized by distinct symptoms, and manifestation of toxicity may be noticeable anywhere from one to seventy-two hours after exposure but typically twelve to twenty-four hours after exposure. Visual disturbances, including blurred vision, sensitivity to light, witnessing a snowstorm, and in some cases partial or total loss of light perception, are commonly present in an individual presented in the emergency room with suspected methanol toxicity. Nausea and vomiting may also be present but may not be seen in all patients.

The major complication of methanol poisoning is loss of vision, including partial or total blindness. Methanol toxicity may also be fatal. The lethal dose of methanol in humans is not fully established. Although it is assumed that ingestion of anywhere from 30 to 100 mL of methanol may cause death, fatality from methanol may occur even after ingestion of 15 mL of 40 percent methanol. In contrast, there is a published report that neither death nor blindness occur after the consumption of even 500 mL of methanol. However, cases of visual impairment and blindness are more common with methanol ingestion, and blindness may result from consuming at little as 4 mL of methanol.[25]

How methanol causes blindness is not fully understood. Animal experiments indicate that formic acid, a metabolite of methanol, is responsible for most of the damage. An enzyme very similar to alcohol dehydrogenase, known as retinol dehydrogenase, is present in the human retina, and the metabolism of methanol inside the retina, producing formic acid, causes major methanol-induced retinal toxicity.[26]

Blood methanol levels may vary widely among individuals poisoned with methanol. In general if blood methanol concentration exceeds 20 mg/dL (20 mg of methanol per 100 mL of blood), treatment should be initiated. Wallage and Watterson (2008) reviewed twelve fatal cases of methanol poisoning. Six of the individuals who were found deceased had postmortem methanol concentrations between 84 and 543 mg/dL, and postmortem formic acid levels between 64 and 110 mg/dL. Six other individuals who received therapy prior to death showed blood methanol levels between 68 and 427 mg/dL and formic acid levels between 37 and 91 mg/dL during hospitalization, but their postmortem levels of both methanol and formic acid were significantly lower due to hospital treatment of formic acid toxicity.[27] However, Lushine et al. (2004) described a case where a patient with a blood methanol level of 692 mg/dL on admission was treated with 4-methylpyrazole (fomepizole) and dialysis without any aftereffects.[28]

Methanol is metabolized to formic acid, which makes the blood more acidic by reducing its pH (the measurement of hydrogen ion in a fluid, where pH 7 is neutral). Blood is slightly alkaline in nature, and a delicate balance of a pH between 7.35 and 7.46 is needed for normal physiological function of the human body. Because formic acid is acidic in nature, it lowers blood pH, and the process is an example of metabolic acidosis, where metabolism of the body is responsible for a decrease in the pH of blood, which may be very significant clinically and even life threatening. Metabolic acidosis is secondary to methanol poisoning and is a serious complication of methanol poisoning. Meyer et al. (2000) reported that there was no correlation between blood methanol level and clinical outcome of methanol poisoning, but blood pH of 7 or lower was a strong predictor of death or poor outcome from methanol poisoning.[29]

Another complication of methanol poisoning is lactic acidosis, which may also become life threatening. Lactic acid, a product that is generated in our body during exercise and other activities, is found in small amounts in our blood. The muscles of trained athletes can even use lactic acid as a fuel. Although lactic acid levels in blood may be elevated after exercise, our body can readily convert lactic acid into other products, and lactic acid levels return to normal levels within an hour. However, if lactic acid builds up in our body, it can be harmful, because it can reduce the pH of our blood and cause acidosis (often termed lactic acidosis), which may severely disrupt the body's normal functions. If untreated, severe lactic acidosis may cause death.

Laboratory Diagnosis of Methanol Toxicity

In the clinical laboratory a patient with suspected methanol poisoning is tested for the presence of methanol in the blood. In addition, sometimes formic acid levels are also analyzed along with other volatiles—such as ethanol, acetone, and ethylene glycol—in a single analytical step using a sophisticated technique known as headspace gas chromatographic analysis. Although blood is usually collected from a vein for analysis of blood methanol levels and other tests, a blood sample from an artery (arterial blood) may also be collected to measure the pH of the blood to see if pH is below the normal range. Another indirect indication of methanol poisoning is the increased anion gap in the serum, which can be easily separated from blood cells by centrifugation. The anion gap is defined as the difference between the measured level of positively charged ions (cations) in the blood and negatively charged ions (anions) in the blood.

Anion Gap = Concentration of sodium − (Concentration of chloride + Concentration of bicarbonate)

The concentration of potassium is often ignored because it is very small. The normal anion gap is 8 to 16 mmol/L (millimolar per liter), but in methanol poisoning this anion gap may increase significantly. Anion gap may increase in many pathological conditions, such as renal failure, lactic acidosis, and also in common poisoning, such as salicylate poisoning. Methanol poisoning also increases serum osmolality, another complex analytical measurement of total amounts of dissolved chemicals in serum. In serum, sodium, potassium, chloride, bicarbonate, urea, and glucose together make up 95 percent of total osmolality. Serum osmolality is measured by a principle called "freezing point depression" using an osmometer and is called "measured osmolality." Osmolality can also be calculated from measured concentrations of sodium, potassium, chloride, glucose, and urea.

Osmolar gap = Measured osmolarity − calculated osmolarity

Measured osmolarity should be close to calculated osmolality unless compounds like methanol, ethanol, acetone, ethylene glycol, or related compounds are present in serum. These compounds would increase serum osmolality. For example, if methanol is present in 50 mg/dL, it would increase serum osmolality by 15.6, and in the case of methanol poisoning, osmolar gap would be increased. However, poisoning with ethanol, isopropyl alcohol, ethylene glycol, acetone, and other organic solvents could also increase osmolar gap.

Treatment of Methanol Toxicity

Methanol poisoning can be treated using a variety of agents, such as ethanol, 4-methylpyrazole (fomepizole), and sodium bicarbonate, as well as dialysis. The outcome of methanol poisoning appears to be related more to the interval of time between exposure and initiation of treatment and to degree of acidosis rather than to the initial blood methanol level. Early and aggressive therapy with bicarbonate and ethanol and subsequent initiation of hemodialysis are strongly recommended whenever methanol is detected in blood, especially in patients who also have metabolic acidosis and demonstrated anion gap.[30] Sodium carbonate is a basic compound (a basic compound can neutralize an acid) and can bring the blood pH back to normal in the case of metabolic acidosis. Intravenous administration of sodium bicarbonate, which reduces the acidity of blood, is often initiated if the pH of blood is 7.2 or below. Intravenous administration of ethanol using a 10 percent solution of ethanol is also initiated if blood methanol concentration is more than 20 mg/dL or when ingested methanol amount is 30 mL or more.[31] Ethanol is an effective antidote for methanol poisoning, and the sooner the therapy can be initiated, the better the outcome. Ethanol is a preferred substrate for alcohol dehydrogenase, and in the presence of ethanol, metabolism of methanol to toxic formic acid metabolite is greatly reduced. Because the human body can effectively handle small amounts of formic acid, converting it to carbon dioxide, methanol toxicity can be greatly reduced by ethanol therapy.

Another effective therapy for methanol overdose is hemodialysis. Methanol is a small molecule with a molecular weight of only thirty-two. Methanol can be effectively removed from circulation using hemodialysis. Usually hemodialysis, along with ethanol therapy for methanol poisoning, should be initiated if the blood methanol level is 50 mg/dL or more. Hemodialysis may also be initiated if an individual has ingested 30 mL or more of methanol or based on other clinical indications as determined by the physician treating such overdose.[32]

Recently, fomepizole (4-methylpyrazole), a potent competitive inhibitor of alcohol dehydrogenase has been used as an antidote to treat methanol poisonings. This antidote has the capability of slowing down the formation of formaldehyde from methanol. Formaldehyde is toxic and responsible for toxic effects due to methanol ingestion, and small formaldehyde buildup can be secreted in urine. Bicarbonate therapy can also be used with fomepizole therapy to correct metabolic acidosis caused by methanol.[33]

Case Report

An adult male presented to the emergency room with central blindness after ingesting methanol. His blood pH was 7.19, indicating severe metabolic acidosis, and his blood methanol level was 97 mg/dL. The patient was treated aggressively with ethanol, fomepizole, and hemodialysis. Further methanol metabolism was totally blocked by fomepizole and the patient recovered from this life-threatening methanol poisoning; fourteen days after this episode he recovered his vision completely.[34]

ETHYLENE GLYCOL: COMMERCIAL USE AND HOUSEHOLD PRODUCTS

Ethylene glycol is a colorless and relatively nonvolatile liquid that has a high boiling point of 193.7°C. It has a sweet taste, which is why children and pets tend to ingest it, causing ethylene glycol toxicity. An adult may drink ethylene glycol as a substitute for ethanol or in a suicide attempt. Because of the low melting point and high boiling point, ethylene glycol is used as a major ingredient in automobile antifreeze. Ethylene glycol is also an ingredient in several domestic products and is also widely used for commercial purposes. Ethylene glycol is used in deicing fluid and as a starting material for preparing various polyester products in industry (see table 12.1). In Germany ethylene glycol was used in the explosives industry during wartime.

Currently ethylene glycol is commercially prepared from ethylene. In the first step, ethylene, a hydrocarbon, is converted into ethylene oxide, and then ethylene oxide is converted into ethylene glycol by using silver as a catalyst and a high temperature, usually 250°C.

Human Exposure to Ethylene Glycol

Because ethylene glycol is relatively nonvolatile, inhalation exposure to it is not generally considered an occupational health hazard. In one study (Gerin et al. 1997), the authors measured ethylene glycol levels in 154 breathing zone air samples and 117 urine samples from thirty-three aviation workers exposed to deicing fluid (basket operators, deicing truck drivers, leads, and coordinators) during forty-two workdays over a winter period of two months at a Montreal airport. Ethylene glycol concentrations in air samples were relatively low, and measurable amounts of ethylene glycol in urine were only found in basket operators and coordinators, but some of them did not wear masks or were accidently sprayed with deicing fluid. However, acute or chronic renal toxicity, the major complication of ethylene glycol exposure, was not found in any of the aviation workers. The authors concluded that health hazards from exposure to ethylene glycol in the form of inhalation is not significant, but other routes of exposure such as the percutaneous route (absorption through the skin) may cause health hazards.[35]

Absorption of ethylene glycol through the skin may cause serious toxicity, especially if there are any skin lesions. Bouattar et al. (2009) reported a case of toxicity in a thirty-eight-year-old man who presented at the hospital with nausea, vomiting, abdominal pain, and worsening of his mental status. The patient also experienced renal failure and was treated with hemodialysis. The renal biopsy revealed the presence of calcium oxalate crystals, a characteristic of ethylene glycol poisoning. It was later discovered that the patient worked in a cement factory and handled ethylene glycol without protective gloves. In addition, the patient had had cutaneous psoriasis for ten years. (Normal skin cells mature and replace dead skin every twenty-eight to thirty days, but in psoriasis, skin cells sometimes mature in less than a week. Because the body can't shed old skin as rapidly as new skin, cells rise to the surface and patches of dead skin develop on the arms, back, chest, elbows, legs, nails, and in other parts of the body and appear as red skin lesions. Psoriasis is a noncontagious autoimmune disease.) The authors concluded that cutaneous contact with ethylene glycol may cause poisoning in the presence of skin lesions.[36] The major route of exposure to ethylene glycol is ingestion of fluids containing ethylene glycol. Ethylene glycol is rapidly and completely absorbed from the intestinal tract after oral ingestion.

How the Body Handles Ethylene Glycol

Ethylene glycol itself is relatively nontoxic, like methanol. But when the body metabolizes it, it produces toxic compounds, which are responsible for its adverse effects. The peak blood ethylene glycol concentration (highest ethylene glycol level) occurs within one to two hours after ingestion. Ethylene glycol is also metabolized by the same enzyme systems that metabolize ethanol and methanol. The half-life of ethylene glycol in blood (half-life is the time required for blood concentration to reduce half of its initial concentration) is three to five hours. Ethylene glycol is primarily metabolized in the liver (approximately 80 percent) while another 20 percent is excreted in the urine unchanged. Metabolism of ethylene glycol by the liver is a four-step process. Ethylene glycol is first metabolized to glycoaldehyde by alcohol dehydrogenase, and

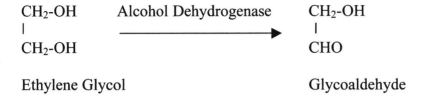

Ethylene Glycol   Glycoaldehyde

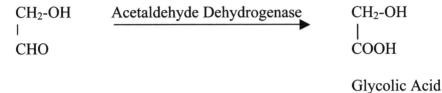

Figure 12.2.   **Metabolism of ethylene glycol to glycolic acid**

then glycoaldehyde is further metabolized by aldehyde dehydrogenase into glycolic acid (fig. 12.2).

The conversion of ethylene glycol in two steps to glycolic acid occurs relatively rapidly, but then glycolic acid is further transformed to glyoxalic acid and then further transformed to the metabolite oxalic acid. Oxalic acid binds with calcium-forming calcium oxalate, the end toxic metabolite of ethylene glycol. The mechanism of conversion of glycolic acid to oxalic acid is not fully understood, but it has been established that lactate dehydrogenase enzymes present in hepatocytes (major cells in the liver) catalyzes this transformation (fig. 12.3).[37]

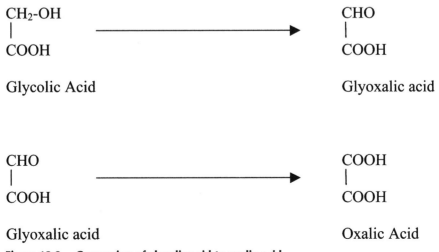

Figure 12.3.   **Conversion of glycolic acid to oxalic acid**

ETHYLENE GLYCOL TOXICITY

Ethylene glycol toxicity in humans occurs in several stages. The first stage is the neurological stage where mild euphoria, like ethanol poisoning, may be observed within thirty minutes of ingestion of ethylene glycol. Other neurological symptoms may include nystagmus, ataxia, seizure, and even coma, and these symptoms may be observed between thirty minutes and up to twelve hours after ingestion of ethylene glycol. The next stage of ethylene glycol poisoning is cardiac symptoms, including mild hypertension and tachycardia. Finally, between twenty-four to seventy-two hours after exposure, symptoms of renal failure may be observed, especially in patients who are not treated (table 12.2).

Major complications of ethylene glycol poisoning are metabolic acidosis and renal failure, and these complications may be fatal. The lethal dose of ethylene glycol is usually assumed as 100 mL, but there are reports of fatality from ethylene glycol poisoning even from ingestion of only 30 mL.[38] Death from ethylene glycol poisoning may follow if symptoms are untreated within eight to twenty-four hours after poisoning. On the other hand, prognosis of ethylene glycol poisoning is good if treated in a timely fashion. A thirty-six-year-old man with a history of depression consumed a massive amount of ethylene glycol (3 liters) in a suicide attempt. On admission, his blood ethylene glycol level was 1889 mg/dL, a very high ethylene glycol level that is potentially fatal. Despite ingesting a lethal amount of ethylene glycol, this patient survived due to prompt medical attention and aggressive treatment using hemodialysis.[39]

The blood level of ethylene glycol in fatal poisoning may vary widely among different individuals. Rosano et al. (2009) reviewed twelve medi-

Table 12.2. Common Symptoms of Methanol and Ethylene Glycol Toxicity

Compounds	Symptoms of Toxicity
Methanol	
Early symptoms	Inebriation (appear drunk/intoxicated), drowsiness
Delayed symptoms (12–24h)	Vomiting, dyspnea (difficulty in breathing), Kussmaul respiration (deep, slow, and labored breathing characteristic of metabolic acidosis), vertigo, blurred vision, absent light perception, partial to total blindness
Ethylene glycol	
Early symptoms (Neurological; 30 min–6 h)	Euphoria, appear intoxicated, stumbling, increased thirst
Intermediate symptoms (Cardiopulmonary; 6 h–24 h)	Vomiting, decreased body temperature, tachycardia, deep, slow, and labored breathing
Late symptoms (Renal: 24–72 h)	Low urine output, renal failure, coma

cal examiners' cases where fatality was due to ethylene glycol poisoning and observed that the ethylene glycol concentrations ranged widely from only 5.8 to 779 mg/dL with a mean value of 183 mg/dL. The concentration of glycolic acid, a metabolite of ethylene glycol, varied from 81 mg/dL to 177 mg/dL. Calcium oxalate crystals were detected in renal tissues.[40] In another case report, an adult male died from ethylene glycol poisoning with a blood ethylene glycol level of 25 mg/dL. Acute renal failure was the cause of death, and calcium oxalate crystals were identified in renal cells (tubular epithelial cells) using confocal laser scanning microscopy.[41] Garg et al. (2009) reported a case where a person who died from ethylene glycol poisoning showed a very high level of ethylene glycol in postmortem blood (2340 mg/dL) but without elevated concentration of any ethylene glycol metabolites. In addition, oxalic acid crystals were not detected in the urine.[42]

Although most cases of ethylene glycol poisoning are due to accidental ingestion or suicidal attempts, there is an interesting case where ethylene glycol was used in a homicide in which a thirty-six-year-old female caregiver poisoned a seventy-five-year-old man suffering from both diabetes and hypertension. On postmortem investigation, the causes of death were established as acute poisoning by ethylene glycol and recent blunt impact injuries to the head, trunk, and extremities. A trial by jury involving the female caregiver resulted in her conviction, and she was sentenced to twenty-three years to life in prison.[43]

Ethanol protects the human body from the toxic effect of ethylene glycol unless a person injects both ethylene glycol and ethanol at the same time. Usually laboratory findings of ethylene glycol poisoning, such as osmolality and anion gap, are not present and may obscure the diagnosis of ethylene glycol poisoning.[44] However, concurrent ingestion of methanol and ethylene glycol is dangerous. Arai et al. (1983) reported a fatal case of poisoning by a mixture of methanol (80 percent) and ethylene glycol (20 percent) in a seventy-two-year-old man who was found semicomatose and subsequently hospitalized. It was estimated that he drank between 150 to 200 mL of fluid containing both methanol and ethylene glycol. Despite aggressive therapy, the man died from the complications of toxicity from both of these agents.[45]

Ethylene glycol poisoning often results in acute renal failure, especially if treatment by doctors at a medical facility is delayed. The mechanism of ethylene glycol toxicity was thought to be due to accumulation of toxic metabolites, such as glycoaldehyde, glyoxylate, and oxalic acid. However, more recent investigations reveal that the accumulation of calcium oxalate crystals—mostly calcium oxalate monohydrate—accounts for most major toxicity and acute renal failure due to ethylene glycol poisoning. Calcium oxalate crystals are found in both calcium oxalate monohydrate (one molecule of water is incorporated in the structure of calcium oxalate) or calcium oxalate dihydrate (two molecules of water are incorporated).[46] However, another major complication of ethylene glycol poisoning is caused by glycolic acid.

Oxalic acid is found in high amounts in some poisonous plants and is also present in significant amounts in various foods, such as beets, spinach, and certain fruits (table 12.3). Our bodies also produce oxalic acid on their own, for example, from degradation of vitamin C (ascorbic acid). It is assumed that more than 80 percent urinary excretion of oxalic acid is due to endogenous production (the body's production of oxalic acid), while another 20 percent derives from food. Some individuals have a genetic defect in producing more oxalic acid endogenously and also have a higher rate of intestinal absorption of oxalic acid. These individuals are at greater risk of developing kidney stones, because almost 80 percent of all kidney stones are due to the formation of calcium oxalate crystals. Intestinal absorption of oxalic acid makes a substantial contribution to oxalic secretion in urine, and this absorption can be modified by decreasing oxalate intake or increasing the intake of calcium, magnesium, or fiber.[47]

Laboratory Diagnosis of Ethylene Glycol Poisoning

Treatment for ethylene glycol poisoning is an important issue because early diagnosis based on symptoms (central nervous system depression, cardiopulmonary complications, and renal insufficiency) and laboratory tests are crucial for treatment. Early diagnosis can prevent mortality as well as avoid complications from ethylene glycol poisoning. Laboratory findings of ethylene glycol poisoning include increased anion gap, metabolic acidosis (blood pH significantly lower than 7.35), increased osmolar gap, oxalic acid crystals in the urine, and detectable ethylene glycol level in the blood.[48] For example, if ethylene glycol is present in the blood in an amount of 50 mg/dL, it would increase the measured serum osmolality by 8.1, thus increasing the osmolar gap.

Table 12.3.   Food Containing High or Moderate Amount of Oxalic Acid

Oxalic Acid Content	Food
High oxalic acid	Beets, coca, figs, parsley, poppy seeds, spinach, lime peel, nuts, Brussels sprouts
Moderate oxalic acid	Green beans, blackberry, blueberry, carrot, celery, strawberry, green onions, okra, green peppers, sweet potatoes, lettuce, carrots, cauliflower, broccoli
Low oxalic acid	Corn, tomato, squash, peas, onion, potato, kale, apple, asparagus, apricots

Blood levels of ethylene glycol are usually measured by headspace gas chromatography, either singly or in combination with other volatile compounds, such as methanol, acetone, and isopropyl alcohol. In addition, there are some enzymatic methods available for rapid determination of blood ethylene glycol levels using an automated analyzer in the clinical laboratory setting.

Treatment of Ethylene Glycol Poisoning

Toxicity from ethylene glycol is mostly due to ingestion, because unlike methanol, ethylene glycol is relatively nonvolatile and inhalation is not a route of exposure that may cause toxicity. Many ethylene glycol poisonings are the result of using ethylene glycol as a cheap alcohol substitute or in attempted suicide. Children and animals often consume large amounts of ethylene glycol because of its sweet taste. In an attempt to prevent ethylene glycol poisoning, denatonium benzoate may be added to ethylene glycol, because this agent has a bitter taste. In eight states the addition of a bittering agent to antifreeze formulations containing ethylene glycol is compulsory (table 12.4).

Ethylene glycol poisoning is treated by using bicarbonate, ethanol, fomepizole, and hemodialysis. The sooner the treatment is initiated, the better the outcome. If treatment can be started early enough after ingestion, simple administration of ethanol intravenously may be sufficient for full recovery from ethylene glycol poisoning. In one report (Karlson-Stiber and Persson 1992), the authors treated four patients with ethylene glycol poisoning and ethylene glycol blood levels varying from 62 mg/dL to 124 mg/dL with ethanol alone. These patients demonstrated minimal metabolic acidosis, and none of them developed any kidney damage.[49] In another report (Velez et al. 2007), the authors treated a thirty-three-year-old man who drank half a gallon of antifreeze and an unknown amount of beer with fomepizole alone. His blood ethylene glycol level was 70.6 mg/dL, but fortunately this patient presented to the hospital within one hour of ingestion of ethylene glycol and beer. Over the next three days the patient was treated, but no further complications, such as metabolic acidosis or renal insufficiency, developed in this patient. This report indicates that early initiation of treatment has a favorable outcome in ethylene glycol poisoning.[50]

Table 12.4.   States Where the Addition of a Bittering Agent Is Compulsory in Antifreeze Containing Ethylene Glycol

Arizona	New Mexico	Virginia
California	Oregon	Washington
Maine	Tennessee	

Hemodialysis to correct metabolic acidosis, along with ethanol or fomepizole infusion and bicarbonate therapy, may also be needed in treating patients with more serious ethylene glycol toxicity. This is a clinical decision made by the attending physicians based on symptoms, laboratory values, and many other factors. In general, patients with severe metabolic acidosis, high serum potassium values, seizure, or coma during admission show poor outcomes from ethylene glycol poisoning. A patient may also die from ethylene glycol poisoning despite aggressive therapy, including hemodialysis.[51]

Propylene glycol, which is similar to ethylene glycol, is used as an industrial solvent and can also be used in antifreeze formulations. Propylene glycol is significantly less toxic than ethylene glycol and is preferred for antifreeze used in motor homes and recreational vehicles. Propylene glycol is also used as a diluent for oral, topical, or intravenous pharmaceutical preparations so that active ingredients can be dissolved properly in the formulation.

TOXICITY WITH ISOPROPYL ALCOHOL, ACETONE, AND RELATED COMPOUNDS

Although less common, toxicity may result from other organic solvents used in many domestic products. Isopropyl alcohol is also known as rubbing alcohol, which is a 70 percent aqueous solution of isopropyl alcohol. Isopropyl alcohol is slowly metabolized by alcohol dehydrogenase to acetone. Acetone is also found in many domestic products, for example, nail polish remover. Neither isopropyl alcohol nor acetone can cause metabolic acidosis, and poisoning from these compounds may be less life threatening than methanol or ethylene glycol poisoning, but there are reports of death from isopropyl alcohol poisoning. The lethal dose of isopropyl alcohol in an adult is estimated to be 240 mL, which is significantly higher than the lethal dose of either methanol or ethylene glycol. Acetone concentration is often higher than isopropyl alcohol in patients, and acetone can cause ketosis, a life-threatening illness. Using sponges soaked in rubbing alcohol to clean neonates can cause burning and even death in premature neonates following excessive cleaning. A twenty-one-day-old baby boy was presented to the hospital with isopropyl alcohol poisoning secondary to the mother applying gauze pads or cotton balls soaked with isopropyl alcohol to the umbilicus with every diaper change. The isopropyl alcohol concentration in the serum was 8 mg/dL and acetone concentration was 203 mg/dL. The patient was discharged from the hospital after three days.[52] An eighteenth-month-old child was wrapped in towels soaked with isopropyl alcohol by her mother to control a high fever (104°F). The towel was wrapped around the child's waist for approximately four hours and the child became lethargic. She was admitted to the ICU in a comatose condition and had a high serum osmolar gap. Eight hours after exposure, her serum isopropyl alcohol level was 162 mg/dL and her acetone level was 180 mg/dL. She responded to supportive care and was discharged from the hospital after three days in stable condition.[53]

Sometimes isopropyl alcohol is used along with propyl alcohol in topical antiseptic solution. Propyl alcohol is also metabolized by alcohol dehydrogenase to propyl aldehyde and then to propionic acid by acetaldehyde dehydrogenase. Because propionic acid can lower blood pH, ingestion of propanol may cause metabolic acidosis. Blanchet et al. (2007) reported a case where a hospitalized patient drank two 100 mL bottles of a topical antiseptic solution containing both isopropyl alcohol and propyl alcohol on two separate days. Eight hours after the second ingestion, his blood isopropyl alcohol concentration was 37 mg/dL, propyl alcohol concentration was less than 10 mg/dL, and acetone concentration was 227 mg/dL. The patient was treated with fomepizole. This case points out the need to limit access to alcohol containing antiseptic solutions on wards where alcoholic or psychotic patients are hospitalized.[54] There are other reports of similar ingestion of isopropyl alcohol and propyl alcohol. Death may even occur from such solvent ingestion. Alexander et al. (1982) reviewed fifty-seven cases of fatality from isopropyl alcohol poisoning.[55]

SOLVENT AND GLUE SNIFFING

Although it is not within the scope of this book to discuss solvent and glue abuse, because of the gravity of the problem, a brief description is provided here. Solvent (inhalant) abuse is common among adolescents, not only in the United States but also worldwide. In the United States, approximately 20 percent of adolescents have tried inhalants at least once by the time they reach eighth grade. Abused inhalants include solvents, glues, adhesives, paint thinners, fuels, and propellants (petroleum products). Inhalant abuse includes breathing directly from a container or soaking a rag with the solvent and then placing it over the nose and mouth, as well as pouring the solvent in a plastic bag and then breathing the fumes. Abuse of inhalant can produce euphoria, just like other abused drugs. When an abuser becomes hypoxic by rebreathing from a bag, the euphoric effect may even intensify.[56]

Various easily available household products that are abused include glue, adhesives, nail polish, nail polish remover, cigarette lighter fluid, butane gas, gas (petrol), air fresheners, deodorant, hair spray, pain-relieving spray, typewriter correction fluid, paint thinners, paint removers, and a variety of other agents. These household and office products contain toxic solvents such as toluene (paint, spray paint, adhesives, paint thinner, shoe polish), acetone (nail polish remover, typewriter correction fluid, and markers), hexane (glue, rubber cement), chlorinated hydrocarbon (spot and grease removers), xylene (permanent markers), propane gas (gas to light the grill, spray paints), butane gas (lighter fluid, spray paint), and fluorocarbons (hair spray, analgesic spray, and refrigerator coolant such as Freon).

Solvent abusers often present with nonspecific symptoms, but long-term abusers may come to the hospital with a wide range of neuropsychiatric symptoms. The most serious consequence of solvent abuse is death, which may occur after aspiration or asphyxia. Nearly 50 percent of deaths from solvent abuse are due to sudden sniffing death syndrome. Steffee et al. (1996) reported two cases of fatal volatile solvent inhalation abuse; gasoline sniffing in a twenty-year-old man and aerosol air freshener inhalation in a sixteen-year-old girl.[57] Pfeiffer et al. (2006) reported two cases where individuals sniffed cigarette lighter fluid containing isobutane for euphoria and hallucinations and died due to cardiac arrhythmia and other complications. Isobutane was detected in heart blood and brain tissue of both individuals.[58] Although death from solvent vapor inhalation in most cases is intentional abuse to get high, there is a case report of an adult male who unintentionally inhaled excessive amounts of paint thinner vapor and then died due to multiple organ failure.[59]

CONCLUSION

Methanol, ethylene glycol, and related alcohols are not made for human consumption but are widely used in domestic products. Such products must be kept completely out of reach of children, because ingestion of these products by children may cause life-threatening toxicity and may even be fatal. Ethylene glycol, in particular, should be kept out of reach of children and animals, because both children and animals (especially dogs, because cats do not have sweet taste buds) are drawn to ethylene glycol due to its sweet taste. Intentional or accidental poisoning of methanol or ethanol glycol require prompt medical attention because the sooner the therapy can be initiated, the better the outcome. Although symptoms of methanol toxicity, especially neurologic symptoms, may appear within thirty minutes of ingestion of ethylene glycol, symptoms of methanol toxicity may not be apparent for a period of twelve to twenty-four hours. Both methanol and ethylene glycol are relatively nontoxic, but severe toxicity from both these agents are due to their toxic metabolites: formic acid for methanol and calcium oxalate for ethylene glycol. Both methanol and ethylene glycol poisoning can be effectively treated with sodium bicarbonate, ethanol, fomepizole, and hemodialysis. Isopropyl alcohol, which is commonly used as rubbing alcohol, is less toxic than methanol or ethylene glycol, but excessive use of pads soaked with rubbing alcohol in cleaning newborn babies may cause significant toxicity or may burn the delicate skin of a newborn. Solvent abuse is a significant problem among adolescents, and such abuse is dangerous because it may cause severe toxicity, multiple organ failures, and even death.

NOTES

1. L. E. Davis, D. Hudson, B. E. Benson, L. A. Jones Easom, et al., "Methanol Poisoning Exposures in the United States: 1993–1998," *Journal of Toxicology: Clinical Toxicology* 40, no. 4 (2002): 499–505.

2. A. C. Bronstein, D. A. Spyker, L. R. Cantilens, J. R. Green, et al., "2007 Annual Report of the American Association of Poison Control Centers' National Poison Data System (NPDS): 25th Annual Report," *Clinical Toxicology* 46, no. 10 (December 2008): 927–1057.

3. C. Scheutz, P. Kjeldsen, J. E. Bogner, A. De Visscher, et al., "Microbial Methane Oxidation Process and Technologies for Mitigation of Landfill Gas Emission," *Waste Management Research* 27, no. 3 (August 2007): 409–55.

4. K. Knittel and A. Boetius, "Anaerobic Oxidation of Methane: Progress with an Unknown Process," *Annual Review of Microbiology* 63 (October 2009): 311–34.

5. A. S. Hakemian and A. C. Rosenzweig, "The Biochemistry of Methane Oxidation," *Annual Review of Biochemistry* 76 (July 2007): 223–41.

6. J. Schrader, M. Schilling, D. Holtman, D. Sell, et al., "Methanol-Based Industrial Biotechnology: Current Status and Future Perspective of Methylotrophic Bacteria," *Trends in Biotechnology* 27, no. 2 (February 2009): 107–15.

7. Giles Clark, "Oxford University Discovers New Methanol Process," November 5, 2008, *Biofuel Review*, http://www.biofuelreview.com/content/view/1770.

8. T. B. Reed and R. M. Lerner, "Methanol: A Versatile Fuel for Immediate Use," *Science* 182, no. 4119 (December 1973): 1299–1304.

9. Indycar.com staff, "Ethanol Will Fuel the Indycar Series: Renewable, Responsible Energy Recognized by President Bush," http://www.indycar.com/news/?story_id=4102.

10. "Toshiba Launches Portable Fuel Cell for Mobiles," http://physorg.com.

11. M. Givens, K. Kalbfleisch, S. Bryson, and R. Carl, "Comparison of Methanol Exposure Routes Reported to Texas Poison Control Center," *Western Journal of Emergency Medicine* 9, no. 3 (August 2008): 150–53.

12. V. S. Bebarta, K. Heard, and R. C. Dart, "Inhalation Abuse of Methanol Products: Elevated Methanol and Formate Levels without Vision Loss," *American Journal of Emergency Medicine* 25, no. 6 (October 2006): 725–28.

13. M. L. Frenia and J. L. Schauben, "Methanol Inhalation Toxicity," *Annals of Emergency Medicine* 22, no. 12 (December 1993): 1919–23.

14. A. Downie, T. M. Khattab, M. I. Malik, and I. N. Samara, "A Case of Percutaneous Industrial Methanol Toxicity," *Occupational Medicine* (London) 42, no. 1 (February 1992): 47–49.

15. P. Hantson, J. Y. Lambermont, and P. Mahieu, "Methanol Poisoning during Late Pregnancy," *Journal of Toxicology Clinical Toxicology* 35, no. 2 (March 1997): 187–91.

16. M. Belson and B. W. Morgan, "Methanol Toxicity in a Newborn," *Journal of Toxicology: Clinical Toxicology* 42, no. 5 (August 2004): 673–77.

17. A. Paine and A. D. Davan, "Defining a Tolerable Concentration of Methanol in Alcohol Drinks," *Human and Experimental Toxicology* 20, no.11 (November 2001): 563–68.

18. Y. D. Hang and E. E. Woodams, "Influence of Apple Cultivar and Juice Pasteurization on Hard Cider and Eau-de-Vie Methanol Content," *Bioresources Technology* 101, no. 4 (February 2010): 1396–98.

19. B. A. Magnuson, G. A. Burdock, J. Doull, R. M. Kroes, et al., "Aspartame: A Safety Evaluation Based on Current Use Levels, Regulations and Toxicological and Epidemiological Studies," *Critical Review in Toxicology* 37, no. 8 (August 2007): 629–727.

20. A. Zehetner and M. McLean, "Aspartame and the Internet," *Lancet* 354, no. 9172 (July 1999): 78.

21. W. Lindinger, A. Taucher, A. Jordon, A. Hansel, et al., "Endogenous Production of Methanol after Consumption of Fruit," *Alcoholism: Clinical and Experimental Research* 21, no. 5 (August 1997): 939–43.

22. C. Turner, P. Španěl, and D. Smith, "A Longitudinal Study of Methanol in the Exhaled Breath of 30 Healthy Volunteers Using Selected Ion Flow Tube Mass Spectrometry, SIFT-MS," *Physiological Measurement* 27, no. 7 (July 2007): 637–48.

23. J. A. Kruse, "Methanol Poisoning," *Intensive Care Medicine* 18, no. 7 (July 1992): 391–97.

24. F. C. Johlin, C. S. Fortman, D. D. Nghiem, and T. R. Tephly, "Studies on the Role of Folate-Dependent Enzymes in Human Methanol Poisoning," *Molecular Pharmacology* 31, no. 3 (May 1987): 557–61.

25. J. A. Kruse, "Methanol Poisoning," *Intensive Care Medicine* 18, no. 7 (July 1992): 391–97.

26. C. D. Garner, E. W. Lee, T. S. Terzo, and R. T. Louis-Ferdinard, "Role of Retinal Metabolism in Methanol-Induced Retinal Toxicity," *Journal of Toxicology and Environmental Health* 44, no. 1 (January 1995): 43–56.

27. H. R. Wallage and J. H. Watterson, "Formic Acid and Methanol Concentrations in Death Investigations," *Journal of Analytical Toxicology* 32, no. 3 (April 2008): 241–47.

28. K. A. Lushine, C. R. Harris, and J. S. Holger, "Methanol Ingestion: Prevention of Toxic Sequelae after Massive Ingestion," *Journal of Emergency Medicine* 24, no. 4 (May 2004): 433–36.

29. R. J. Meyer, M. E. Beard, M. W. Ardagh, and S. Henderson, "Methanol Poisoning," *New Zealand Medical Journal* 113, no. 1102 (January 2000): 11–13.

30. S. C. Pappas and M. Silverman, "Treatment of Methanol Poisoning with Ethanol and Hemodialysis," *Canadian Medical Association Journal* 126, no. 12 (June 1982): 1391–94.

31. B. R. Ekins, D. E. Rollins, D. P. Duffy, and M. C. Gregory, "Standardized Treatment of Severe Methanol Poisoning with Ethanol and Hemodialysis," *Western Journal of Medicine* 142, no. 3 (March 1985): 337–40.

32. A. Gonda, H. Gault, D. Churchill, and D. Hollomby, "Hemodialysis for Methanol Intoxication," *American Journal of Medicine* 64, no. 5 (May 1978): 749–58.

33. K. E. Hovda, K. S. Anderson, P. Urdal, and D. Jacobsen, "Methanol and Formate Kinetics during Treatment with Fomepizole," *Clinical Toxicology* (Philadelphia) 43, no. 4 (April 2005): 221–27.

34. M. L. Sivilotti, M. J. Bruns, C. K. Aaron, K. E. McMartin, et al., "Reversal of Severe Methanol-Induced Visual Impairment: No Evidence of Retinal Toxicity Due to Fomepizole," *Journal of Toxicology: Clinical Toxicology* 39, no. 6 (June 2001): 627–31.

35. M. Gerin, S. Patrice, D. Begin, M. S. Goldberg, et al., "A Study of Ethylene Glycol Exposure and Kidney Function of Aircraft De-icing Workers," *International Archives of Occupational and Environmental Health* 69, no. 4 (March 1997): 255–65.

36. T. Bouattar, N. Madani, H. Hamzaqui, Z. Alhamany, et al., "Severe Ethylene Glycol Intoxication by Skin Absorption," *Nephrologie and Therapeutique* 5, no. 3 (June 2009): 205–9.

37. P. R. Baker, S. D. Cramer, M. Kennedy, D. G. Assimos, et al., "Glycolate and Glyoxylate Metabolism in HepG2 Cells," *American Journal of Physiology and Cell Physiology* 287, no. 5 (November 2004): C1350–1365.

38. A. D. Walder and C. K. G. Tyler, "Ethylene Glycol Antifreeze Poisoning: Three Case Reports and a Review of Treatment," *Anesthesia* 49, no. 11 (November 1994): 964–67.

39. B. Johnson, W. J. Meggs, and C. J. Bentzel, "Emergency Department Hemodialysis in a Case of Severe Ethylene Glycol Poisoning," *Annals of Emergency Medicine* 33, no. 1 (January 1999): 108–10.

40. T. G. Rosano, T. A. Swift, C. J. Kranick, and M. Sikirica, "Ethylene Glycol and Glycolic Acid in Postmortem Blood from Fatal Poisonings," *Journal of Analytical Toxicology* 33, no. 8 (October 2009): 508–13.

41. C. Pomara, C. Fiore, S. D'Errico, I. Riezzo, et al., "Calcium Oxalate in Acute Ethylene Glycol Poisoning: A Confocal Laser Scanning Microscopy Study in a Fatal Case," *Clinical Toxicology* (Philadelphia) 46, no. 4 (April 2008): 322–24.

42. U. Garg, C. Frazee, L. Johnson, and J. W. Turner, "A Fatal Case Involving Extremely High Levels of Ethylene Glycol without Elevation of Its Metabolites or Crystalluria," *American Journal of Forensic Medicine and Pathology* 30, no. 3 (September 2009): 273–75.

43. E. J. Armstrong, D. A. Engelhart, A. J. Jenkins, and E. K. Balraj, "Homicidal Ethylene Glycol Intoxication: A Report of a Case," *American Journal of Forensic Medicine and Pathology* 27, no. 2 (June 2007): 151–55.

44. K. A. Ammar and P. S. Heckerling, "Ethylene Glycol Poisoning with a Normal Anion Gap Caused by Concurrent Ethanol Ingestion: Importance of the Osmolar Gap," *American Journal of Kidney Disease* 27, no. 1 (January 1996): 130–33.

45. H. Arai, H. Ikeda, M. Ichili, M. Lino, et al., "A Case of Poisoning by a Mixture of Methanol and Ethylene Glycol," *Tohoku Journal of Experimental Medicine* 141, no. 4 (December 1983): 473–80.

46. K. McMartin, "Are Calcium Oxalate Crystals Involved in the Mechanism of Acute Renal Failure in Ethylene Glycol Poisoning?" *Clinical Toxicology* 47, no. 9 (November 2009): 859–69.

47. R. P. Holmes, H. O. Goodman, and D. G. Assimos, "Dietary Oxalate and Its Intestinal Absorption," *Scanning Microscopy* 9, no. 4 (April 1995): 1109–18.

48. A. F. Eder, C. M. McGarth, Y. G. Dowdy, J. E. Tomaszewski, et al., "Ethylene Glycol Poisoning: Toxicokinetics and Analytical Factors Affecting Laboratory Diagnosis," *Clinical Chemistry* 44, no. 1 (January 1998): 168–77.

49. C. Karlson-Stiber and H. Persson, "Ethylene Glycol Poisoning: Experiences from an Epidemic in Sweden," *Journal of Toxicology: Clinical Toxicology* 30, no. 4 (December 1992): 565–74.

50. L. I. Velez, G. Shepherd, Y. C. Lee, D. C. Keyes, "Ethylene Glycol Ingestion Treated Only with Fomepizole," *Journal of Medical Toxicology* 3, no. 3 (September 2007): 125–28.

51. B. Hylander and C. M. Kjellstrand, "Prognostic Factors and Treatment of Severe Ethylene Glycol Intoxication," *Intensive Care Medicine* 22, no. 6 (June 1996): 546–52.

52. P. M. Viver, W. J. Lewander, H. F. Martin, and J. G. Linakis, "Isopropyl Alcohol Intoxication in a Neonate through Chronic Dermal Exposure: A Complication of a Culturally Based Umbilical Care Practice," *Pediatric Emergency Care* 10, no. 2 (April 1994): 91–93.

53. M. Arditi and M. S. Killner, "Coma Following Use of Rubbing Alcohol for Fever Control," *American Journal of Disease in Children* 141, no. 3 (March 1987): 237–38.

54. B. Blanchet, A. Chrachon, S. Lukat, E. Huet, et al., "A Case of Mixed Intoxication with Isopropyl Alcohol and Propanol-1 after Ingestion of a Topical Antiseptic Solution," *Clinical Toxicology* (Philadelphia) 45, no. 6 (September 2007): 701–4.

55. C. B. Alexander, A. J. McBay, and R. P. Hudson "Isopropanol and Isopropanol Deaths: Ten Years' Experience," *Journal of Forensic Sciences* 27, no. 3 (July 1982): 541–48.

56. C. E. Anderson and G. A. Loomis, "Recognition and Prevention of Inhalant Abuse," *American Family Physicians* 68, no. 5 (September 2003): 869–74.

57. C. H. Steffee, G. J. Davis, and K. K. Nicol, "A Whiff of Death: Fatal Volatile Solvent Inhalation Abuse," *Southern Medical Journal* 89, no. 9 (September 1996): 879–84.

58. H. Pfeiffer, M. Al Khaddam, B. Brinkmann, H. Kohler, et al., "Sudden Death after Isobutane Sniffing: A Report of Two Forensic Cases," *International Journal of Legal Medicine* 120, no. 3 (May 2006): 168–73.

59. S. A. Zaidi, A. N. Shaw, M. N. Patel, V. V. Shah, et al., "Multi-organ Toxicity and Death from Acute Unintentional Inhalation of Paint Thinner Fumes," *Clinical Toxicology* (Philadelphia) 45, no. 3 (May 2007): 287–89.